History of Periodontology

The authors and publisher wish to acknowledge the generous financial support from the companies listed below. Their support has made this publication possible.

**OraPharma, Warminster, Pennsylvania**

**G. Hartzell & Co., Concord, California**

# *History of Periodontology*

**Fermín Carranza**, Dr Odont, FACD
Professor Emeritus of Periodontology
University of California, Los Angeles
Los Angeles, California

**Gerald Shklar**, DDS, MS, FACD
Charles A. Brackett Professor Emeritus of Oral Pathology
Harvard School of Dental Medicine
Boston, Massachusetts

*with a contribution by*

**Ray C. Williams**, DMD
Professor of Periodontology
University of North Carolina School of Dentistry
Chapel Hill, North Carolina

quintessence books

**Quintessence Publishing Co, Inc**
Chicago, Berlin, Tokyo, Copenhagen, London, Paris, Milan, Barcelona, Istanbul, São Paulo, New Delhi, Moscow, Prague, and Warsaw

# *Dedications*

*To Bernardo Blitzer, dear friend and colleague,*
*a man of intellect, integrity, and wit.*
—FC

*To all our contemporary colleagues who witnessed*
*with us the last half century of unprecedented*
*progress and the coming of age of our specialty.*
—FC and GS



**Library of Congress Cataloging-in-Publication Data**

Carranza, Fermín A.
History of periodontology / Fermín Carranza, Gerald Shklar.
p. ; cm.
Includes bibliographical references.
ISBN 0-86715-424-1 (pbk.)
1. Periodontics—History.
[DNLM: 1. Periodontics—history. WU 11.1 C312h 2003] I. Shklar, Gerald. II. Title.
RK361 .C373 2003
617.6'32—dc21

2002154335

quintessence books



Quintessence Publishing Co, Inc
551 Kimberly Drive
Carol Stream, IL 60188
www.quintpub.com



Editor: Arinne Dickson
Production: Angela Kreeger and Susan Robinson
Cover design: Dawn Hartman
Printed in Canada

# Table of Contents

# *Foreword*

Drs Fermín Carranza and Gerald Shklar have presented us with a labor of love, and I have the pleasure of writing the foreword. Having taught periodontics in all parts of our country for half a century, I have always been amazed at how little our students know of the history and culture of our profession. If we included questions about the history of our specialty on our board examination, how many of our candidates would pass? And yet we stand on the shoulders of these pioneers. Could we understand the biology of microbes if not for the groundbreaking work of Leeuwenhoek and Pasteur? Could we comprehend the mechanism of union of oral tissues to metal if not for the pioneering work of those who struggled with the question of epithelial attachment to tooth structure? I think not.

But there is more to history than reciting names and dates. History represents memory, and without memory, a society cannot exist. As Greek thought taught us, a society and a culture create a common history, a common ethos, a common world view, and a common ethics, resulting in a common action based on these values. Thus, memory is more than nostalgia for the good old days. Rather, it represents a bridge between the past and the present, and hopefully the future.

Drs Carranza and Shklar have presented us with an extensive memory of accomplishments by individuals who initiated thought about periodontics, thereby opening new avenues of inquiry for us. I remember Balint Orban once telling me (I was fortunate to be one of his first students at the University of Illinois), "Sig, when you graduate, I do not expect you to repeat me and my teaching but rather to challenge the truth of my views." The individuals mentioned in this book all chose to analyze and challenge the ideas of their predecessors and mentors and move forward with their own findings.

I salute the authors for this outstanding contribution to the history of periodontics. Reading it now, I remember vividly the vitality and spirit of Orban and Goldman, of Glickman and Schluger, and of so many others, who, at the scientific meetings, not only presented their findings but engaged in verbal duels that made lasting impressions on those privileged to be present. It gave the audience a sense of the presenters' personalities, and in many ways, that was the greatest teaching. Similarly, the authors of this book not only describe the scientific accomplishments of the pioneers and creators of modern periodontics, but also give us a sense of their personalities, of the times they lived in, of their human condition.

I hope this volume will be of great interest to all periodontists, and I particularly hope it will open the window of our profession's heritage to those entering the field.

S. Sigmund Stahl, DDS, MS
Professor of Periodontology and Executive Associate Dean
Nova Southeastern University College of Dental Medicine
Fort Lauderdale, Florida

# *Preface*

*The longer you can look back, the farther you can look forward.*
*—Winston Churchill, 1944*

The growth of a scientific discipline is marked by its advancement in research concepts and techniques, the development of new therapeutic approaches, the clarification of its mission, and the broadening of its purposes. The maturity of a scientific specialty is marked by a knowledge of its roots, an understanding of its historical past, and a recognition of the role of its forefathers in attaining its present status. The realization that current knowledge is but a fleeting phase in the development of science and technology clarifies why understanding the origins of this knowledge helps to more accurately and intelligently look into the future.

An intensive search of the literature failed to find a book that covers the entire scope of the history of periodontology. This book attempts to achieve this by providing a broad look at the evolution of concepts, from ancient times to the present, that led to our present understanding and treatment of periodontal diseases. We have presented the landmark contributions to periodontics in relation to the basic sciences and clinical developments of the times and in the context of each period's social and political events. We have also highlighted the accomplishments of the pioneers and included fascinating insights about their lives.

The philosophical basis for this book is the recognition that periodontology is rooted in the medical sciences and, in the greater picture, is related to biology and technology. The medical scientific revolutions of the nineteenth century—the development of the germ theory of disease by Pasteur and Koch and its clinical application by Lister; the introduction of general anesthesia by Wells and Morton, and local anesthesia by Koller and Halstead; the discovery of X rays by Röntgen; and the introduction of clinical and microscopic pathology by Virchow—are the hallmarks of the birth and growth of periodontology as a specialty. Research in the last decade linking periodontal health with the cardiovascular, respiratory, and endocrine systems (among others) lends credible scientific support to the concept that periodontology is integral to the medical sciences. This concept is stressed from a historical point of view.

Both of us have been interested in the history of periodontology and dentistry in general since we were students together in Prof. Irving Glickman's periodontal postdoctoral program at Tufts University in 1951. After years of collaborating on the periodontal history chapter for *Glickman's Clinical Periodontology* and its successive editions, we decided that a book on the subject would be useful for new and experienced periodontists to learn about their predecessors and understand the origins of their profession. To our benefit, one of us has studied the pre-Renaissance era while the other is interested in more recent centuries, which made the division of work an easy task.

It is our hope that this book will be informative and inspiring for periodontal scholars, teachers, students, and practitioners in their continuous endeavors to improve our discipline, and that it will be of interest to dentists, physicians, and allied professionals, as well as medical and science historians.

Throughout the writing of this book, numerous individuals provided valuable assistance at the different stages of its development. We would like to acknowledge George Bernard, Bernardo Blitzer, Jorge Preloran, Robert Rockney, S. Sigmund Stahl, and Henry H. Takei for their helpful critiques and constant support of our project.

The following people generously provided information on several topics and helped to solve various problems: Eugenio Auil, of Santiago, Chile; Lavin Flores-de-Jacoby, of Münster, Germany; Rolf Mustchelknauss, of Stuttgart, Germany; Michael Newman, Sascha Jovanovic, and Jackie Kaslow, of the University of California at Los Angeles; and Alice de Forest, of the American Academy of Periodontology. We are also grateful to Mrs. N. M. Keim for graciously providing information about John Oppie McCall.

We are particularly indebted to Ray C. Williams for writing the excellent chapter on "The Future of Periodontics" and to S. Sigmund Stahl for writing the foreword.

The commercial sponsorship of OraPharma (Mr. Russell Secter) and G. Hartzell & Son (Mr. Andrew McIver Hartzell) is especially appreciated.

The confidence and support of Quintessence Publishing Co, particularly of Ms. Tomoko Tsuchiya, is gratefully acknowledged. The help of our editor, Ms. Arinne Dickson, and her attention to every detail have contributed greatly to improving the quality of this book.

Last but not least, we wish to thank our wives, Rita and Se-Kyung Oh, for their constant support and understanding.

# *Part I*

# *The Prehistoric Era and Early Civilizations*

# 1

# The Prehistoric Era, and Early Middle Eastern and Egyptian Civilizations

## The Prehistoric Era

The widespread existence of oral diseases in early humans has been well established through the recovery and study of human skeletal remains in many regions of the world. Paleopathology has developed into a significant discipline that not only studies disease in ancient skeletal remains, but also attempts to relate the type of pathologic entities to other known facts about the cultural background of the society in which the subjects lived. Many sophisticated laboratory techniques, such as carbon-14 dating, are now available for the dating of skeletal remains and the tools and artifacts found with them.

Because teeth are highly calcified structures, they are well preserved in their natural state for thousands of years, and the maxilla and mandible are often found in a reasonably undamaged state with the embedded teeth. Entire skulls are sometimes unearthed still containing numerous teeth in their alveolar sockets, and teeth that have fallen out of the alveolus are often located nearby, allowing the original dentition to be reconstructed. The anatomy of the roots of teeth can be analyzed directly, and those still embedded in the jaws can be seen radiographically. Physical anthropologists concentrate on the teeth to determine whether a prehistoric skeleton represents an early human or an apelike creature.

The study of dental tissues in prehistoric humans has also developed into a special discipline, *paleostomatology*, or *paleopathology*,[10,11,15] of the teeth and jaws. Examination of teeth can disclose excessive wear of enamel related to diet, dental caries, or developmental malformations such as enamel hypoplasia. The jaws may reveal evidence of gross deformities such as cleft palate or osteoporosis. Examination of alveolar bone can disclose evidence of chronic periodontal disease or periodontal abscesses (Fig 1). Radiographic studies of teeth can reveal features such as internal resorption, root resorption, abnormal dentin development, hypercementosis, and formation of reparative dentin. Radiographs of jaws may disclose the presence of alveolar apical abscesses, cysts, or possible tumors or tumorlike lesions. Studies of the temporomandibular joint may suggest the occurrence of arthritic pathology. Various types of metabolic bone disease may also be suggested by the overall features of the craniofacial complex and by the radiographic appearance of the trabeculae and cortical regions of the jaws.

Diseases of organs, as well as probable etiologic agents, can be detected when soft tissues are preserved, such as those in ancient Egyptian mummies. Even microscopic studies can be carried out both on hard and on soft tissues that have been preserved for thousands of years.

Through pictorial representation researchers have also begun to obtain evidence of disease and possible medical practice in paleolithic humans. Some ancient pictures drawn on the walls of caves remain for study. Pictorial records in other types of dwellings have not been preserved.

Dental caries and enamel hypoplasia have been found in the oldest paleolithic remains, and evidence of chronic periodontal disease and chronic abscesses, as well as dental caries and developmental malformations, has been found in the extensive paleolithic material available.[1,12]

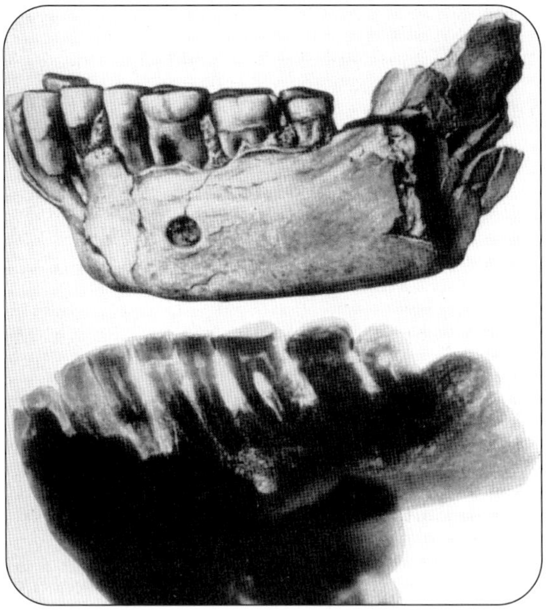

**Fig 1** Periodontal disease in a pre-Neanderthal mandible (found at Ehringsdorf, near Weimar, Germany, by Hans Virchow).

Skeletal studies also disclose the presence of osteoarthritis of the temporomandibular joint, fractures, infections, and possible jaw tumors and cysts. Cranial injuries are also commonly found, probably resulting from assaults with the developing hand axes and other weapons of the era.[15]

From the Neolithic period there is extensive evidence of trepanning, a surgical operation that employed a flint knife with a relatively sharp edge to cut holes in the skull; the holes are often regularly shaped with smooth edges. The purpose of these operations is obscure. It is likely that they were carried out to permit evil spirits to escape from the skull—evil spirits that were causing severe headaches or possibly mental or neurological disorders such as depression or convulsions. Many early societies, in some way, had made the association between the brain and the vitality, or even the personality, of the individual.

## Sumer, Assyria, Babylonia

In Mesopotamia, the land between the Tigris and Euphrates Rivers, a number of ancient civilizations developed, starting with the Sumerians around 3200 BC and ending with the Babylonians and Assyrians.

Sumeria is one of the three oldest civilizations, together with the Indus valley civilization (in the region that is now part of Pakistan) and the early dynasties of Egypt. The Sumerians, with the Egyptians, are credited for originating metallurgy. They worked with gold, silver, lead, and various bronzes, and they developed glazes for use on pottery and tiles. The development of writing was one of the most significant features of the Sumerian civilization, for it recorded history on clay tablets with imprinted cuneiform figures. Researchers continue to learn more about life in this period as understanding of these figures increases.

The Sumerians were overtaken by the Babylonians, probably around 1830 to 1531 BC. Evidence shows that the Euphrates changed its course around this period, and Babylon, on its new bank, was able to develop rapidly, at the expense of the Sumerian cities on the earlier banks of the river. With trade and consolidation came military power, and the Babylonians defeated the Sumerians and destroyed their cities. The Babylonians, however, were impressed with the greatness achieved by the older, Sumerian civilization and assimilated the Sumerian religion and language to their own culture. The Babylonians advanced the cuneiform writing of the Sumerians and left vast numbers of clay tablets with written records on topics ranging from governmental edicts and laws to religious charms and medical prescriptions. Much of our knowledge of Babylonian and Assyrian medicine comes from these tablets.

The Assyrian people coexisted with the Babylonians for over seven centuries; the Assyrian capital, Nineveh, was less than 300 miles north of Babylon. The Chaldeans lived south of Babylon in the old Sumerian city of Ur. All of these societies had a common religious and cultural background, spoke the same, or similar, languages, and wrote in the same cuneiform script. For most of the time, the Babylonians were preeminent, both militarily and culturally. They developed agriculture, trade, and commerce, as well as sciences such as mathematics, geometry, and astronomy. Babylonian astronomers accurately recorded some planetary rotations and were able to forecast eclipses.

The Assyrians, meanwhile, developed an advanced society of their own and had considerable military capability. They captured Babylon around 1100 BC. Large libraries were built, and scribes were commissioned to copy all the classics of Sumerian and Babylonian literature. More than 30,000 tablets have been catalogued from this vast treasure of early writings.

Probably the most significant work of Babylonia-Assyria that has been preserved is the Code of Laws of Hammurabi, the oldest known codification of laws.[9] Many of the laws are related to the practice of medicine, indicating that physicians and surgeons were practicing their arts at this time. One law, for example, established surgical fees for successful treatment and penalties for unsuccessful treatment, depending on the social status of the patient.

Almost all of our knowledge of Babylonian and Assyrian medicine comes from the clay tablets of the great library of Ashurbanipal, king of Assyria. Because this is a vast accumulation of older writings, the exact age or period of any tablet or set of tablets is difficult to assess. Of the 30,000 tablets in the British Museum, some 800 are either medical texts or incantations for the relief of disease. Religion was strong and pervasive in these early societies, and doctors, lawyers, and other professionals were probably of the priestly class. The cure of any disease, to a large extent, depended on driving out the demons thought to cause that disease. Thus, the incantations had religious overtones, although they were considered to be medical prescriptions and surgical procedures.

Thompson[14] was able to translate many of the drugs and ingredients used in the medical tablets from Ashurbanipal's library. He found some 250 vegetable substances and 120 minerals, as well as a variety of ingredients to be used as vehicles, including wines, oils, honey, wax, animal fat, and milk. Many of the agents mentioned (such as aloes, anise, asafetida, belladonna, cannabis, cardamom, cassia, castor oil, cinnamon, colocynth, coriander, garlic, henbane, juniper, licorice, mandragora, mint, mustard, myrrh, pomegranate, and poppy) not only had some therapeutic value, but also became the basic pharmacopoeia of succeeding civilizations. Most of these medicaments appear in the great collection of Dioscorides, a Greek pharmacologist, whose writings served as the basis for European medicine until the sixteenth century. As in all primitive societies, many of the medicaments involved human and animal excrement, presumably to force out the demons with the disgusting nature of the concoction.

Diseases of the eyes, mouth, and teeth were common, and many of the tablets offer approaches to the management of oral and dental diseases. Dental caries was thought to be caused by a "tooth worm," a concept also found in ancient Chinese and Indian cultures. Ashurbanipal's library includes a number of remedies for periodontal disease. For example:

> If a man's teeth are loose and itch (painful) a mixture of [myrrh, asafetida, and opopanax as well as pine-turpentine] shall be rubbed on his teeth until blood comes forth and he shall recover.[14]

Discolored teeth were considered a problem, and remedies were provided for them:

> If a man's teeth have become yellow ... you shall mix together salt, ammi, Lolium, pine-turpentine; you shall rub his teeth with this mixture using your finger.[14]

## Ancient Egypt

Ancient Egypt has been considered the classic ancient civilization, for many reasons. For instance, historians of succeeding civilizations, such as Greece and Rome, wrote about Egypt's ancient monuments. Herodotus, the famous Greek historian, revealed facts about ancient Egyptian life that Egyptian documents did not disclose. The massive temples and monuments of ancient Egypt still exist, and most of them are in a reasonable state of repair. The dry climate of Egypt has preserved large numbers of artifacts that convey many details about the everyday life of the Egyptians—their occupations, their furniture, their games, their children's toys, their clothes, and their ornaments. Finally, the Egyptians developed hieroglyphics, which emerged as a written syllabic language. A considerable number of documents and books written on papyrus scrolls have survived, describing various aspects of Egyptian life. In addition to papyri, temple walls, coffins, and buildings were used for recording documents, history, and religious texts. The result of all these remnants is that more is known about ancient Egypt than about other ancient civilizations.

Pre-dynastic Egypt dates back to 4000 BC; the First Dynasty started around 3400 BC. Pre-dynastic Egypt developed metallurgy, as did Sumer-Akkad, and used gold, silver, lead, and copper. Glazes for pottery were also developed during this era.

The Old Kingdom is represented by the third through the sixth dynasties (ca 3000–2500 BC). During this period, architecture and sculpture reached their first peak of development. The capital city of Egypt at the time was Memphis, and the great pyramids of Cheops and Chefren, together with massive sculptures, were the major architectural legacy of the age.

The Middle Kingdom, represented by the eleventh through thirteenth dynasties (ca 2160–1700 BC), developed after several hundred years of anarchy following the end of the sixth dynasty. The New Empire emerged with Thebes as the capital and lasted from the eighteenth through twenty-fourth dynasties (ca 1580–712 BC). Many of the kings of this period are well-known historically; Thutmosis and Amenophis made Egypt a major world power through military superiority and subjugated many neighboring states in the Middle East.

Akhnahton is well-known as the founder of a new religion, replacing the traditional, complex polytheism with a form of monotheism. The single deity worshiped was the sun god. Akhnahton's capital was moved to El Asmarna. His reign was a period of great artistic accomplishment; the famous statue of his beautiful wife, Nefertiti, is one of the symbols of this age.

The fame of the Egyptians as physicians is recorded in numerous ancient epics and texts. Homer's *Odyssey* states that the physicians of Egypt were skilled beyond those of all other lands. Herodotus' work repeatedly mentions the doctors of Egypt, stressing their reputation for excellence and pointing out that the profession was composed of specialists for different types of diseases.

> The art of medicine among them is distributed thus: each physician is a physician of one disease and no more; and the whole country is full of physicians, for some profess themselves to be physicians of the eyes, others of the head, others of the teeth, others of the stomach and others of the more obscure ailments.[7]

Hippocrates and his school were aware of Egyptian medical practice, and we now know that many of their remedies and surgical approaches were copied from Egyptian practice of the time or from Egyptian texts that may have been available to them.

Egyptian medicine was, to a large extent, based on magic or religion, as was much of the culture, art, and architecture in general. Knowledge of Egyptian medicine has become reasonably comprehensive in recent years, with the translation of a number of medical treatises written on papyrus.[2–6,13] Two of these papyri are worthy of mention. The Edwin Smith papyrus,[2] which is primarily a surgical treatise, is the most impressive of all the medical papyri in terms of its rational and modern approach to patient diagnosis and management. The Ebers papyrus[3,4] is the longest and most complete of all the Egyptian medical treatises, and deals with the medical management of many diseases, organizing the diseases by sites of involvement. It is more a compendium of recipes than an organized medical text.

In addition to these well-known medical papyri, numerous other papyri in major museums of Europe and America occasionally refer to diseases and their management, but they are primarily magical in content.

From studies of the various papyri, it is apparent that Egyptian medical practice was strongly influenced by religion in terms of its theoretical understanding of disease. Diseases were considered to be the "possession" of a patient by a demon. Common beliefs were that either the demon was present in the patient's body or the demon was able to project some poison or noxious substance or evil emanation into the patient. Therapy involved some magical spell to drive out the demon or to rid the body of whatever noxious substance had been forced into it. Diseases were treated both by incantations and by the use of some medication or charm. The medication in many cases appeared to have some rational or empirical basis.[5] It would seem that some of the physicians had learned not to rely entirely on magic words and charms, but had learned instead to use medicaments that were found by experience to have some value. These physicians had a better chance of treating diseases successfully.

Among the drugs mentioned in the Ebers papyrus and other medical papyri were many plant remedies such as acacia, anise, barley, cassia, caster bean, coriander, cucumber, cumin, date, fennel, fig, garlic, juniper, leek, lettuce, lotus, peas, poppy seeds, saffron, sunflower, styrax, terebinth, wheat, willow buds, white thistle, and wormwood. Minerals used included copper, feldspar, iron oxide, limestone, red ochre, sodium carbonate, sodium bicarbonate, salt, and sulfur. Resinous materials such as frankincense, myrrh, styrax, turpentine, and mucilaginous substances such as acacia gum had antiseptic qualities and were used to coat abrasions and ulcerations. Beer, milk, wine, and honey were commonly used as vehicles or binding substances for plant or mineral remedies; animal fat and grease were often used, as were animal tissues and animal excrement.

Much of this materia medica became the basis for later Greek and Roman compendia, such as the materia medica of Dioscorides and Galen. Many of the remedies can be found in later books of the sixteenth and seventeenth centuries, having been taken from the Greek and Latin texts to form the basis of Renaissance medicine.

The Edwin Smith papyrus suggests that alongside the magical approach was a highly rational approach to therapy based on proper diagnosis, as well as surgical skills and medical knowledge when necessary. This papyrus is the first example of a modern medical textbook. It includes some knowledge of anatomy, physiology, and pathology, and discusses patient management in terms of clinical findings, diagnosis, choice of therapy, and prognosis. The book methodically discusses forty-eight patients with a variety of surgical problems. Each case description includes a summary diagnosis, an extensive diagnosis, a prognosis, a choice as to whether therapy is indicated, and in several cases, a description of actual therapy. The difference between benign and malignant tumors was understood. Benign tumors were treated with surgery, while malignant tumors could not be successfully treated. Cauterization was used for some tumors and ulcers. Surgical therapy was described in some detail. The presence of a pulse was noted, and the heart was recognized as the center of the vascular system. This document also contains the earliest descriptions of linen swabs and bandages, the suturing of wounds, the use of splints for setting fractures, and the use of antiseptic and astringent medicaments for infected wounds.

The Ebers papyrus presents a more complicated picture of Egyptian medicine. Some remedies are rational, such as astringent mouthrinses for gingival disease, while others are merely magical and have little or no rational basis for their use. This papyrus is a compilation, as indicated by its writer, and although it was apparently written around 1600 BC, many of its prescriptions and recipes probably date back as far as 3000 to 2500 BC. The writer identifies three types of medical men: the physicians, who used both external and internal remedies; the surgeons, who treated wounds and fractures; and the sorcerers, who used magic in the form of exorcisms and spells or amulets and charms.

Little is known about the practice of dental medicine in ancient Egypt, apart from the medical papyri and their diagnostic and therapeutic features. Tooth extraction with forceps is mentioned, but extraction of a tooth with fingers alone obviously refers to a tooth rendered mobile by periodontal disease. Prescriptions to "strengthen" the teeth presumably refer to periodontally diseased teeth. Several such prescriptions appear in the Ebers papyrus[6]:

> *A prescription to strengthen the teeth:* One part each of Powder of the fruit of the palm, Green lead and Honey. To be mixed and the teeth rubbed with it.
>
> *Another prescription to strengthen the teeth:* One Part each of Powder of flint stones, Green lead and Honey. To be rubbed on the teeth.

There are many other prescriptions for diseases of the mouth and teeth, using mixtures of many agents that to date cannot be translated from the original hieratic script of the Ebers papyrus. From recent studies of mummies, it is apparent that periodontal disease was common among upper-class Egyptians. It is not surprising that there were many remedies used to treat the painful condition.

## References

1. Begg PR. Stone Age man's dentition. Am J Orthodont 1954;40:273,298,452,517.
2. Breasted JH. The Edwin Smith Surgical Papyrus, vol 2. Chicago: University of Chicago Press, 1930.
3. Bryan CP. The Papyrus Ebers. New York: Appleton, 1931.
4. Ebbell B. The Papyrus Ebers: The Greatest Egyptian Medical Document. Copenhagen: Levin and Munksgaard, 1937.
5. Estes JW. The Medical Skills of Ancient Egypt. Canton, MA: Science History Publications, 1969.
6. Guerini V. History of Dentistry. Philadelphia: Lea & Febiger 1929.
7. Herodotus. Cary H (trans). New York: Harper & Row, 1872.
8. Jastrow N. The medicine of the Babylonians and Assyrians. Proc Roy Soc Med Sect Hist Med 1914;7:109–176.
9. Johns CHW (trans). The Oldest Code of Laws in the World. Edinburgh: T. and T. Clark, 1903.
10. Moodie RL. Paleopathology. An Introduction to the Study of Ancient Evidences of Disease. Urbana: University of Illinois Press, 1923.
11. Moodie RL. Studies in palæodontology. J Am Dent Assoc 1928;15:1826.
12. Parma C. Research on prehistoric jaws. Paradentologie 1948;2:123.
13. Ranke H. Medicine and surgery in ancient Egypt. Bull Inst Hist Med 1933;1:237-257.
14. Thompson RC. Assyrian Medical Texts. Proc Roy Soc Med Sect Hist Med 1925;19:29–77.
15. Williams HU. Human palæopathology. Arch Path 1929;7:839.

# 2

# Ancient India and China

## India

The first civilization on the Indian subcontinent was the Harrapan (ca 2500–1500 BC), located in the Indus River Basin in what is now Pakistan. It is primarily known through the extensive excavations of its two chief cities, Mohenjo-Daro and Harrapa. These were large, well-designed cities with elaborate brick buildings, well-planned streets, and sophisticated sewage systems draining homes and large buildings with brick-built conduits. Harrapan religion had a strong fertility component, the script was pictographic, and the craftsmanship was of a high order. This was an advanced society, roughly contemporaneous with Egypt and Mesopotamia. However, there is insufficient documentation to provide much insight into the culture and science.

Around 1600 BC the Harrapan civilization was overtaken by invading Aryan-speaking tribes from the Iranian plateau. Despite their aversion to much of Harrapan culture, the Aryan tribes absorbed parts of it. It is with the coming of these Aryan tribes that Indian history begins. They laid the foundations of Indian culture by developing a new language, Sanskrit. Sanskrit not only became one of the great languages of antiquity, but it has survived to the present.

Indian medicine has been divided into the Vedic period (1500–800 BC) coinciding with invasion of the Hindus, the Brahman period (800 BC–1000 AD), and the Mongol period, starting in 1000 AD.

The Vedic Period is the time of the writing of the great books of Indian knowledge, such as the Rig-Veda. Medicine in the Vedic period was primarily magic or supernatural with diseases treated by prayers and incantations. Physicians are mentioned in the Rig-Veda; they had medicine chests and herbal remedies. There were also surgeons. The Atharva-Veda mentions various diseases, including tumors, abscesses, diarrhea, jaundice, convulsions, heart disease, hemiplegia, venereal diseases, and skin diseases. Diseases of the eyes and of the teeth are also mentioned. Artificial limbs, artificial eyes, and artificial teeth are mentioned, indicating the existence of prosthetic therapy.[5,6]

The Brahman Period was the great age of Indian medicine, and two major books have survived to give us some idea of the heights reached by the Brahman physicians and surgeons. The books are the *Susruta Samhita*[7] and the *Charaka Samhita*.[1] The *Susruta Samhita* is the greatest medical work in Sanskrit and probably dates to the sixth century BC, with numerous revisions in later years. The *Charaka Samhita*, named for its Indian-physician author, was written between 120 and 162 AD.

The *Susruta Samhita* is particularly impressive for its sections on surgery; Susruta himself was known primarily as a surgeon. He studied anatomy, using dissection of human cadavers. Like all Indian writers, he classified, counted, and assigned a numerical value to every subject of investigation. The body had 300 bones, 700 blood vessels, 900 ligaments, 500 muscles, and 107 vital parts. Susruta's physiological sections reveal his concept of the body as composed of various humors that produce the important fluids and secretions. In medicine and pathology,

Susruta provides descriptions of diabetes, anginal cardiac pain, tuberculosis, and leprosy among other diseases. Among 760 medicinal plants used as drugs were opium, aconite, pomegranate, castor oil, cinnamon, ginger, and cannabis. Minerals used were antimony, mercury, silver, and various salts.

Susruta describes his surgery in detail, including the instruments used and the actual technical procedures. There were 101 surgical instruments, classified into various groups. Forceps, knives, small forceps, probes, and tongs were further subdivided. Silk thread was used for suturing wounds. Likewise, Susruta outlines six basic types of operations: excision, scarification, aspiration, extraction, evacuation, and suturing. Suture needles could be straight or curved, depending on the requirement. Incision and extraction of bladder stone is carefully described. Plastic surgery, particularly rhinoplasty, was developed by Susruta, using pedicle flaps from the cheek to replace the skin of the nose and severing the cheek attachment once the nasal tissue had taken hold. Two small tubes were placed in the nostrils to facilitate breathing and to help hold the flap in proper position.

Susruta's many sections on oral diseases are of considerable interest. He describes a disease in which "the gums of the teeth suddenly bleed and become putrefied, black and slimy, and emit a fetid smell."[7] Although this description is more appropriate for acute necrotizing ulcerative gingivitis, it is often cited to indicate Susruta's understanding of scurvy. Susruta offers an accurate description of periodontitis, referring to tooth mobility and suppuration from the gingiva. Apart from the detailed treatment of oral diseases, Susruta devotes a section to preventive dentistry, with instructions for proper tooth brushing and the use of mouthwashes to cleanse the tongue.

Charaka's work is less interesting than that of Susruta. Its medicine is often a mixture of magic and religion, with disease treated by charms and incantations. Yet Charaka's anatomy and physiology are fairly similar to Susruta's. There is the same numbering of bones (306 in this case) and the same three vital humors, often interpreted as air, bile, and phlegm. Diseases are classified according to their causes by the different humors and then further classified as they relate to different tissues of organs.

Charaka devotes several sections to the mouth, oral hygiene, and the management of oral diseases. He advocates a toothbrush to cleanse the teeth and mouthwashes for the treatment of periodontal disease. In addition, his study reveals that caries was thought to be caused by worms, and decayed teeth were extracted, if necessary.

Some descriptions from the *Susruta Samhita* are of interest to the history of periodontology.

> Sitada [Scurvy]. The gums of the teeth suddenly bleed and become putrefied, black, slimy and emit a fetid smell. They become soft and gradually slough off. The disease has its origin in the deranged condition of the local blood and Kapham.
>
> Danta-Veshtaka. The teeth become loose in the gums, which exude a discharge of blood and pus. This disease is due to the vitiated blood of the locality.
>
> Maha-Saushira. The disease in which the teeth become loose, the palate marked by sinuses or fissures, the gums putrefied.
>
> Paridara. The disease in which the gums become putrefied, wear off and bleed [bleeding gums]. The disease has its origin in the deranged condition of the blood.
>
> Upakusa. The disease in which the gums become marked by a burning sensation and suppuration and the teeth become loose and shaky [in their gums] in consequence and bleed at the least shaking. There is a slight pain, and the entire cavity of the mouth becomes swollen and emits a fetid smell; this disease is due to the vitiated condition of the blood.
>
> Danta-Vaidarbha. The disease which is consequent upon the friction of the gums marked by the appearance of a violent swelling about the portion (so rubbed and in which) the teeth become loose and can be moved about, which is due to an extraneous cause such as a blow etc.

> In the case of Danta-Sarkara [Tartar-calcareous deposits on the teeth], the deposit should be removed in such a way as not to hurt the roots of the tooth, after which the part should be dusted (Prati-sarana) with powdered Laksha with honey.

From Chapter XXIV:

> *Tooth-Brushing:* A man should leave his bed early in the morning and brush his teeth. The toothbrush (Danta-Kashtha) should be made of a fresh twig of a tree or a plant grown on a commendable tract and it should be straight, not worm-eaten, devoid of any knot, or at most, with one knot only (on one side), and should be twelve fingers in length and like the small finger in girth. The potency and taste of the twig (toothbrush) should be determined by, or vary according to, the season of the year and the preponderance of any particular Dosha in the physical temperament of its user. The twig of a plant possessed of any of the four tastes as sweet, bitter, astringent and pungent should be alone collected and used. Nimba is the best of all the bitter trees; Khadira of the astringent ones; Madhuka of the sweet; and Karanja of the pungent ones.
>
> The teeth should be daily cleansed with (a compound consisting of) honey, powdered Tri-katu, Trivarga, Tejovati, Saindhava and oil. Each tooth should be separately cleansed with the preceding cleansing paste applied on (the top of the twig bitten into the form of) a soft brush, and care should be taken not to hurt the gum anywise during the rubbing. This tends to cleanse and remove the bad smell (from the mouth) and the uncleanliness (of the teeth) as well as to subdue the Kapha (of the body). It cleanses the mouth and also produces a good relish for food and a cheerfulness of mind.

## China

Chinese civilization began in the Yellow River valley, far from the co-existent Egyptian, Mesopotamian, and Harrapan cultures. Although later influenced by other civilizations, Chinese culture retained an autonomous and inward-looking character.

Chinese medicine can be divided into an ancient or legendary period, from approximately 3000 to 1122 BC, and a historical period, from 1121 BC to 960 AD. The latter period is often referred to as the golden age of Chinese medicine. Following the historical or golden period, the medieval period led to the modern age.

The ancient period stretches from prehistory to the end of the Shang dynasty and offers little historical data but many legends and myths. The historical period starts with the Chou dynasty and ends with the T'ang dynasty. During the Chou dynasty, medicine was closely associated with the philosophical teachings of the time. The Chou era was first marked by a period of royal power, stability, and the maturation of a feudal system (ca 1027 BC–771 BC). This period was followed by chronic warfare and political fragmentation, with the role of the Chou kings gradually reduced to the performance of religious rites (ca 722 BC–221 BC). Despite these difficulties, cities grew, technology and transportation improved, trade increased, and the later part of the Chou dynasty witnessed the golden age of Chinese philosophy.

The Han dynasty, which followed, was an age of science and medicine. Medicine came into the realm of science, and direct observation of patients was emphasized. While ancient Chinese concepts of physiology were nascent, some statements suggest an understanding of the continuous circulation of the blood controlled by the heart.

Gradually medicine became more sophisticated, and individual physicians of note have been identified and written about. A number of detailed case histories evidence a well-organized protocol including the patient's name, disease, and circumstances under which the disease was contracted, treatment prescribed, and discussion of diagnostic reasoning based on knowledge of the time. Outcome of therapy is also noted. Among the diagnostic procedures was evaluation of pulse, indicating a level of understanding comparable to that of contemporary Greek medicine.[3,4,9] The *Nei Ching*, the great classic of ancient Chinese medicine, has been translated as the *Yellow Emperor's Textbook of Medicine*. The *Nei Ching* represents a whole system of medicine, classifying disease on the basis of diagnosis.[8]

*Treatment of dental and oral disease.* Treatment of oral diseases, as well as other diseases, was to be effected either by drugs or by the use of acupuncture, a uniquely Chinese approach to therapy. Drugs were used in various prescriptions, either for local or systemic effect. Locally, drugs were applied in powders, tablets, ointments, or lotions. Ingredients of the various mixtures consisted of herbs, minerals, or, often, esoteric agents such as ground-up mouse bones and urine of a child. Plants used in many Chinese prescriptions included garlic, mint, horseradish, and rhubarb. Among the minerals were calcium carbonate and sodium bicarbonate.

A remedy for toothache is described as follows:

> one roasts a bit of garlic, crushes it between the teeth, and afterwards mixes it with chopped horseradish seeds, reducing the whole to a paste with human milk; one then forms it into pills; these are to be introduced into the nose on the side opposite to that where the pain is felt.[2]

Surgery was practiced, and tooth extraction was often advised for toothache, particularly if the tooth was loose and the gums greatly swollen, with extension of swelling to the cheek. Diseases of the gingiva and underlying periodontal tissues are described in detail. The following is from Dabry[2]:

> *Ya-heou* was a condition with red, soft and swollen gums and a fetid, purulent material exuding from them. [The description is suggestive of necrotizing gingivitis.]
>
> *Ja-suen* was a condition in which the gums were swollen, but gradually destroyed by ulceration, leaving the roots of the tooth exposed. [The description is suggestive of chronic destructive periodontitis.]
>
> *Tchuen-ya-kan* was a condition of swollen gums without ulceration, lasting for a few days and frequently seen in young children. [The description is suggestive of herpetic stomatitis.]
>
> *Ya-ting* was described as a localized swelling of the gingiva with the formation of a tumor-like mass which bursts and exudes blood. [The description is suggestive of a periodontal abscess.]
>
> *Tso-ma-ya-kan* was described as severe ulceration of the gums with black color and fetid breath in children following small-pox. [This would have been the necrotizing gingivitis or gangrenous stomatitis occasionally seen after the severe debilitation following a systemic infection.]

Dentistry, among the Chinese, was practiced as a specialty of medicine, and most of the major medical works of Chinese antiquity devote chapters to diseases of the teeth and diseases of the mouth and gingiva.

Toothache is referred to, in general terms, as *ya-tong*, and several different varieties are distinguished[2]:

> *Fong-je-tong* was associated with red, swollen gingiva and discharge of purulent material. [It would probably refer to a tooth with an alveolar abscess and draining fistula.] The pain was intense or acute and there could also be swelling of the cheek.

*Fong-lan-tong* also connoted a toothache with intense pain but without red, swollen gingiva. [This probably referred to the pain of an acute pulpitis, prior to apical extension into the alveolar bone.]

*Ye-tong* referred to tooth pain with red, swollen gums. Eventually the gums become black and the teeth become loose. [The description here is suggestive of periodontitis.]

In general, Chinese classical medicine and dentistry were based on theories that are no longer accepted as scientifically valid. Chinese knowledge of anatomy and physiology was in its early stages, and its concepts of medicine were magical rather than scientific. Two natural principles, *Yang* and *Yin*, were said to control the body's health, and their equilibrium was essential to normal function. A disequilibrium caused disease.

## References

1. Charaka. The Charaka Samhita. Kaviratna AC (trans). Calcutta: Kaviratna, 1896–1913.
2. Dabry P. La Medicine chez les Chinois. Paris: Plon, 1863.
3. Dawson P. Su-wen, the basis of Chinese medicine. Ann Med Hist 1935;7:59–64.
4. Morse WR. Chinese Medicine. New York: Hoeber, 1938.
5. Mukhopadhyaya G. The Surgical Instruments of the Hindus (2 vols). Calcutta: University Press, 1914.
6. Sarma PJ. Hindu medicine and its antiquity. Ann Med Hist 1931;3:318.
7. Susruta. The Susruta Samhita (3 vols). Bhishagratna KKL (trans). Calcutta: Bhishagratna, 1907–1916.
8. Veith I. Huang Ti Nei Ching Su Wen, The Yellow Emperor's Classic of Internal Medicine. Baltimore: Williams and Wilkins, 1949.
9. Wong KC, Wu LT. History of Chinese Medicine. Tientsin, China: Tientsin Press, 1932.

# 3

# Later Middle Eastern and Mediterranean Civilizations

## The Hebrews

The Jews are the "people of the book." The first five books of the Old Testament are said to have been written by Moses or, according to legend or doctrine, taken as dictation from God Himself. The Pentateuch, as these five books are often referred to by Christians, is the holy Torah, or Law, of the Jews. The development of a unique monotheistic religion, and with it a state in the land that is now Israel, is among their contributions to civilization.

All we know about Hebrew medicine and dentistry comes from the Old Testament and the later Talmud, the rabbinical laws founded on tradition. Despite rule by a priestly class and belief in a demonic theory of disease, the ancient Jews did have practicing physicians, called *rophe* in Hebrew, and these physicians were either general practitioners or specialists such as internists, surgeons, ophthalmologists, and dentists. Magic, of course, played an important role in early Hebrew medicine. God could easily inflict disease, as he did against the Egyptians, giving them plagues of pox and death to the firstborn children.

Indeed, the Old Testament describes a large number of diseases, including epilepsy, gout, cancer, goiter, hypergonadism, venereal disease (gonorrhea), dropsy, and apoplexy. There is a good description of angina pectoris and possible references to diabetes, diphtheria, and bubonic plague.[1,2,5]

Yet the Hebrew physician had a limited knowledge of anatomy because dissection was forbidden by Hebrew law, as a violation of the dead. Anatomical knowledge was presumably gained by careful observation of the exterior of the body and by dissection of animals.

The Hebrews had a materia medica but references are often confusing. Honey was often mixed with various plants and other substances. Salves and plasters are mentioned. The major medical contribution of the Hebrews is presumably to public health and sanitation. In Leviticus, Moses laid down his treatise on hygiene; it has been summarized as "pure food, pure water, pure air, pure bodies, and pure dwellings."

No individual physicians have come down to us by name and no medical treatises were written or, at least, have survived. Since the Jews were prohibited from pictorial representations, no illustrations of disease or physicians have been found. However, the background of Hebrew medicine was probably instrumental in determining that many Jews in later years would become famous physicians, both in Middle Eastern and in Western European countries.

Much of our knowledge of Hebrew medicine and stomatology comes from the Talmud rather than the Bible. The Talmud is essentially a juridical compilation that advances the laws of the Old Testament.

The teeth and digestion are often mentioned in the Talmud by various commentators:

> When a man loses his teeth, his nutrition is diminished, as said the prophet Camos.
>
> Until 40 years solid nourishment is primary, after this age it is drink (liquid nourishment) that is primary.

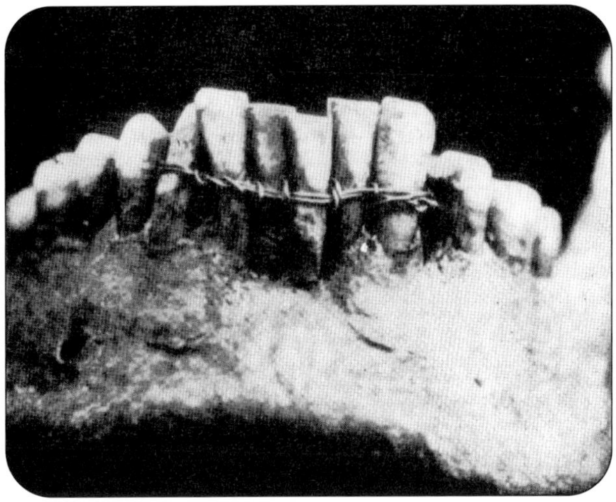

**Fig 2** Phoenician specimen dated fifth century BC, with gold wire ligature to immobilize teeth loosened due to periodontal bone loss. This specimen was found by Charles C. Torrey in 1901, in an excavation site in the city of Sidon in Southern Lebanon.

Presumably this is due to early loss of teeth and inefficient mastication or to periodontal disease and tooth mobility requiring a soft diet.

Aging and tooth loss is described metaphorically by Rabbi Yohoua ben Hananya. He is said to have told the emperor Hadrian that in age

> The mountains are covered with snow
> The roads to the entrance are covered with ice
> The dogs are not barking
> The mills are not turning

The first scene refers to the white head, the second to the gray beard, the third to a feeble voice, and the fourth to the absence of teeth so no grinding can occur.

Other rabbis describe periodontal disease, with some of its features. The Hebrew materia medica for disease was relatively primitive, but pepper, salt, ginger, and cannel were used to calm dental pain. Vinegar was to be put on the finger and then applied to the side of the painful tooth. A mouthwash of vinegar was not considered as beneficial.

Oral hygiene was carried out with dentifrices such as fine salt. A toothpick (*qesem*) was used to clean the interdental spaces. Halitosis was considered a severe problem that required treatment; pepper was suggested, among other remedies.

## The Phoenicians

The Phoenicians were a Semitic people who established a number of seaports along the Asian coast of Palestine-Syria. They were a seafaring people and traded in dyes, glass, cedar, wine, metal, and ivory ornaments and artworks. They were among the first people to develop a written alphabet and they influenced the written languages of later civilizations, including Greece and Rome. The Phoenicians explored the western Mediterranean from their base at Tyre and established a number of colonies, of which Carthage became preeminent.

Phoenician artifacts indicate that they excelled in working with gold, and teeth bound together by gold wire are described, the latter appliance presumably constructed to support loose, periodontally involved teeth[3] (Fig 2).

## The Etruscans

The Etruscans flourished in central Italy from about the eighth to the first centuries BC. Their origin is still debated, but the Greek historians thought they came from Asia Minor. Their language was not Indo-European and they left no literature. The Etruscans had excellent harbors and were famous for their seamanship. Thus they accumulated considerable wealth through trade, as well as from mineral resources. In addition, they were fine artists whose work reflected considerable technical skill. Because they traded with the Phoenicians and Egyptians, the Etruscans are thought to have acquired many of these skills during their travels. Eventually the Etruscans merged with Rome, and their culture was absorbed.

Dental appliances have been found in Etruscan tombs. The appliances, discovered in tombs at Orvieto and Cerveteria, are gold bands that appear to have attached to natural teeth to support tooth replacements. These gold frames were constructed to hold loose teeth, to steady others, and to contain artificial teeth. Frames were cast and neatly soldered and rivets were placed to hold the artificial teeth.[6,7] These specimens may be seen in various museums in Italy.

## The Scythians

The Scythians, a tribe of Iranian-speaking nomads, populated the steppes north of the Black Sea during the seventh to fourth centuries BC. Fierce warriors, they penetrated into the Middle East but were eventually driven out by the Medes. The Scythians are notable for their elaborate tombs in Crimea and their magnificent gold weapons and ornaments. A Scythian vase of electrum (gold-silver alloy) was discovered in Crimea and appears to depict a physician or dentist examining the mouth of a patient.[4]

Unfortunately no written records remain to show whether the Phoenicians, Etruscans, or Scythians had an understanding of oral or dental diseases and whether they carried out any treatment.

## References

1. Asbell MB. Practice of dentistry among the ancient Hebrews. J Am Dent Assoc 1941;28:1098–1107.
2. Brim CJ. Medicine in the Bible. New York: Froben, 1936.
3. Clawson MD. A Phoenician dental appliance of the 5th century BC. Trans Am Dent Soc Europe 1933;142–160.
4. Eames WH. Scythian dentistry. Indep (Dent) Pract 1886;7:290–292.
5. Kaufman I. Medicine and surgery in the time of the Bible and the Talmud. J Am Dent Assoc 1944;31:777–784.
6. Weinberger BW. Ancient dentistry in the old and new world. Ann Med Hist 1934;6:264–279.
7. Weinberger BW. An Introduction to the History of Dentistry. St. Louis: Mosby, 1948.

# 4

# Pre-Columbian America

The rituals and religious beliefs of early North American Indians bear many similarities to those of other ancient cultures. There was usually a primary Creator or Great Spirit, and numerous lesser figures, often symbolized by celestial bodies, winds, clouds, fire, lightning and thunder, oceans or rivers, mountains, animals, fish, birds, and even plants and flowers. The more developed a society, the more elaborate its religious rituals and priestly hierarchy. Much of the evidence of Pre-Columbian American civilization is essentially religious-ritualistic in nature.

## Mayas and Aztecs

The Mayas (33–1400 AD) developed a highly sophisticated civilization with large cities, spectacular monuments, and a writing system composed of a form of hieroglyphic characters. Each of the glyphs had an independent meaning: they were ideographic rather than alphabetic figures constructing language. The Mayan record can still be seen on many stone monuments in Copan and Palenque; however, a vast number of books, with hieroglyphs and colored illustrations on paper made from the fiber of the agave plant, were destroyed by order of the conquering Spanish and their religious advisors. Only three of these books have survived: the Dresden Codex, the Perez Codex in Paris, and the Tro-Cortesiano in Spain. These books deal primarily with religion and the calendar.

The Aztecs overtook the Mayas and absorbed most of their culture. Then in 1521 the Aztec empire fell to the Spanish conquerors. Many fragments of writing and illustration remain from the Aztec civilization, and these offer a relatively broad picture of the culture, religion, and scientific and medical accomplishments.[1,2,4]

Medicine, as in other early societies, was closely allied to religion, and disease was considered a form of punishment for one's transgressions or the whim of a powerful and unkind deity. Legions of gods controlled the heavens and the earth and all the functions of man and nature around him.

Experience taught, however, that some diseases could be cured or their symptoms alleviated by certain medicinal plants. Disease could also be prevented by appropriate dances, rituals, incantations or prayers, and amulets or charms. The most important extant manuscript is the *Badianus Manuscript* or *Codex Barberini*, in the Vatican Library.[3] It was written by an Aztec, Martinus de la Cruz, a physician of the College of Santa Cruz, and translated into Latin by another Aztec, Joannes Badianus, and is often referred to as the *Aztec Herbal*. Although it was written as late as 1552, during early Spanish rule, and dedicated to the Spanish viceroy of Mexico, it represents a true picture of early Aztec medicine. The manuscript makes up an extensive materia medica, listing diverse animal, plant, and mineral remedies for the treatment of various diseases. Animal remedies were extracted from various organs including the brain, concretions or pathologic calcifications found in various organs (kidney stones, etc), and ashed bone or horn. One hundred eighty-five of the plant remedies are, fortunately, illustrated in the manuscript, so identification is possible for most of those listed. Among the important remedial plants were a species of datura that contained the drugs atropine, hyoscyamine, and scopolamine; peyote, containing a pain-relieving agent; tzompalti, containing a hypnotic drug; and tobacco, used as a depressant. Minerals included jasper, pearl, salt, red ochre, gypsum, saltpeter, alum, amber, and gold.

The *Aztec Herbal* evinces use of astringent lotions and mouthwashes, as well as purgatives such as cascara. Aztecs burned incense to drive away diseases such as epilepsy, that were assumed to be associated with evil spirits. One hundred one diseases are mentioned in thirteen sections, beginning with ailments of the head and progressing to those of the feet. Pulmonary and cardiac problems are mentioned as well as urinary problems, dysentery, and various ailments of skin.

The text investigates diseases of the mouth, including tooth pain, ulceration of mouth and oropharynx, and periodontal problems. Remedies for dental and oral diseases are presented, as are several prescriptions for toothache and various dentifrices to clean and shine the teeth.[3]

The following exerpts are taken from the fifth chapter:

> *Cure of Festering or Swelling Gums.* Pains of the teeth and gums are allayed by scarifying and properly purifying the gums, while the seeds and root of the nettle, rubbed up with yolk of egg and white honey, are applied to the festered part.
>
> *Tooth Polish to Shine the Teeth.* Rough teeth are to be diligently made smooth; the dirt being removed, they are to be rubbed with white ashes in white honey, using a small cloth, whereby elegant cleanness and real brightness will stay.

## The Inca Empire

The Incas of Peru represent another advanced civilization, flourishing from 1000 AD or earlier until they were conquered by the Spaniards under Pizarro in 1532. The Incas had developed a sophisticated urban society with carefully planned cities, highways, public buildings, and dwellings of different styles. There was an organized system of government, advanced agriculture, and obvious technological accomplishments necessary for the construction of cities of stone, and highways that traversed the mountainous region of Peru. The Incas might have held complex ideas regarding philosophy and government, but they did not develop a written language, and except for some pottery, little pictorial evidence remains.

Inca medicine and science may have been fairly advanced but research reveals little of it. The shapes and forms of water jugs in various museums show operations such as childbirth or figures with obvious pathology. Archeological studies have revealed further information about diseases and surgical practice. Skull trepanning was practiced with skilled technique, evidenced by the round, smooth holes in the skulls of mummies, but whether the procedure was performed as a religious rite or for the relief of headaches or mental and neurological problems is not known. Explorers' and conquerors' records note that the Incas had an extensive materia medica. Many of the drugs were new to Europeans, but quinine and coca soon became popular for their unusual qualities. Curare was also used in Peru, as was balsam, ipecac, and guaiaic.

Dental studies of Inca remains reveal extensive wear of molar teeth due to the coarse grains that formed their major diet. Abrasion of the buccal surfaces of the molar teeth was also commonly seen. Unusual features in Inca teeth are inlays applied to maxillary anterior teeth for decorative purposes. The cavities were carefully drilled to permit the insertion of jade or gold fillings. The absence of caries in this region of the anterior teeth suggests a cosmetic rather than therapeutic purpose for these inlays.

## References


1. Boone EH. The Codex Magliabechiano. Berkeley: University of California Press, 1983.
2. Cooper CJ. Codex Mendoza, 3 vols. London: Waterlow & Sons, 1938.
3. Gates W. De La Cruz-Badiano Aztec Herbal of 1552. Baltimore: The Maya Society, 1939.
4. Nuttal Z. The Book of the Life of the Ancient Mexicans. Translation and Commentary. Berkeley: University of California Press, 1903.

# Part II

# Classical and Medieval Ages

# 5

# Greece, Rome, and Byzantium

## Greece

Greek civilization remains one of the astonishing achievements. One small city-state, Athens, was to foster the greatest talent that ever existed, in fields as diverse as philosophy, literature, drama, painting, sculpture, architecture, and science. Above all, among extant documents from various ancient cultures, the Greek records stand out as the first to convey abstract ideas. The Greeks created theoretical systems, often complete to the smallest details, and these made possible their elaborate philosophical systems—systems essentially free of the magic and religious constraints of the Asiatic and Egyptian civilizations. Political and ethical philosophy flourished, but science also advanced as abstractions and theories were tested in the realm of the concrete and observable.

A concept of the four elements of the physical world, namely earth, water, air, and fire, was applied to medical thought and practice, and diseases were thought to be an imbalance of the basic elements or qualities of matter in the body. Medicaments were sought to counter the nature of the imbalance. For example, if a disease was thought to be caused by an excess of heat, then cooling agents or drugs would be sought. Thus, early Greek medicine developed from the earlier concepts of philosophy and its views of the physical world.

The chief medicinal agents used by the Greek physicians of the Hippocratic period were barley gruel or *ptisan, hydromel* (a mixture of water and honey), *oxymel* (a mixture of wine and honey), and *melicrate* (possibly a kind of mead).[15] The barley gruel was the major medicament used in all acute diseases and its preparation was rigidly outlined. It could be mixed with water, milk, or wine and then honey, salt, or herbs could be added to produce a mixture known as *cyclon*. Each of the possible additives was supposed to produce a different medicament, such as cooking or astringent or laxative or purgative. The gruel was usually administered with meals in increasing doses until the fever was lowered. Herbs were also used for a variety of purposes. Black hellebore was a commonly used laxative. Hyssop, together with vinegar and salt, was a common emetic (if it did not work, it could be helped by placing a finger down the throat). Topical applications were used to dress wounds and relieve the discomfort or pain of open wounds. Chamomile mixed with beeswax and olive oil appears to have been an effective ointment. Pitch could be added for an analgesic effect.

The most significant figure in ancient Greek medicine was Hippocrates (460–377 BC) (Fig 3). He has been revered as the Father of Medicine and until recently his code of medical ethics was part of the graduation ceremony for medical students. Hippocrates was a prolific writer, producing over sixty separate treatises in his field of interest.[1]

Hippocrates' contributions to modern medicine are threefold. First, he showed the importance of clinical observation of the patient; second, he recognized the value of letting nature help the healing process rather than instituting various procedures that may be damaging ("Above all, do no harm"); and third, he introduced the concept of disease prevention through proper nutrition and a healthy environment.

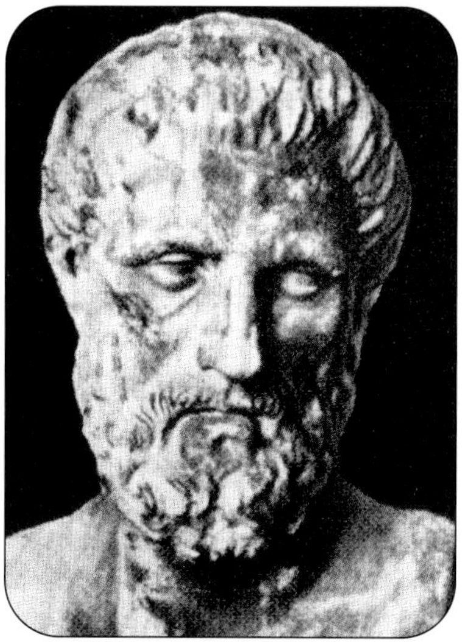

**Fig 3** Bust of Hippocrates dated to fourth century BC, found in Odeion of Cos in 1929, and now at the Museum of Cos.

In relation to pathology of the mouth and jaws, Hippocrates describes dislocations and fractures of the mandible (On Joints, Section 30) and accurately details epidemic parotitis or mumps, including the orchitis that may occur as a complication (On Epidemics, Book 1, Section 1). He also notes that the mouth could be affected by ulcers in many types of systemic diseases (On Epidemics, Book 3, Section 7).

Democritus (ca 460–370 BC), an eminent pre-Socratic philosopher, developed a theory of atomism. The world was made up of basic, indivisible particles of matter moving through empty space. The particles (atoma) had shape, mass, and motion but no other qualities, such as color or flavor. These were subjective and were supplied by the observer. Democritus applied his theory to the variety of taste sensations in the mouth, offering the first approach to the physiology of taste.

Aristotle (384–322 BC) was the leading scholar, teacher, and philosopher of ancient Greece, and possibly the most influential philosopher in the history of Western thought. His career encompassed political advisor as well as teacher. He was a student and, later, a teacher in the Academy of Plato. After Plato's death he joined the court of King Philip II of Macedonia and became tutor to Alexander. Later he returned to Athens and founded his own school, the Lyceum, with a broader curriculum than the Academy, particularly in the study of nature and natural phenomena. Aristotle was apparently a genius with universal knowledge spanning the disciplines, and wrote learned treatises on philosophy, politics, and science.[19]

Aristotle investigated oral disease, particularly in a treatise called *Problems.* He talks about the causes of periodontal disease and dental caries and discusses the nature of occlusion and the shapes of the teeth for this purpose.

> *Problemata, Book 22.* Why do figs, which are soft and sweet, destroy the teeth? Do they, owing to their stickiness, penetrate into the gums, and, because they are soft, insinuate themselves into the spaces between the teeth, and, being hot, quickly cause decay? Perhaps also, owing to the hardness of the seeds, the teeth are quickly caused to ache in the process of chewing them up.[19]

## Rome

While the civilization of Greece was intellectual and esthetic, that of Rome was based mainly on practical considerations of governing and maintaining an empire. Rome was a formidable military power and developed legal and technological expertise to maintain its imperial strength. A vast network of roads was necessary for the armed legions and they were constructed so well that many still exist today. Great wealth was expended to import Greek art and to copy the style. The greatest of Greek minds came to work in Rome, and many of the important treatises produced in Rome were written in Greek. Roman citizens lived in luxury; technological advances improved the quality of material life enormously. Water was brought from long distances by aqueducts[9] and introduced into homes through metal pipes. Personal cleanliness was now not only possible but extolled as a virtue. The result was that Roman citizens' health improved. Sewage systems were developed for the urban areas, made possible by the running water in houses.[9] The city of Rome used advanced technology to build a sprawling metropolis with great public buildings and elaborate homes.

Roman law is still essentially the law that governs all our basic legal transactions. Romans, with wealth and leisure, could indulge their artistic and intellectual desires. They became great encyclopedists, gathering the knowledge of the past, and their compilations were of great help in education. Many of these treatises were still in use hundreds of years later.

A world empire required not only a strong leadership, but a strong army with well trained soldiers and effective weapons. It required highways to move the army rapidly and the technology to build camps rapidly to maintain the troops. One of the Romans' major achievements was to establish hospitals throughout the empire, to care for ill and wounded soldiers.[20] Essential, too, were the well-trained doctors who looked after them. In addition, technological advances resulted in the manufacture of superior surgical instruments.[20] Although more crude in design, many Roman instruments are similar to those still used today.

Rome, with its enormous wealth, attracted the best of Greek physicians, scientists, artists, and architects. Many Romans were similarly educated and therefore able to carry on the Greek tradition of scholarship. Romans began to write in Latin rather than Greek, and Latin would become the language of scholars for the next 1,200 years. Rome also fostered its own poets and dramatists in the Latin language. But it was in scholarship that the Roman mind excelled, particularly in vast encyclopedias that were meant to set down all the available knowledge in a particular field. Strabo wrote the first world geography, and Vitruvius the first work on architecture. Pliny the Elder wrote a vast work on natural history, quoting hundreds of authors.[18] Although many inaccuracies exist, the amount of solid information is enormous. Lucretius produced a long poem, *On The Nature of Things*, a work of science with many advanced ideas, but still incorporating much of the traditional Greek philosophy on the nature of the physical world.

Celsus (25 BC–50 AD) wrote a large work on medicine—a comprehensive review of medical knowledge of the time. Celsus stresses the importance of learning anatomy by dissection but cannot accept some of the cruelty of the age. "To open the bodies of the living is, moreover, cruel and useless; but those who devote themselves to medicine, cannot dispense with the dissection of the dead." Celsus' *De Re Medicina*[7] became one of the basic texts of Renaissance medicine along with other classic works, such as the *Canon* of Avicenna. Celsus was a timeless writer in many ways. His descriptions are clear to twenty-first-century readers. His materia medica classifies drugs according to their actions. They are described as stomachics, calefacients, emollients, irritants, inflators, refrigerants, nutritives, cauterants, purges, and so on.

Celsus originated the concept of compounding different agents in proper ratio and used weights and measures in these prescriptions. Their mode of administration was also presented, such as plasters, salves, pastilles, powders, and so on.

Celsus offers treatment for a number of periodontal conditions:[7]

> If blood escapes from the gums, it suffices to chew purslane; if from the mouth, undiluted wine should be held in it; if this does no good, then vinegar. … If the gums have retracted from the teeth, the same antherae are of service. It is also useful to chew pears and apples which are not too ripe, and to hold the juice in the mouth. Vinegar that is

> not too sharp can also be held in the mouth to similar advantage. … In the mouth too some conditions are treated by surgery. In the first place, teeth sometimes become loose, either from weakness of the roots, or from disease drying up the gums. In either case the cautery should be applied so as to touch the gums lightly without pressure. The gums so cauterized are smeared with honey, and swilled with honey wine. When the ulcerations have begun to clean, dry medicaments, acting as repressants, are dusted on.

Dioscorides (40–90 AD) was a Greek physician and surgeon born in Anazarba, Cilecia, who served as an army surgeon in the legions of the Emperor Nero. He wrote a number of treatises on medical subjects but is famous for a magnificent *Materia Medica,* or herbal, that was the basis for all work on the subject until the sixteenth century. Dioscorides' herbal represented the knowledge in the field up to his time and not only was the authoritative work, but also served as the textbook for medical education in this field until modern times. Much of the book is a compendium of drugs, many of which appear to be original to Dioscorides. Over 600 plants are described in terms of preparation, storage, use, doses, pharmacological effects, and the diseases that can be prevented or alleviated by these drugs. Book I deals with spices, salves, and oils. Book II deals with agents of animal and vegetable derivation such as milk, honey, and various grains. Books III and IV deal with plants and roots. Book V deals with wines and minerals. The important drugs include acacia, aloes, alum, ammonia, anise, apocyanum, cannabis, cantharides, cardamom, cassia, colchicine, colocynth, copper, coriander, croton oil, gentian, gold, hellebore, hemlock, hyoscyamus, iron, lead, lily, mercury, mandragora, mustard, myrtle, nutgalls, opium, peppermint, roses, saffron, salt, silver, solanum, starch, thyme, tragacanth, and vinegar.[8]

One of Dioscorides' more important contributions was to use drugs as pain killers, sedatives, or analgesics. Opium was used for relief of pain and the soporific effects of opium, mandragora, and hyoscyamine are noted. The famous passage in Chapter 76 of Book IV suggests a concept of anesthesia.[5] The wine of mandragora was to be used

> upon those being sleepless and those in great pain and upon whom they wish to produce anesthesia [Dioscorides' word] while being cut or cauterized.

Memphis stone was to be used for local anesthesia:

> It is said that this being beaten small and smeared upon the places to be cut or cauterized, produces anesthesia without danger.

The number of drugs used for specific diseases was very large, possibly indicating relatively low effectiveness in many cases.

Chapter 77 sheds light on contemporary treatment of the mouth[5]:

> Loose teeth and spongy gums are made tight if the following is used as a mouth-wash and kept in the mouth for some time: a decoct of the leaves of the olive tree, ass' milk, the juice of pickled olives, gum myrrh with wine and oil as a mouth-wash, bituminous coal boiled with wine, planetree leaves boiled with vinegar, vinegar of squills, chewed blackberries; equally as good is mallow root; iron rust placed dry thereon, in the same manner pomegranate flower, fissile alum and myrrh mixed, or without myrrh with vinegar and honey; further, in the same manner burned sory, gum styrax mixed with salt and placed thereon. Or myrrh, pompholyx, starch powder, equal parts, finely powdered and dry. Or pomegranate peeling, nutgalls, chalcanthon mixed with vinegar as a mouth-wash; or ten frogs, one-half chus, vinegar, four drams chalcanthon, six drams mandragora root boiled down to one-third as a mouth-wash. For the toothache the following remedy is also of service: four drams aloes, one dram gum thus, four drams fissile alum to be mixed with honey and rubbed thereon.

Chapter 78 suggests some mouthwashes to be used remedially[5]:

> Against swelling, proud flesh, and gangrene of the gums the following are good remedies as mouth-washes and held in the mouth: The juice of garden purslane, a decoct of the root of tragacanth in wine, the juice of pickled olives, oil pressed from unripe olives, quince oil, and the oil of mastic. To be held in the mouth: Myrrh with wine and oil, gum cedar with vinegar and sediment of oil, also a decoct of nutgalls, a decoct of the bark and the leaves of mulberry, vinegar of squills.

Aretaeus of Cappadocia was a physician in the second century AD. Little is known of his life, but he left a remarkable legacy in clinical medicine, with excellent descriptions of many diseases, including cholera, tetanus, pneumonia, diphtheria, and diabetes. He wrote about a variety of neurological diseases, including epilepsy, migraine, and paraplegia.[4]

Galen is one of the supreme figures in the history of ancient medicine. Clinician, thorough observer and researcher, and prolific writer,[10–14] his complete works in the 1821–1833 edition of Kuhn take up twenty-two volumes.[20] In addition to the eighty-three genuine works on medicine that exist in published form, at least another forty have been lost. In the entire medical literature, Galen's works were used most widely and for the longest period of time. Galen's reputation has suffered only from the fact that his writings were used as major textbooks until the eighteenth century. Many doctrines and observations that were acceptable and even advanced for his own times became outdated and were viewed as filled with errors in the new scholarly and scientific approaches of the Enlightenment in Europe. One can hardly fault Galen that his works were revered and unquestioningly accepted as medical dogmas by succeeding generations of physicians for some 1,300 years. The ignorance and superstition that followed the fall of Rome and lasted for a thousand years can be blamed for the dogmatic acceptance of Galen's writings. In actuality, Galen's treatises contain many superb observations and a well systematized approach to medicine generally, even though his writings on dental and periodontal topics are not particularly original.

In addition to those mentioned above, other contemporary physicians contributed information on dental medicine at this early time: Soranus of Ephesus (ca 98–138 AD),[21] Caelius Aurelianus,[6] and Scribonius Largus. Their writings primarily deal with dental caries and the management of toothache.

## Byzantium

Despite the strong efforts of the emperors Diocletian and Constantine, the Roman Empire in the West could not overcome the stress of constant warfare with northern barbarians and the resultant economic and cultural decline.

The Byzantine Empire rose when the Roman emperor Constantine adopted the Christian religion and founded the city of Constantinople, which was to become the capital of the new empire. Its language was Greek, and the many scholars of theology and medicine, as well as the poets, wrote in that language. From its beginning in the fourth century until the eleventh century the Byzantine empire was the major power in Europe in strength and prestige. It was heir to the Greco-Roman civilization and it developed a high level of architecture, art, music, and literature, as well as science and medicine. Constantinople occupied a position similar to that previously held by Rome, and its university became the center of Byzantine learning. The empire under Justinian, from 527 to 565, exerted its influence over most of the Mediterranean region, including Greece, Turkey, and parts of Spain, Italy, the Middle East, and North Africa.

The Byzantine Empire was constantly at war with Persians from the east, Slavs from the north, Lombards in Italy, and other tribes in the west.

Perhaps the greatest achievement of Justinian's reign was the reorganization and reformation of the Roman legal system. The task of rendering Roman law clear, coherent, and suitable for a Christian society was assigned by Justinian to a body of ten prominent legal authorities. The result was the Justinian Code, which played an important role in the development of modern law. The eventual decline of the empire resulted from struggles with the developing Arabic civilization and the competing sea-faring powers such as Venice.

There were four major medical writers of the Byzantine era—Oribasius,[16] Aetios of Amida,[2] Alexander of Tralles,[3] and Paul of Aegina.[17]

Among the four outstanding Byzantine writers, Oribasius (ca 325–?) was physician to the Emperor Julian and, although he made few original discoveries, wrote an encyclopedia of medicine in seventy volumes that preserved the works of many early writers. He has a number of sections on toothache and gingival inflammation.[16]

> TREATMENT OF TOOTHACHE; OF TEETH THAT SUFFER FROM COLD AND ARE MOBILE
>
> Mash the roots of plantain or boil them and use as a mouthwash (decoction); use similarly as a mouthwash myrtle branches boiled in vinegar, or roots of cinquefoil boiled in wine, or black hellebore with vinegar, or mash the skin of the caper root. For the toothache that results from cold, use the root of pyrethrum, warm wine, hyssop, wild raisin, pennyroyal with oxymel, the grains and leaves of henbane with vinegar, or with donkey's milk; all this will restabilize the mobile (loose) teeth. Heat the outside part with pouches of burnt salt in the form of small pellets. Heat the tooth itself: dip a dry branch of oregano in boiling oil and apply it on the crown of the painful tooth.

Aetios of Amida (502–575) compiled a large corpus of material.[2] Book VIII of his *Tetrabiblion* has thirty-one sections devoted to diseases of the mouth and their management. Sections 22 through 27 are devoted to diseases of the gingiva and bear the following titles: About Inflammation of the Gums, About Bleeding Gums, About Purulent Gums, About Rotten Gums, About Parulis, and About Epulis.

For example, the following excerpt details his approach to a common problem:

> ABOUT THE GRINDING OF TEETH
>
> Because the teeth are loose and mobile, if we want the lower teeth not to come into contact with the upper teeth, we take a file and we grind that tooth, which is necessary to avoid this from happening. On the day that the grinding is done, we suggest to the patient to avoid eating hard food.

Alexander of Tralles (525–605) practiced in Rome and traveled widely. He has been described as the greatest scholar in medicine between Galen and the Renaissance. His twelve books on medicine[3] were translated into Latin and Arabic and were widely studied in the medical schools of the middle ages. They were also an important foundation for the development of Arabic medicine.

Paul of Aegina (625–690) was the last of the great Byzantine physicians and left an extremely large body of work in twelve volumes that were translated into English in 1844 by Francis Adams.[17] Paul was familiar with the Greek and Roman writings on medicine and expanded and clarified their work. He wrote extensively on disease of the mouth and on surgical procedures of the oral tissues, such as ankyloglossia and its surgical management. Paul also devoted many sections of his work to diseases of childhood, discussing the problems of the emerging dentition and describing a variety of oral lesions such as aphthae, epulis, and parulis. The record shows he also excised tonsils and extracted cataracts. In his texts he suggests some preventive measures as well as treatments for tooth decay and gum disease:

*Preservatives of the teeth.* The teeth will not decay if the following things be attended to: in the first place, to avoid indigestion, and frequent repetitions of emetics. Guard against such food as is hurtful to the teeth, as dried figs, honey boiled, so as to become very hard, dates which are difficult to rub down, and all glutinous substances; likewise such things as are difficult to break, and may thereby loosen the teeth; in like manner also, such substances as set the teeth on edge, and everything which is cold and putrid. The teeth also ought to be cleaned after supper.

*A dentifrice.* The burnt roots of birthwort, burnt hartshorn with some mastich.—Another: White salts mixed with honey, and wrapped in the leaves of the fig-tree, and burnt until reduced to ashes.—Another: Buccinae filled with salt and burnt; land snails burnt with honey; unwashed wool burnt with a little salts. With each of these, for the sake of fragrance, let there be mixed the schaenanth, or spikenard, Indian leaf (malabathrum), or cyperus, or iris.

*An application which will whiten the teeth, repress swelling of the gums, and produce fragrant breath.* Of pumice-stone, of roasted salts, of iris, of each, dr. iv; of cyperus, dr. v; of spikenard, dr. j; of pepper, dr. vj; pulverize, and use.

*For corroded gums.* Of the flowers of roses, dr. viij; of galls, dr. iv; of myrrh, dr. ij. Erosions and running from the gums are cured by washing with asses' milk, the decoction of olive leaves, or vinegar of squills; or by the following dry applications: the rust of iron, and flowers of the cultivated pomegranate. For swelling and fungous flesh of the gums, the juice of purslain retained in the mouth, the brine of pickled olives, warm oil of unripe olives, or lentisk oil, or oil of apples, or lees of oil, are applicable; and the following powders: the rust of iron or copper, the roots of birthwort, the seed of plantain, diphryges, calcined copperas, pomegranate flowers.

## References


1. Adams F (trans). The Genuine Works of Hippocrates, 2 vols. New York: Wood, 1886.
2. Aetios of Amida. Aetii Amideni. Libri medicinales V-VIII. Alexander Olivieri (ed). Berlin: Corpus Medicorum Graecorum, 1950.
3. Alexander of Tralles. Practica, 2 vols [German translation]. Puschman T (trans). Vienna: Braumuller, 1878.
4. Aretaeus. The Extant Works of Aretaeus, the Cappadocian. Adams F (trans). London: Sydenham Society, 1856.
5. Berendes J. The home remedies of Dioscorides. Dent Cosmos 1915;15:642–644.
6. Caelius Aurelianus. On Acute Diseases and on Chronic Diseases. Drabkin IE (trans). Chicago: University of Chicago Press, 1950.
7. Celsus. De Medicina, 3 vols. Spencer WG (trans-ed). Cambridge, MA: Harvard University Press, 1948.
8. Dioscorides. The Greek Herbal of Dioscorides. Goodyer J (trans). Gunther RT (ed). New York: Hafner, 1959.
9. Frontinus. The Two Books on the Water Supply of the City of Rome of Sixtus Julius Frontinus. Herschel C (trans). New York: Longman Green, 1913.
10. Galen. The Natural Faculties. Brock AJ (trans). Cambridge, MA: Harvard University Press, 1916.
11. Galen. Hygiene. Green RM (trans). Springfield, IL: Charles C. Thomas, 1951.
12. Galen. Anatomical Procedures. Singer C (trans). London: Oxford University Press, 1956.
13. Galen. Medical Experience. Walzer R (trans). London: Oxford University Press, 1944.
14. Galen. On the Usefulness of Parts of the Body. May MT (trans). Ithaca, NY: Cornell University Press, 1968.
15. Lund FB. Greek Medicine. New York: Hoeber, 1936.
16. Oribasius. Oevres d'Oribase, 6 vols [French translation]. Daremberg, Bussemaker (trans). Paris: Imprimerie Nationale, 1851–1876.
17. Paulus Aeginata. The Seven Books of Paul of Aegina. Adams F (trans). London: Sydenham Society, 1844.
18. Pliny. The Natural History, 10 vols. Rackham H, Jones WHS, et al (trans, eds). Cambridge, MA: Harvard University Press, 1979.
19. Ross WD. The Works of Aristotle, 10 vols. London: Oxford University Press, 1908–1930.
20. Shklar G, Chernin D. A Sourcebook of Dental Medicine. Waban, MA: Maro, 2002.
21. Soranus. Gynecology. Temkin O (trans). Baltimore: Johns Hopkins University Press, 1955.

# 6

# Arabian Medicine

The rise of Islam was a complex political and religious phenomenon. Arabian science and, particularly, Arabian medicine were not only among the great attainments of the eastern world in the Middle Ages, but represented to a large extent the impetus for the rise of European medicine in the later Middle Ages and Renaissance. In the early medical schools of Salerno and Montpellier, texts were the renowned Arabic treatises in Latin translation. Much of medieval and Renaissance stomatology and dentistry was derived from Arabic writings, particularly the medieval treatises of Avicenna and Abulcasis.

Arabic medical texts evolved, to a large extent, from Greek, Roman, and Byzantine sources. As Browne pointed out many years ago, Arabian science and Arabian medicine really represent "the body of scientific and medical doctrine which is enshrined in books written in Arabic language, but which is for the most part, Greek in origin, though with Indian, Persian, and Syrian accretions, and only in a very small degree the product of the Arabian mind."[5] Translation of Greek texts into Arabic was one of the most important intellectual ventures carried out under the patronage of the early Abbasid Caliphate at Baghdad between the years 750 and 850 AD. These classical treatises were later translated back into Latin during the Middle Ages because the Greek originals were unavailable.

The Arabic empire was to encompass the entire Middle East and extend throughout northern Africa and into Spain. The capital of the empire was Baghdad and this city became a central seat of learning as well as a thriving metropolis with hospitals and other modern institutions. Eventually Baghdad shared intellectual and medical eminence with Cordoba, in Spain, and thus they epitomized the greatness of both the eastern and the western Caliphate.

By the tenth century Cordoba was the most modern city in Europe, with 70 libraries, 900 public baths, and 50 hospitals, as well as an outstanding university. The empire lasted until 1250 AD, when destruction of Baghdad by the Mongols was so complete that little of the Islamic culture survived, although the eastern Caliphate, in Spain, continued for another 200 years.[7]

The three great names in eastern Arabian medicine are Abu Bakr Muhammed, ibn Zakariyya al Razi (ca 841–926), Ali ibnu'l Abbas al Majusi (d. 994), and Abu Ali al-Hussain ibn Sina (980–1037), known in Western literature as Rhazes, Haly Abbas, and Avicenna, respectively.[5,6] Rhazes, possibly the most well-known and most original of the three, wrote on a variety of subjects but excelled in medicine. Rhazes became physician-in-chief at the famous Baghdad hospital and taught medicine in terms of clinical cases, complete with patients' names, symptomatology, therapy, and results. Of Rhazes' surviving works the largest is *Al Hawi*, an encyclopedic work on medicine and surgery, in twenty-five volumes. Among the specific achievements of Rhazes, in addition to case report teaching, was the first accurate description of smallpox and measles among the infectious diseases[10] and an extensive materia medica including mercurial ointments.

Haly Abbas composed an extensive treatise on medicine, known as *al-Maliki*, which was regarded as the standard text on the science and practice of medicine until it was superseded by the *Canon* of Avicenna around 1010 AD. Haly Abbas, born in Persia, wrote with clarity, style,

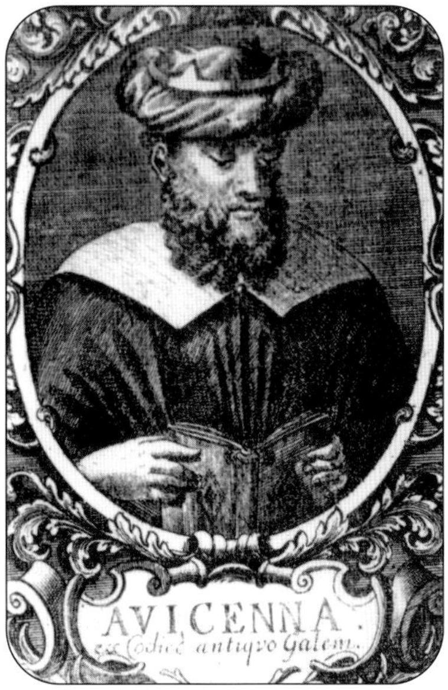


Fig 4 Avicenna.

and organization unequaled among his contemporaries. Haly Abbas credits his predecessors but evaluates their work critically, pointing out that Hippocrates is often too concise and obscure, while Galen tends to be verbose. He criticized Rhazes' work for being too verbose and obscure.

Among Haly Abbas' discoveries is a capillary system between veins and arteries, the blood vessels being distinguished by an absence or presence of pulsation. Detailed descriptions are offered of catheterization, laryngotomy, suturing of blood vessels before sectioning, and excision of tumors. Pleurisy is described as well as many dermatologic disorders such as eczema, scabies, seborrheic dermatitis, and alopecia areata.

Haly Abbas' *Kitabu'l-Maliki* recommends methods for cleaning the mouth, in a section on oral diseases[12]:

> Dentifrices should be used that give a nice smell to the mouth such as musk seeds. Wipe the gums in the morning and evening using a rough piece of cloth and clean with fermenting juice and grease the gums with rose oil if the gum was hot (inflamed). Or one can use elder balsam if it was cold and humid and chewing cloves and mastic with some stavesacre and pyrethrum.

Avicenna, while perhaps not the greatest of Arabian physicians, was certainly the greatest intellect of Islam (Fig 4).[3,4] His knowledge and attainments were almost unbelievable in scope. By the time he was 18 years old, he had exhausted all the known sciences, treated the Sultan of Bukhara, and completed his study of ancient texts. By age 21 he had composed an encyclopedia of all the sciences except mathematics. His fame rests on two great works: the *Canon*, a comprehensive treatise on medicine, and the *Shifa*, an encyclopedia of Aristotelian philosophy and science. He made many contributions to mineralogy, chemistry, astronomy, and the physics of heat, light, and sound.

The *Canon* is possibly the longest lasting medical text of all time, having been in continuous use for almost 600 years. Among its contributions are concise descriptions of meningitis, tuberculosis, and chronic nephritis.

Avicenna's contributions to stomatology consisted primarily of the diagnosis and systematization of oral disease.[11] He used an extensive materia medica for oral and periodontal diseases and rarely resorted to surgery. Venesection and other primitive procedures were performed. However, Avicenna insightfully discusses dental problems such as tooth mobility.

He understood that tooth decay was caused by putrefaction. Treatment consisted of cleaning out the carious areas and preventing further decay through use of appropriate drugs, usually astringent in nature. Discoloration of teeth was treated with abrasive pastes. Various drug combinations were used in dentifrices and mouthwashes. Anesthetic drugs were used in cases of toothache.

The *Canon* of Avicenna[3] is comprehensive. Sections on the oral cavity and its problems are as follows:

### Mouth and Tongue

1. Anatomy of the Mouth and Tongue
2. Diseases of the Tongue and Treatment
3. Abnormalities or Loss of Taste and Treatment
4. Paresis of the Tongue and Difficulty of Articulation
5. Spasms and Paralysis of the Tongue and Treatment
6. Enlarged Tongue [Macroglossia] and Treatment
7. Binding of the Tongue [Tongue-tie] and Treatment
8. Swellings of the Tongue and Treatment
9. Problems in Locution [Speech Defects]
10. Ranula and Treatment
11. Inflammation of the Tongue [Glossitis]
12. Treatment of the Fissures of the Tongue
13. Protrusion of the Tongue
14. Mouth Eruptions and their Treatment
15. Malignant Ulcers and their Treatment
16. Excessive Salivation and Treatment
17. The Removal of Horrible [Bad] Odors
18. Bleeding from the Mouth [Hemorrhage] and Treatment
19. Halitosis and its Treatment
20. Mouth Breathing

### The Teeth

1. General Discussion of the Teeth
2. Dental Hygiene and Conservation of the Teeth
3. General Discussion of Treatment of Dental Problems
4. Toothache, Its Signs and Treatment
5. Medicines [Drugs] used in the Treatment of Dental Pain
6. Stupefying [Anesthetic] Drugs
7. Loose Teeth and Their Treatment
8. Corrosion [Caries] of the Teeth
9. Breakdown of the Teeth from Decay and Treatment
10. Discoloration of the Teeth and Treatment
11. Facilitating the Eruption of the Teeth
12. The Regimen for Extraction of Teeth
13. Extraction of Decayed Teeth without Pain
14. Worms in the Teeth
15. Causes of Grinding of the Teeth and Treatment
16. Elongation of Teeth
17. Teeth on Edge and Treatment
18. Sensitive Teeth and Treatment
19. The Treatment of Debilitated [Weak] Teeth

### Concerning the Gingiva and Lips

1. Diseases of the Gums and their Treatment
2. Bleeding Gums and Treatment
3. Fissures of the Gums
4. Ulcers of the Gums
5. Enlargement of the Gums and Treatment
6. Recession of the Gums and Treatment
7. The Treatment of Softness [Looseness] of the Gums
8. Diseases of the Lips
9. Fissures of the Lips and Treatment
10. Swellings and ulcers of the Lips
11. Hemorrhoids [Varicosities] of Lips
12. Tremors of the Lips

### Tooth Mobility[12]

The mobility of the teeth may be due to a fall, weakness of the nerve, decay of the root, enlargement of the socket, break in the gum (recession or ulceration) or atrophy of the teeth due to dryness such as in old people, or people in convalescence who have remained for a long period of time with poor nutrition, and could also be due to the shortness of the dental papillae.

*Treatment*

1. Avoid chewing on the mobile teeth.
2. Talk less.
3. Avoid touching the mobile teeth with the tongue.
4. If the cause of the mobility was decay, treat the decay using astringent, gargle, and massaging drugs.

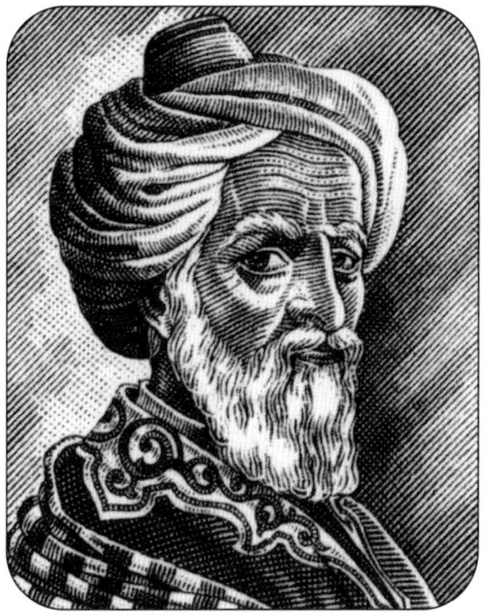

**Fig 5** Abulcasis (from a Syrian stamp issued in 1964).

5. If the cause was atrophy give good nutrition, but this type of mobility is difficult to manage. Use refreshing substances for adherence and massage. Also, place drops of nightshade juice and rose oil in the ear.
6. If the cause of the mobility was atrophy, nutrition does not give good results because it does not make it large quickly so we have to use a cold-producing astringent.

If the cause of the mobility was due to a fall or a hit use the same treatment. If it was due to a relaxing humid use a hot astringent such as water which has been cooked with cypress leaves and sultana wine with dill and salt or water cooked with sagapenum. From the adherent substances use 2 d of alum, 1 d of salt, and place on the root of the tooth. One may use copper rust with olive oil and lilly roots, cypress bark, 4 d of each with one part of dill. One may use tamarisk ashes or salt or burnt deer horn and salt mixed with burnt honey, burnt fruit, 10 d of each, myrrh, saffron, spike, mastic, 2 parts each. Saffron dry herb of grace with sumach and pomegranate blossom, 3 parts each. From this mixture prepare a dentifrice and adherent substance. Astringent mixed with aloes and colcothar (rouge) is a good dentifrice for this purpose. Another prescription is cyperus, rose, nard, and rock salt, (karnarge) burnt deer horn, equal parts of each. In cases of deficiency of dental papillae use burnt vitriol blue, and aloe mixed with cypress, pomegranate blossom, and sumach.

Abulcasis, or Albucasis, (b. 936) (Fig 5) was the greatest physician of the western Caliphate. Born in Cordoba, he became physician to the Caliph and composed a thirty-section encyclopedia titled *Al Tasrif*, or *The Method*, the definitive treatise of medicine and surgery. The last section is on surgery and represents the first illustrated surgical text, containing figures of several hundred surgical instruments and their use.

Among Abulcasis' contributions are descriptions of hemophilia, operation for cancer of the breast with metastases, use of ligatures and cautery for bleeding vessels, and lithotomy. Contributions to dentistry and stomatology also number among his achievements. In periodontology he understood that calculus deposits on the teeth were the major etiologic factor in periodontitis. He described in detail the technique of scaling the calculus deposits from the teeth with a set of instruments he developed (Fig 6).[1,2,8,9,11]

His instructions for the removal of teeth are similar to those used today and represent considerable sophistication in technique as well as instrumentation. Abulcasis also practiced orthodontics, correcting gross occlusal abnormalities. Teeth were filed if prominent in the arch and extracted if they erupted completely behind other teeth.

Gold or silver wires were used to splint loose anterior teeth that had been injured by a blow or a fall. The loose teeth were fastened to a stable tooth on each side and the wires carefully adapted—twisted and cut to avoid injuring the oral mucosa. Replacement of teeth was also suggested, using bone of cattle carved to the exact shape and size and wired into the appropriate position.

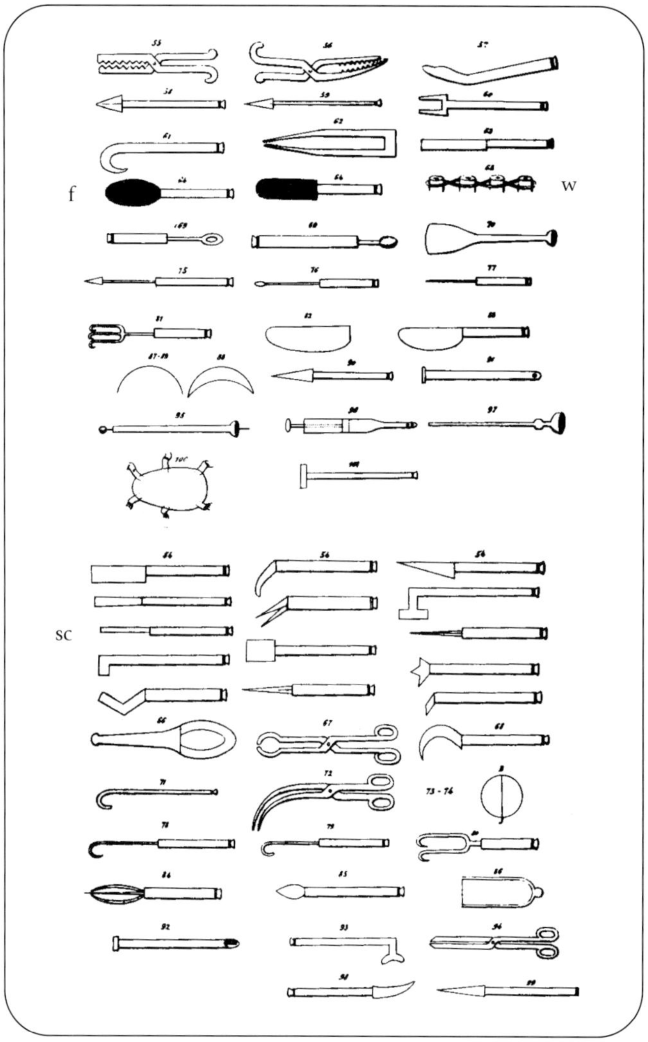


**Fig 6** Abulcasis' periodontal instruments showing files (f), scalers (sc), and the wiring (w) of loose teeth. A comparison of the many published editions and codices of Abulcasis' *De Chirurgia* reveal considerable differences in the number and shapes of the instruments represented. These renditions, from the 1532 edition, being more carefully drawn, more closely resemble the drawings and description in the original text. Some instruments are double-edged, and therefore serve a twofold purpose to facilitate scaling of several surfaces. Many resemble those now in use. Each handle has a row of elevations and depressions designed to afford a better grip of the instrument.

Abulcasis offers detailed descriptions of a frenectomy, of mucous cysts, and of tumor-like growths on the gingiva.[1]

### Excision of Fleshy Growths of the Gums
(Chapter XXVIII)

The gums are frequently the site of fleshy excrescences, which the ancients have named epulis. They must be lifted with a retractor or taken hold of with tongs and be excised at their base. The blood or fluid should be left to drain; then the area should be covered with green, powdered vitriol, or some other astringent, desiccative powder. If the growths should recur after operation, a frequent happening, they should be excised a second time and the area cauterized. They will cease to recur after cauterization.

### On the Scraping of Teeth
(Chapter XXIX)

Coarse, irregular concretions sometimes become deposited on the internal or external surface of the teeth, or between the gums: the teeth take on a black, yellow, or green color, then the gums become altered and this in turn is followed by exfoliation of the teeth. To treat this condition, have the patient sit in front of you and place his head on your knees. Scrape the teeth and the molars [the molars are always distinguished from the other teeth and designated by the word "dhirs," plural form being "adhras"] which present these concretions or gravel-like deposits, until none remain. Also scrape every black, green, yellow, or otherwise colored area, until they are completely cleared up. It is possible that a single scraping will suffice. If not, begin a second, third or fourth time until you have fully reached your goal.

Know that scraping of the teeth is done with instruments of varied shape, according to the purpose for which they have been designated.

The scrapers used for scraping the inside of the teeth are different from those used for the outside, or from those used to scrape the interdental surfaces.

Such is the assortment of scrapers which you must have at your disposal [(See Figure)].

### On the Filing (Sawing) of Prominent Teeth (Chapter XXXII)

Sometimes certain teeth develop abnormally and produce a deformity; this is most often seen in women and slaves. You must then examine whether these teeth grew behind the others. In such a case they can be neither sawed nor filed, they must be removed. If they are adherent to neighboring teeth, the adhesion must be severed with an instrument resembling a little saw, which is as follows, [(See Figure)].

The instrument must be of Indian iron with a very sharp cutting edge. Sectioning will require several days on account of the hardness of the teeth. If the prominence is such that it can be filed, this should be done with a file of Indian iron of the following shape [(See Figure)].

The entire instrument should be constructed of Indian iron. The handle shall be small for a better grip. It shall be similar to the files with which we make needles. You shall use it to file the tooth little by little, in several sessions, and with care to avoid loosening it, for it could fall out and in the process take with it an adjacent tooth. You should also scrape the tooth with a scraper such as we have described.

Should there be any chipped tooth which injures the tongue while speaking, it should be filed until the chip has been removed, and the area is smooth and polished, so that it will not further injure the tongue or harm one's speech.

### On the Consolidation (or Enmeshing) of Loose Teeth, Using Gold or Silver wires (Chapter XXXIII)

If the anterior teeth are loose, if they have been injured by a blow or in a fall, if the patient cannot chew anymore and astringent drugs have been of no value in the treatment, one is left with no other choice than splinting the teeth with either gold or silver wires. Gold is preferable. Indeed, silver will change and become green in a few days, whereas gold is not attacked and will always remain preserved in the same state. The wire will be of an average gauge and proportioned according to the available interdental space. The wire network is established as follows. Introduce the bent wire between two healthy teeth. With the free ends fasten the loose teeth, either one or several, and extend this network past the loose teeth until you reach healthy teeth. From there you continue your interlacing back to the starting point. Tighten carefully and skillfully so that the teeth will no longer rock. Keep the wires at the base of the teeth so that they will not become displaced. Cut the extra wire with pliers. Twist the free ends and tuck them between healthy teeth in such a way that they will not injure the tongue. Leave the teeth thus bound as long as they will remain in place. Should a wire loosen or break, it should be replaced with a new one, which must be constantly retained.

We are showing you here the teeth and the network which binds both the healthy and the loose teeth together [(See Figure)].

When one or two teeth have fallen out they can be replaced and consolidated in the same manner we have just explained, and they will be maintained. For this, one needs a light and a trained hand.

Sometimes, teeth can be replaced by pieces of cattle bone whittled to the shape of teeth, which are positioned in the space occupied by the teeth that have fallen out and fastened into place as we have just described, and one gets along quite well.[1]

## References


1. Albucasis. La Chirurgie. LeClerc L (trans). Paris: Balliere, 1861.
2. Albucasis. On Surgery and Instruments. Spink MS, Lewis GL (trans-eds). Berkeley: University of California Press, 1973.
3. Avicenna. Canon Medicinae. Venice, 1507. Facsimile by: Hildesheim, Germany: Georg Olms Verlagsbuchhandlung, 1964.
4. Avicenna. Autobiography. In: Arberry AJ. (trans) Avicenna on Theology. London: John Murray, 1949.
5. Browne EG. Arabian Medicine. Cambridge: University Press, 1921.
6. Campbell D. Arabian Medicine, 2 vols. London: Kegan Paul, Trench, Trubner, 1925.
7. Elgood C. A Medical History of Persia and the Eastern Caliphate. Cambridge: University Press, 1951.
8. Khalifah ES. Dentistry in the 12th century as revealed in the medical writings of Maimonides. Br Dent J 1938; 67:133-139.
9. Khalifah ES, Haddad SI. Dental gleanings from Arabian medicine. J Am Dent Assoc 1937;24:944-955.
10. Rhazes. Treatise on Smallpox and Measles. Greenhill WA (trans). London: Sydenham Society, 1848.
11. Shklar G. Stomatology and dentistry in the golden age of Arabian medicine. Bull Hist Dent 1969;17:17.
12. Shklar G, Chernin D. A Sourcebook of Dental Medicine. Waban, MA: Maro, 2002.

# 7

# The Middle Ages

Historians have used the term *Middle Ages* to refer to the period between the decline and fall of Rome in 410 AD and the rebirth of civilization in the beginning of the fifteenth century. It can also be looked upon as the period between the end of the ancient era and the beginning of the modern age. Within this historical period unique developments in architecture, art, music, literature, science, and medicine took place.

The Middle Ages can be divided into two periods. The early Middle Ages, following the invasion and sack of Rome by the Visigoth barbarians from the north, has traditionally been seen as an age of ignorance, superstition, disease, and fear; it has been called the Dark Ages, although historians now frown on the use of this term. Western Europe, at the time, was broken up into a large number of warring barbarian kingdoms or duchies, and the frontiers were devastated by Vikings from the north, Muslims from the south, and Magyars from the east.

Through all these changes in Europe and the decline of Roman civilization, Christianity flourished. Indeed, the early Middle Ages have been called the Age of Faith. Learning was maintained in the numerous monasteries built throughout Europe. The monks carefully guarded whatever books from the Greek and Roman culture they were able to save and also maintained whatever knowledge of science and medicine did not conflict with theology. The monasteries developed herb gardens, and the monks used classical herbal remedies for the treatment of disease. Many of the monasteries became famous as centers of learning, and scholars were able to develop in this environment, with its relative stability and its access to some of the texts of the classical age. Women, too, such as Hildegard of Bingen (1098–1179), became noted scholars in the early Middle Ages, when they were able to study and teach in convents.[12]

During the second part of the Middle Ages, from 900 to 1400, important changes began to occur, including the rediscovery of classical civilization with its great philosophers such as Aristotle, the emergence of the Gothic style with the building of the great European cathedrals, and innovations in music, sculpture, and painting—precursors of their magnificent expressions in the Renaissance.

Science and medicine developed slowly during the Middle Ages.[2,6,8,11] The late Middle Ages were marked by the founding of the first universities and medical schools. The medieval church, with its doctrine that "God is the Supreme Educator," supervised education and all matters relating to it. Schools of higher learning, called *studium generale,* were developed by some of the religious orders, and these eventually became the early universities. The medical school of Salerno was founded as early as the tenth century, and the law schools of Padua, Ravenna, Verona, and Bologna were founded during the eleventh century. In the thirteenth century the University of Paris became preeminent and brought students from many countries to be taught by the greatest scholars of the age, such as Roger Bacon and Albertus Magnus. Oxford and Cambridge were founded shortly thereafter, organized in a manner similar to that of the University of Paris. The medical school of Montpellier was founded in 1289 and received the official right to grant diplomas by Pope Nicholas IV, thus giving it official status as a medical faculty.[3]

Medicine in the earlier Middle Ages was practiced by a number of educated monks who were, essentially, herbalists.[10] Their herbals were largely compilations from Dioscorides and others, but there were also original botanical observations and therapeutic suggestions. Platearius was an early herbalist in Salerno. Rufinus wrote an herbal in the thirteenth century. Surgeons of the twelfth and thirteenth centuries made a number of original contributions. In 1170 Roger of Salerno wrote a book on surgery that became a standard text for the next century in the medical schools of Europe. Roland of Parma, a student of Roger, extended his teaching in a book on surgery presented in 1250. Hugo Borgognoni of Lucca (died ca 1258) lectured in Bologna, on surgery, and is known primarily for the teachings of his son Theodoric, who recorded his surgical principles and made a number of refinements. Theodoric (1205–1296) understood the difference in the flow of blood from arteries and from veins, and he recommended firm binding of wounds to stop hemorrhage. He also recommended the suturing of wounds to prevent contamination (this was before any knowledge of infection). He used a "soporific sponge" to relieve the pain of surgery. Theodoric used advanced techniques for setting fractures. In fractures of the mandible he suggested binding the teeth together with gold wire or silk ligatures to bring the bone fragments into proper alignment.[13]

Among the notable physicians and surgeons of the late Middle Ages are Arnold of Villanova (1235–1312), William of Saliceto (1200?–1277),[14] Lanfranck (1250?–1310),[8] Henri de Mondeville (d. 1320),[5] Guy de Chauliac (1300–1370),[1,4,9] and John of Arderne (1307–1390).[7] They made few original contributions to medical and surgical practice but were familiar with the writings of the Arabic as well as the Greek physicians, in their Latin translations, and wrote treatises that incorporated this knowledge for the medical practitioners of the time. They also wrote in the vernacular so nonscholars could understand their works. Guy de Chauliac, for example, wrote his great book of surgery in French. Guy de Chauliac, born in the town of Chauliac near Lyon around 1300, became the most noted surgeon of the Middle Ages. He stood at the crossroads of medicine and surgery of the Greeks and Romans and that of the Renaissance. He led the way to Ambroise Paré, Fabricius, Vesalius, and the great medical advances of the sixteenth century. Guy was not only educated in the basic Greek texts of Hippocrates and Galen; he also knew about the major contributions of Arabic medicine and surgery of the tenth and eleventh centuries, from both the eastern Caliphate based in Baghdad (Rhazes, Avicenna, Haly Abbas) and the western Caliphate in Spain (Abulcasis). Guy studied medicine initially at Montpellier and then at Bologna, two of the major medical schools of the time.

Guy's most significant contribution is a surgery tract[4]; it was the definitive textbook for several hundred years. Published first in French in 1498, it went through several editions and was translated into many of the common languages of the time. At his death in 1368 he was so highly regarded in his specialty that he was called the Father of Surgery by someone as eminent as Fallopius.

The book outlines the importance of surgery and describes various surgical operations and the instruments used at the time, including scissors, speculum, razor, scalpel, needle, and lancet. The surgeon, according to Guy, should have several basic qualifications. He should be educated ("a man of letters"), expert, intelligent, and a man of good habits. Guy recognizes that the role of the surgeon is to assist nature. Furthermore, Guy describes the removal of foreign bodies, the placement and suturing of separated tissues, methods of controlling hemorrhage, treatment of fractures, and surgical excision of cancer. In addition, Guy provides an absorbing description of the bubonic plague that raged Avignon in 1348. His materia medica, however, continued to be that of Galen, as was his approach based on the ancient Greek theory of the four basic humors underlying disease processes by their proportional excess or defect.

Guy's writings on dentistry, dental medicine, and oral surgery are of interest.[9] He discusses a variety of diseases of the tongue and describes frenectomy. He explains tooth caries, the intense pain of pulpitis, and the development of draining dental abscesses (which he considers a positive sign of healing). He mentions that most dental operations are carried out by dentists rather than physicians but feels that physician-surgeons perform these operations with greater safety. His mention of the many instruments dentists use is taken mainly from the work of Abulcasis.

He offers extensive medicaments for the treatment of the various diseases of the teeth, gingiva, and oral mucosa. Most of these herbal remedies make little sense today since they are based on the ancient Greek concept of the four humors: blood, phlegm, yellow bile, and black bile. Health meant the proper proportions of these humors in the body. Illness meant some abnormal proportion that must be corrected by appropriate medication. The remedies were considered to act on the qualities of the elements or humors. Some medicaments were undoubtedly used because of successful prior experience on patients, while others were based on the writings of the Greek and Roman physicians. Certainly wine and vinegar would be appropriate for cleansing surgical wounds. Opiates would definitely relieve pain. Pomegranate juice was an excellent astringent mouthwash, and the pumice powders would be effective in cleansing the teeth of surface film. Tartar was removed by scalers since rinses and tooth powders would not have any effect upon it. In fact, the materia medica of Guy de Chauliac was a significant advance from "witches' brew" types of medicaments with truly disgusting and weird ingredients that have no rationale whatever.

It is appropriate, historically, to consider Guy de Chauliac an early representative of the Renaissance rather than the Middle Ages, since his medicine was essentially a "rebirth" of Greek medicine from both Greek and Arabic sources, with the addition of many advances of the Arabic physicians of the tenth century, particularly in surgery. Guy was also familiar with the surgical teachings of the Salerno school and its major figure, Roger, as well as his immediate predecessors, Saliceto, Lanfranck, and Henri de Mondeville. The following excerpt is from Guy's *La Grande Chirurgie*[10]:

### On Loosened and Weakened Teeth

Sometimes the tooth rocks (is mobile) because of a primary cause, such as a fall or a blow, and sometimes because of a preceding cause, of moisture which softens the nerve and the ligament. Once in a while dryness and lack of food, and at other times corrosion and diminution of gingival tissue are the cause. When dryness and lack of food are the cause, as in old people, and patients with consumption, the disease will not heal; in other cases medicaments will help and with this it is necessary to avoid chewing on the affected teeth (principally hard things) and to reduce the amount of talking. The teeth should not be touched or moved. If corrosion is the cause, it should be cured. When a fall or blow is the cause, after letting blood (as well as having purged and emptied the salivary moisture with mastic and pyrethrum when the cause is due to softening moisture) Galen quotes the advice of Archigenes that alum, with incense, cinnamon, and cypress be put on the root. Rhazes prescribes the following: Rx - pomegranate, roses, galls, galingale, sumac one part of each, and alum, a half part. This is to be applied or rubbed into the gums. In another case he adds acacia, hypocystis, myrobalans, and orders vinegar rinses and the fashioning of troches to be rubbed onto the roots of the teeth. Should this not help, then the diseased teeth can be bound to healthy teeth with a golden chain (wire) as proposed by Abulcasis. Should the teeth fall out, they should be replaced by teeth from someone else, or by teeth carved from cow bone. These, when tied carefully, may last a long time.

## References


1. Brennan WA. Guy de Chauliac on Wounds and Fractures. Chicago: University of Chicago Press, 1923.
2. Corner GW. Anatomical Texts of the Earlier Middle Ages. Washington: Carnegie Institute, 1927.
3. Cooper S. The medical school of Montpellier in the fourteenth century. Ann Med Hist 1930;11:163–170.
4. Guy de Chauliac. La Grande Chirurgie de Guy de Chauliac. Nicaise E (ed). Paris: Alcan, 1890.
5. Henri de Mondeville. Chirurgie de Henri de Mondeville. Nicaise E (ed). Paris: Alcan, 1893.
6. Hunt T. The Medieval Surgery. Woodbridge, England: Boydell Press, 1992.
7. John Arderne. De Arte Phisicali et de Cirurgia. D'Arcy Power (trans). London: John Bale, 1922.
8. Lanfranck. Science of Surgery. New York: C. Scribner, 1894.
9. Shklar G. The dental medicine and surgery of Guy de Chauliac, with extended excerpts from the cyrurgia magna. J Hist Dent 1997;45:113–119.
10. Shklar G, Chernin D. A Sourcebook of Dental Medicine. Waban, MA: Maro, 2002.
11. Singer C. The Evolution of Anatomy. New York: Knopf, 1925.
12. Strehlow W, Hertzka G. Hildegard of Bingen's Medicine. Santa Fe: Bear, 1988.
13. Theodoric. The Surgery of Theodoric. Campbell E, Colton J (trans). New York: Appleton-Century Crofts, 1955.
14. William of Saliceto. Chirurgie de Guillaume de Salicet. Paul Pifteau (trans-ed). Toulouse: Saint-Cyprien Press, 1898.

# Part III

# The Modern Era

# 8

# The Renaissance

The Renaissance, or rebirth, of classical civilization and culture can be said to span three centuries, starting in the fourteenth century in Italy and continuing into the seventeenth century. Historical periods, however, always blend, and the late Middle Ages begin to suggest the changes that will occur in the Renaissance.

As the Middle Ages may be said to be the Age of Faith, the Renaissance can be described as the Age of Humanism. With the revival of classical culture and philosophy came new emphasis on the importance of human values rather than religious dogma. Petrarch (1304–1374), the great poet, scholar, and philosopher who is strongly identified with the early Renaissance, wrote that a person is an autonomous creature capable of reason, whose own complex nature is the only proper test of moral truth and goodness. This was a reaction against medieval scholasticism, which respected only those aspects of classical culture that were not offensive to the tenets of Christianity. The humanism of the Renaissance was reflected not only in music, but also in the spectacular transformation involved in the visual arts—sculpture, painting, and architecture.

Towering figures of the Renaissance in Italy included artists Leonardo da Vinci, Michelangelo, and Raphael, and elsewhere in Europe, writers such as Erasmus in Holland, Rabelais and Montaigne in France, Cervantes in Spain, and Shakespeare in England.

Science and medicine advanced enormously in the Renaissance and led to major discoveries, the science and the medicine of the modern era. Copernicus (1475–1543) dispelled the old notion of Earth as center of the universe. Vesalius (1514–1564)[18,19] offered a comprehensive text of the anatomy of the human body, based on the careful study of dissections.[12,13] This served as a basis for the medical and surgical knowledge of the age. Vesalius also founded the great school of anatomy at Padua. Antonio Benivieni (1443–1502), a pioneer of pathology, based his investigations on the observation of individual case records. Jean Fernel (1497–1558) wrote, in *Universal Medicine*, the first treatises on physiology and pathology. Girolamo Fracastoro (1483–1553) conceived of the idea that diseases spread by infection. Paracelsus (1493–1541) wrote the first book on chemistry and considered the various possible roles of chemical reactions in disease. Ambroise Paré (1510–1590) was the first surgeon to discard the harmful procedures of the past to understand wound healing. Realdo Colombo (1510–1577), a student of Vesalius and his successor at Padua, understood basic physiology and described the circulation of the blood. Fallopius (1523–1562) studied anatomy under Vesalius at Padua and eventually succeeded him to the school's chair of anatomy, following the resignation of Realdo Colombo. Fallopius is responsible for many breakthroughs in anatomy and was the first to discover the primary or deciduous dentition and describe the tooth follicle. Fabricius of Aquapendente (1533–1619) was a great anatomist, surgeon, and teacher. He established the medical faculty at Padua where scholars from all over Europe came to study, including William Harvey. Eustachius (1520?–1574) produced detailed anatomical plates and also wrote the first book devoted to the anatomy of the teeth and the physiology of the dentition. Gaspare Tagliacozzi (1545–1599), the first plastic surgeon, described skin grafting. Thus the Renaissance was an age of exploration in the fields of science and medicine as well as in the fine arts.

Indeed, one of the major advances of the Renaissance was the invention of printing, by Johann Gutenberg (c. 1400–1468) in 1450. This meant books could be produced relatively inexpensively and could be afforded by ordinary citizens, as well as scholars. Therefore it was important to have the book appear in the vernacular so people who had no Latin could read the texts. The Bible was translated into German by Martin Luther so everyone could read it, and many medical books appeared in German, French, and English. The first printed dental book was published in German in 1530, under the title *Artzney Buchlein* or *Zene Artzney* (*The Physician of the Teeth*). The author, Michael Blum, offered little new information but presented all the material on the treatment of diseases of the teeth as compiled by the classical writers of Greece and Rome, as well as the Arabian physicians. Several chapters in this short text are devoted to problems of the gingival and periodontal tissues.[1] An excerpt follows:

OF YELLOW AND BLACK TEETH

> Limositas is when whitish, yellowish or blackish slime settles on the lower part of the teeth and over the gums; some call it tartar ... the natural appearance of the teeth is chiefly retained, or, if lost, brought back, by medicines which dry up and cleanse, which have the power to rub away the uncleanliness and to make clean, as pumice-stone, in Latin spuma, and common salt, etc. ... Black teeth shall be well scraped; then rubbed often ...
>
> Another good powder against black teeth, and which also fastens the loose teeth and makes a good odor from the mouth, is the following: Take half an ounce of burnt alum, cream of tartar, red coral, of each two drams; pumice, two and a half drams; charcoal and rosemary, and cypress stalks burnt, sandal-wood, sarcocolla, of each one dram; triturate together, and rub the teeth therewith.

Ambroise Paré (1510–1590) (Fig 7) is considered the greatest surgeon of the Renaissance. Born in Laval, France, Paré had humble origins and no formal education. He followed his father's profession as a barber-surgeon, obtaining a position at the Hotel Dieu, the largest hospital in Paris. Having served in the French Army during various wars, he gained expertise in the treatment of wounds and developed new treatment methods, which he published in 1545. Paré wrote in French rather than Latin, which made his writings accessible to surgeons who did not have a classic university background. The book was an immediate success and was translated into many languages. Paré wrote several other books and was appointed as surgeon to Kings Henri II, François III, and Charles IX.

Paré understood that wounds would heal better without the use of cauterization, the approach of the previous centuries, and developed a number of dressings to cover the wounds. A pious and religious man, Paré said about his method of treating wounds: "I dress them. God heals them."

Paré also developed and improved surgical instruments as well as oral surgical procedures, including gingivectomy for the removal of hyperplastic gingival tissue. He understood the etiologic significance of calculus in periodontitis and developed a set of scalers to remove them.[10,11,14]

Following is an excerpt from Paré's definitive study[17]:

Chapter 26
OF OTHER AFFECTS OF THE TEETH

> The teeth are also troubled with other preternatural affects. For sometimes they shake by relaxation of the gums, or else become corrupt and rotten, or have worms in them, or else are set on edge. For the first, the gums are relaxed either by an external or primitive cause, as a fall or blow: or else by an internal or antecedent as by the deluxion of acrid or waterish humours from the brain, or through want of nourishment in old bodies. If the teeth grow loose by the means of the decaying gums, the disease is then incurable.[10]

Paracelsus (Theophrastus Bombastus von Hohenheim), born in Switzerland in 1493, continues to be a controversial figure of the Renaissance and of humanism (Fig 8). He wrote extensively

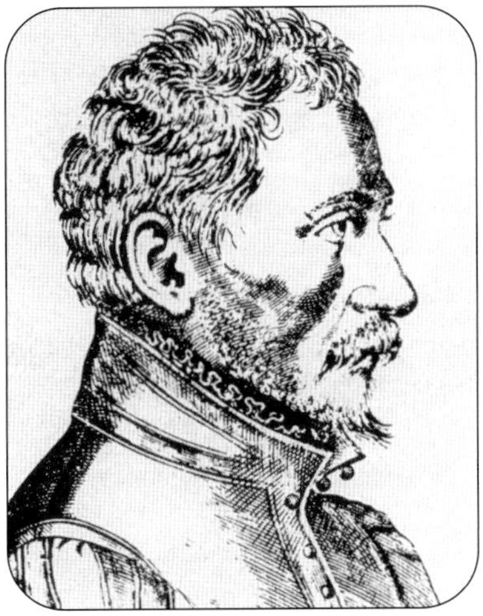

**Fig 7** Ambroise Paré, 1564.

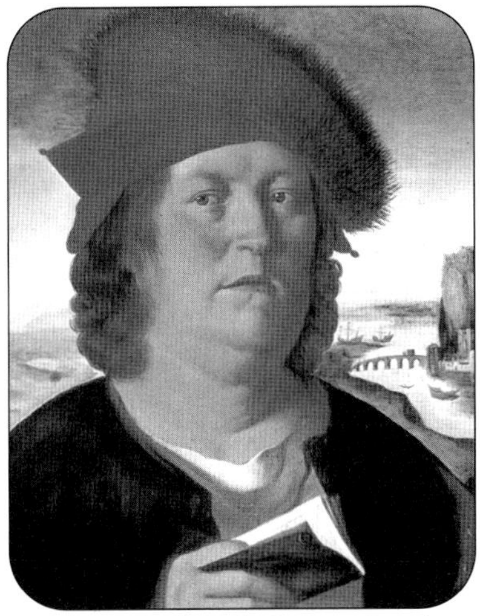

**Fig 8** Paracelsus, by Jan van Scorel.

on a broad range of subjects, and his collected works, fourteen large volumes in the insightful, modern edition of Sudhoff, are repeatedly investigated for ideas ranging from chemistry and the physical world to philosophy and the power of imagination.[5] There are some striking similarities between Paracelsus and his contemporary, Martin Luther. In fact, Paracelsus has been referred to as the Luther of Medicine.

Following early studies in Basel and Wurzburg, Paracelsus traveled widely, to Vienna, Cologne, Paris, Montpellier, and then to Italy, Spain, England, Holland, Denmark, Poland, Russia, Hungary, and many regions in between. After these wanderings, during which he gained knowledge and experience, he settled in Basel where his friend Froben helped him to obtain the position of city physician and professor at the University of Basel.

The name Paracelsus, which he added to his other names and appeared to prefer, was probably meant to establish his superiority to the classical learning of the past as signified by the writings of Celsus on medicine. Paracelsus was an iconoclast with determination and courage. He shocked his medical associates by giving his lectures in German rather than Latin and by publicly burning the *Canon* of Avicenna to demonstrate his contempt for antiquated medical knowledge. Paracelsus was forced to leave his positions and became again a wanderer, traveling to diverse towns and cities where he wrote, lectured, practiced medicine, and quarreled with the medical establishment in each place. He died in 1541, in Salzburg, where his tomb can be seen in the Church of St. Sebastian.

Paracelsus wrote an unusually large number of works, few of which were printed during his lifetime because of his controversial reputation.[6–9] Overall the medical texts have been of greater interest to scholars than have his works on theology, philosophy, alchemy, and astrology. The medical treatises are based, to a large extent, on Paracelsus' own knowledge and experience as a physician and army surgeon.

The *Grosse Wundartzney*, or *Large Book of Treatment of Wounds*, and the *Grosse Chirurgie* present his general approach to medicine and surgery and much of the material is archaic and based on magic potions. He understood that tissues will heal themselves if offered the opportunity, so he was against the use of irritant drugs applied to wounds. He was against the use of sutures and seems to have been frightened of surgery, allowing wounds to suppurate and in this manner eventually discharge foreign materials rather than using surgery to extract them. A treatise titled *Miners Diseases* was the first modern account of occupational disease. Another, *Diseases that Deprive Man of his Reason*, has been hailed as an early psychiatric classic. Despite the fact that his materia medica was based on magic, he did understand the value of many drugs, including that of laudanum as a pain reliever and sulfuric ether as an anesthetic. He used tinctures of alcohol for the administration of numerous drugs and popularized the use of mercury, lead, sulfur, arsenic, iron, and copper sulfate as medicaments.

Among his pathological theories, Paracelsus developed an engrossing hypothesis of disease: the doctrine of tartar. He claimed that pathologic calcification occurs in a variety of organs, and he attributes this process to a metabolic disturbance whereby the body takes nourishment from food and discards the refuse or "tartarus," a material that cannot be broken down and is ultimate matter or "ultima materia." This tartar of ultimate matter, consisting of gravel, mead, and glue was thought to be exogenous and to come from cereals such as barley and peas, milk, meat and fish, and drinks such as wine, beer, and fruit juice. In addition, the tartar content of food was thought to vary in different geographic locations. This material in food could be somehow altered during cooking so that it would be excreted in the feces. In the mouth, saliva served digestion, and some tartar could be found there. In the stomach, other agents served the purpose. Tartar could also be precipitated by the action of salt, which dried up or coagulated mucoid matter in food. The amount of tartar formed depended on the region of the body. Paracelsus recognized the extensive formation of tartar on the teeth and related this to toothache:

> A specific digestive process already takes place in the mouth–and this process is potent enough to sustain life. Its waste products are deposited as Tartar on the teeth–with resulting decay of the gums, wearing down of teeth, pain due to acerbity with which each tartarus is endowed. Toothache is thus comparable to the pain caused by calculus elsewhere.[15]

In addition to specific observations on pathological calcification, his concept of tartar indicates that Paracelsus developed original concepts of disease. A disease could be observed, studied, and its cause determined, rather than considered, as by ancients, a nebulous upset of humoral balance based on the theory of the four humors. Paracelsus conceived of the person as a vital, living being:

> In the anatomy of the dead, you will learn neither nature nor being. It is of little value. It is the living body that teaches the anatomist about health and disease, not the dead one.[6]

This alone distinguishes Paracelsus from his contemporaries, whose major preoccupation was the study of anatomy from the skeleton and gradually from the dissection of human cadavers.

Nevertheless, the anatomists of the Renaissance contributed enormously to the development of modern medicine. Leonardo da Vinci (1452–1519) wrote extensively on all aspects of human anatomy, including the musculature of the face and mouth.[4]

Andreas Vesalius (1514–1564), considered the father of modern anatomy, was a preeminent figure in the development of medicine and modern scientific observation.[12,13,17] Born in Brussels, he studied medicine in Paris but left France for political reasons and earned his medical degree from the University of Padua in 1537, where he subsequently taught anatomy and surgery. In 1543 he published the first modern book on anatomy (*On the Fabric of the Human Body*),[18] which was based on dissection and illustrated with intricately detailed drawings by the Dutch artist Jan Stephen of Calcar, a student of the great Titian. This book remarkably depicted the gross anatomy of teeth.

A contemporary, Bartolomeo Eustachius (1520?–1574) (Fig 9), born in San Severino, Ancona, Italy, studied medicine at the Collegio della Sapienza in Rome, and was appointed professor of anatomy in 1547. Eustachius realized that the Gallenic concepts of anatomy had multiple errors. As physician to the Pope, however, he felt constrained to question them and therefore did not publish his series of anatomic plates, illustrated by Pier Matteo Pini. In the early eighteenth century they were found in the possession of a descendant of Pini, and purchased by Pope Clement XI, who published them in 1714 following the advice of Morgagni. The loss of Eustachius' anatomic studies for more than a hundred years was a significant setback to the advancement of anatomy.

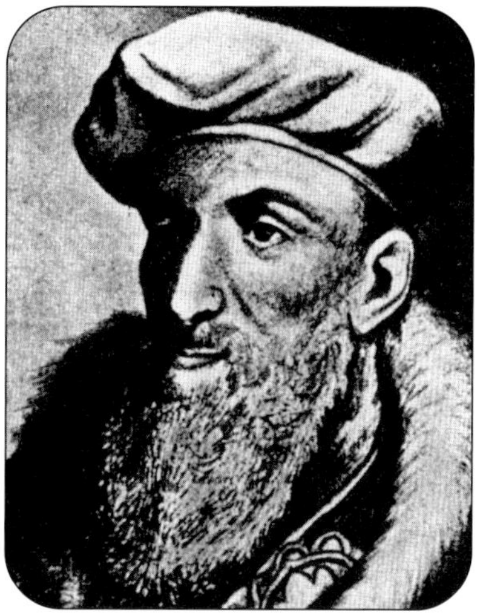

**Fig 9** Eustachius, by Frederigo Baroccio.

Eustachius is credited with publishing, in 1563, the first book on teeth, entitled *Libellus de Dentibus*,[2,16] in which he offered many new concepts, including the first description of the dental pulp and root canals, pointing out that they contain nerves and blood vessels. He was the first to describe the periodontal ligament, referring to it as a type of gomphosis, and he attributed the loosening of teeth in old age to the widening of the periodontal space. He described occlusion in man and animals and introduced the idea that tooth crowns are composed of enamel overlying dentin. In addition, Eustachius noted that permanent teeth develop from dental follicles, not from the roots of the deciduous teeth, as postulated by Vesalius.

Eustachius offered a remarkably modern treatment for periodontal disease, advising both scaling of the calculus and the curettage of the granulation tissue to allow reattachment of the gingival and periodontal tissues.

> Scarcity of nourishment causes the teeth to become weak and loose in old age. The use of astringents to shrink the gums is of limited value. But if the gums diminish and recede, and the teeth, become covered with a hard, cuticle-like substance, reuniting the tooth and gum is as likely as joining the middle and index fingers unless the physician first scrapes the teeth and freshens the gums with a scalpel, and uses medicines that will encourage agglutination [firmness].[2]

Jacques Guillemeau (1550–1613) was one of the great French surgeons of the late Renaissance.[14] Born in Orléans, into a family of surgeons, he studied anatomy with Riolan and surgery with Ambroise Paré. Guillemeau traveled widely with Paré in the various military campaigns where Paré was the chief surgeon. Guillemeau learned a great deal of surgery during these years and was exposed to the ideas of surgeons from many countries. After this apprenticeship he settled in Paris where he became the chief surgeon at the renowned Hotel Dieu Hospital and surgeon to the kings of France. Guillemeau published a treatise on diseases of the eye, in 1585, and his major work on surgery in 1602, *Oevres de Chirurgie.* The latter was widely read and translated into a number of languages, including English. While Guillemeau was an esteemed teacher in his own right, he also served to spread the name of Paré, his teacher. Guillemeau's surgical treatise includes sections on the mouth and the management of dental problems. His description of ligating loose periodontally involved teeth is particularly absorbing[17]:

> And touching the convenience of ligation, or tying of the teeth to join them together and to make fast those teeth that are loose and grow to be moveable and may be waggled up and down, and also to insert any therein which are made by art; all this made conveniently effected in this manner. With a fine gold wire, of fine continental gold, which may easily bend and bow between the aforesaid teeth without any violence. First double

> the wire, laying the same with the duplication between the forward teeth, and then bring both ends to that tooth which is loose, whether it be one or more, until such time as we have drawn unto the sound teeth, one on each side. Then we must reduce the wire unto the sound tooth from which we took our original, gently drawing the wire together close to the roots of the teeth, particularly the loose one. That being done, we must cut both ends of the wire that are together with a pair of shears, and wind the rest thereof round about the bound tooth as close to the root so that it will not perturb or hinder the tongue. If the teeth are not only loose, but being fallen out, we may insert them in their place and tie them with a gold wire, as described before.

During the English Renaissance, a number of well-known British surgeons were concerned with diseases of the teeth and gingiva. Thomas Phaer (1510–1560) wrote the first book on pediatrics, in English, and included chapters devoted to the problems of teething and to ulcers of the mouth. In 1600 Philip Barrough (or Barrow) published the first comprehensive book on medicine, *The Method of Physic, Containing the Causes, Signes, and Cures of Inward Diseases in Man's Body, From the Head to the Foote,* devoting several chapters to dental and periodontal problems. Shakespeare's son-in-law John Hall was a physician and published a small book on diseases of his patients, *Select Observations on English Bodies of Eminent Persons in Desperate Diseases,* in which he mentions a case of a patient "cruelly tormented with pain of his teeth, and very much molested with swelling of his gums." Various mouthwashes cured him. One of the most eminent surgeons of the Elizabethan age was William Clowes (1543–1604). He describes the severe gingival disease in sailors with scurvy: "Their gums were rotten even to the very roots of their teeth."[17]

## References


1. Blum M. Artzney Buchlein. Dent Cosmos 1887;29. Reprinted, Birmingham, AL: Classics of Dentistry Library, Gryphon Editions, 1981.
2. Eustachius. Libellus De Dentibus. Chernin D, Shklar G (trans-eds). Canton, MA: Watson Publishing International, 1999.
3. O'Malley CD. Andreas Vesalius of Brussels 1514–1564. Los Angeles: University of California Press, 1964.
4. O'Malley CD, Saunders JBCM. Leonardo da Vinci on the Human Body. New York: Henry Schuman, 1952.
5. Pachter HM. Magic into Science: The Story of Paracelsus. New York: Henry Schuman, 1951.
6. Paracelsus. Selected Writings. Jacobi J (ed). Guterman N (trans). New York: Pantheon Books, 1951.
7. Paracelsus. Sämtliche Werke, 14 vols. Sudhoff K (ed). Munich: R. Oldenbourg, 1922–1933.
8. Paracelsus. Volumen Medicinae Paramirum. Leidecker K (trans). Bull Hist Med 1949;23(suppl II).
9. Paracelsus. The Hermetic and Alchemical Writings, 2 vols. Waite AE (trans). London: James Elliot, 1894.
10. Paré A. Oevres Completes, 3 vols. Malgaigne JF (ed). Paris: Balliere, 1840–1841.
11. Paré A. The Apologie and Treatise of Ambroise Paré Containing the Voyages Made into Divers Places. Keynes G (ed). Chicago: Univ of Chicago Press, 1952.
12. Saunders JBCM, O'Malley CD. The Illustrations from the Works of Andreas Vesalius of Brussels. Cleveland: World Publishing, 1950.
13. Saunders JB CM, O'Malley CD. A reading from the De Humani Corporis Fabrica of Andreas Vesalius. J Am Coll Dent 1944;11:211–218.
14. Shklar G. Ambroise Paré and Jacques Guillemeau: The contributions to dentistry with their original works translated into English. J Hist Dent 2000;48:85–89.
15. Shklar G. Paracelsus: Renaissance physician, mystic and iconoclast. Oral disease concepts. J Hist Dent 2000;48:123–126.
16. Shklar G, Chernin, D. Eustachio and "Libellus de Dentibus," the first book devoted to the structure and function of the teeth. J Hist Dent 2000;48:25–30.
17. Shklar G, Chernin D. A Sourcebook of Dental Medicine. Waban, MA: Maro, 2002.
18. Vesalius A. The Epitome. Lind LR (trans). New York: Macmillan, 1949.
19. Vesalius A. De Humanis Corporis Fabrica. Basel: Oporinus, 1543. Facsimile, Brussels: Culture et Civilization, 1966.

# 9

# The Seventeenth Century

The seventeenth century was the era of Louis XIV and Cardinal Richelieu in France, along with Pascal (1623–1662), Molière (1622–1673), and Racine (1639–1699); of Oliver Cromwell in England, along with John Milton (1608–1674), and Isaac Newton (1642–1727). It was the Golden Age of Spanish literature with Lope de Vega (1562–1635) and Calderón de la Barca (1600–1681) and painters El Greco (1548–1614), Zurbarán (1598–1664), Diego Velazquez (1599–1660), and Bartolomé Murillo (1617–1682). In addition, cultural life flourished in Holland, with philosopher Baruch Spinoza (1632–1677) and artists Rembrandt (1606–1669) and Jan Vermeer (1632–1675).[3]

The seventeenth century also marked the colonization of the Americas and other parts of the world by European powers. Mexico and Peru had been conquered by Spain in 1523 and 1533, respectively, and Brazil by Portugal in 1549. Champlain established a French colony in Canada in 1603, and the British established colonies in Virginia in 1607 and in Massachusetts in 1620. Holland founded the Dutch East India Company in 1602. These new, distant parts of the world were subjected to diseases from the Old World—smallpox, measles, yellow fever, malaria—but are believed to have, in turn, exported syphilis.[12]

## Medical Sciences

Medical studies in the seventeenth century continued to be based in classical and Arabian texts, and Aristotle, Galen, and Paracelsus were important influences. Medicine continued to be practiced as in the Middle Ages, with the use of antimonium as a panacea and a number of prescriptions with "magical" ingredients such as worms, foxes' lungs, dried vipers, or the moss grown in skulls of people who had died violently. Astrology and alchemy, although somewhat in decline, continued to be important determinants of therapy.[9] The epidemic of bubonic plague (Black Death), which had devastated Europe in the fourteenth century, returned to desolate the city of London in 1665.

A great pharmacological advance was the introduction of quinine in Europe in 1632. This drug was used by the Incas in Peru and taken to the Old World by the Jesuits. The great progress in anatomy, brought about by Vesalius and his followers in the previous century, had as yet had little effect on surgical techniques, and surgeons were still considered to be inferior to physicians.[9]

Scientific research, however, flourished in this century. Investigation in the natural sciences, created by Kepler, Galileo, Descartes, and Newton, stressed the importance of unbiased observation and introduced the concept of experimentation to test a hypothesis, along with mathematical methods to measure the results. Scientific associations were born in this century, such as the Accademia dei Lincei in Rome (1603), the French Academy in Paris (1635), the Royal Society in London (1662), and the Academy of Sciences in Berlin (1700). Moreover the first scientific periodicals appeared.[9]

The application of physics and chemistry to medicine were developed in the seventeenth century, and the leading figures were, in physics, Descartes, Galileo, Sanctorius, and Giovanni

Alfonso Borelli, and in chemistry, Franciscus Sylvius and Thomas Willis.[1,9,14] Similarly, the foremost physicians of the century were Jan Baptista van Helmont (1577–1644) of Brussels, Frenchman François de la Boë, also known as Franciscus Sylvius (1614–1672), Englishmen Thomas Willis (1621–1675) and Thomas Sydenham (1624–1689), and Italians Giovanni Alfonso Borelli (1608–1679) and Marcello Malpighi (1628–1694).

## Dentistry

In general, dentistry made little progress in the seventeenth century. Surgeons and barber-surgeons were still considered inferior practitioners. They trained not in universities but by apprenticeships or in battlefields; many were self-taught. Their practice combined surgery—including tooth extractions—with blood-letting, barber services, and the like. Quacks and charlatans abounded. While some practitioners established themselves in big cities, other, itinerant, peddlers of dentistry and medicine traveled from small town to small town. While the century marked the rise of books that helped some improve their practices, many texts continued to advocate ancient methods based on quackery. Books by the Germans Guilhelmus Fabricius, or Wilhelm Fabry (1560–1634), and Johannes Scultetus, or Johann Schultheiss (1595–1645), to name two examples, describe cases reiterating ancient therapies.[15]

The English surgeon Richard Wiseman (1616–1676) led an adventurous life, serving for many years in various wars before settling in London, where he became surgeon to King George II. In a book published in 1672, entitled *Several Chirurgical Treatises*, he deals with dental problems, citing cases of traumatic injuries to the teeth and mouth, and tumors of the oral cavity.[15]

But the most important dental book of the seventeenth century was Charles Allen's *The Operator for the Teeth*, which was published in English in York in 1686, then in Dublin (1686), and in London (1687).[7] Allen was a barber-surgeon who called himself Professor. His study deals with treatment of dental caries (by filling the cavities with materials he does not describe), tooth extraction, and reimplantation (he rejects transplantation from one human to another, preferring the use of teeth of dogs, sheep, or baboons).

Barthélemy Martin (ca. 1604–1682) was a French surgeon who in 1679 published a book entitled *Dissertation sur les dents*, in which he rejects the notion that primary teeth have roots, and recommends that to avoid diseases of the primary dentition, a nursemaid of the proper temperament and character—preferably blonde—be chosen, and that teeth be cared for by gargling every morning with one's own urine and cleaned with dung of wild cats.[7]

## History of Microscopy

The history of microscopy begins early in the seventeenth century. Hans Jansen, his son Zacharias, and Hans Lipperskey, makers of spectacles in Middelburg, The Netherlands, are thought to have developed the first microscope, which Italian physician-naturalist Giovanni Fabbri named in 1625.[1] The new instrument took two forms: one, the precursor of the present-day light microscope, was the compound microscope, which combined two or more lenses in a tube. The other, the simple microscope, was just a powerful magnifying glass.[16]

The first microscopists began to use the new technology to study insects. They were Englishmen Robert Hooke (1635–1702) and Nehemiah Grew (1641–1712); Italians Marcello Malpighi (1628–1694) and Francesco Redi (1626–1698); and Dutchmen Jan Swammerdam (1637–1680) and Antony van Leeuwenhoek (1632–1723). Hooke published *Micrographia* in 1665; in it he describes lice and other insects, and the structure of wood; he was the first to use the word *cell* to describe pores in wood.[4] Grew studied mostly plants.[5] Malpighi's important

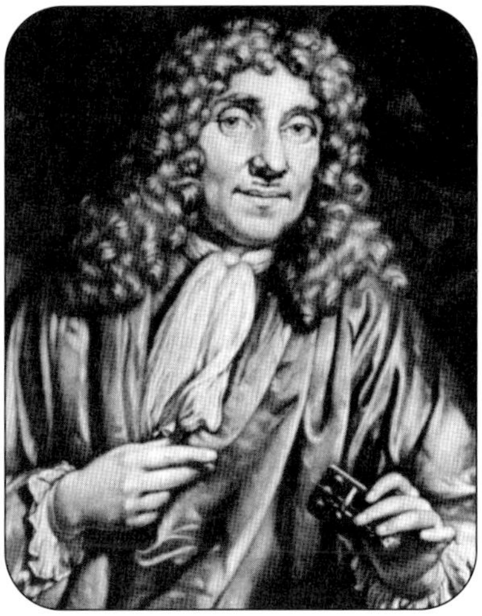

**Fig 10** Antony van Leeuwenhoek. (Oil painting by Johannes Verkolje, 1686.)

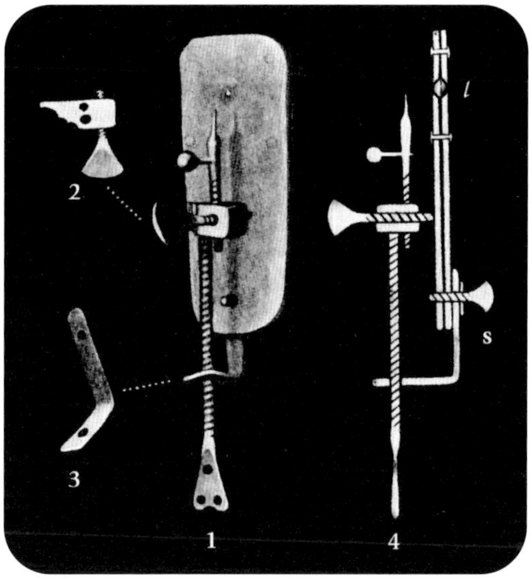


**Fig 11** Leeuwenhoek's microscope. (1) The whole instrument fitted and ready to use; (4) diagrammatic longitudinal section; (l) the biconvex lens mounted; (s) screw to adjust lens. (2) and (3) are mechanisms used to move the specimen into focus at the end of the short rod in front of the lens (l).

discoveries (discussed later in this chapter) in the area of animal microanatomy make him the first histologist in history.[8,11] Redi focused mainly on parasites and was the first to suggest that spontaneous generation did not occur. Swammerdan studied the anatomy of bees and other insects and small animals, using a surprising dissection technique, initially with bare eyes and later with loupes. Leeuwenhoek made astounding discoveries. He and Malpighi made the most important findings in the areas of microbiology and histology, which are crucial to the development of periodontology.

Antony van Leeuwenhoek[2,6,13,17] (Fig 10) was born in Delft, Holland, on October 24, 1632, to a middle class family, typical of the so-called Golden Age of the Dutch Republic. He had no scientific training, having learned only the draper trade; however, he occupied several prestigious administrative positions in the city of Delft, where he lived all his life. Leeuwenhoek was a contemporary and most probably a friend of the famous painter Jan Vermeer (1632–1675), also of Delft.[18]

Around 1659, Leeuwenhoek started to devise his own simple microscope, which consisted of one biconvex lens mounted between two oblong metallic plates, usually made of brass. The instrument was rather small, and since the lens had a very short focus, it had to be placed next to the eye. The instrument had the creative advantage of a sample holder that could be moved in all directions, while the lens remained fixed (Fig 11).[2,13]

The success of Leeuwenhoek's microscope stemmed from the way he prepared and polished the glass lenses, a technique he never revealed. For more than a century after his death, nobody could construct an instrument as good as his. It has been calculated that Leeuwenhoek obtained magnifications of 270 diameters with a resolution of 1.4 microns, although Henniger's observations suggest magnifications of 500 diameters and resolutions of 1.0 micron.[6,17] If the microscopic observation presented great difficulties, the preparation and fixation of the sample[17,19] required ingenious systems and great manual dexterity to microdissect the samples.

In 1673, the Dutch physician Reinier de Graaf, of Delft, already famous for the discovery of the ovarian follicle that still bears his name, wrote to the secretary of the Royal Society of

London to recommend his friend Leeuwenhoek, "a very ingenious man," who had developed microscopes "better than those made by Eustachio Divini." Graaf's letter prompted correspondence between Leeuwenhoek and the Royal Society that would continue for half a century and result in the publication of surprising discoveries. Leeuwenhoek's letters, which continued until his death, would amount to several hundred.

Leeuwenhoek only wrote letters, never books or other types of scientific communication. His style was simple: he wrote as if he were talking, including personal impressions, blended with narratives of his daily life. He wrote only in Dutch, and in simple sentences, sometimes with poor syntax and grammatical errors. Probably by instinct, because he lacked scientific training, Leeuwenhoek was very careful in separating his factual observations, to him indisputable, from his speculations and opinions.

*Microbiologic observations.* Leeuwenhoek's most important discovery was of the existence of microorganisms.[2,10] His first observations were made in fresh water, as described in a letter dated September 7, 1674. He detailed various particles of different shapes moving swiftly in the water. Leeuwenhoek assumed that mobility was synonymous with life and therefore called the minute objects he saw moving under his microscope *little animals* or *animalcules* (*diertgens* in Dutch).[2] He wrote about thirty letters* with descriptions of bacteria and protozoa, and established a method for determining their size, comparing them with a grain of coarse sand (870 microns), a hair from his beard (100 microns), a human erythrocyte (7.2 microns), or bacteria in peppered water (2 to 3 microns).[2,6,17]

*Observations on dental plaque.* Leeuwenhoek discovered microorganisms in the oral cavity. In addition, his letters describe what is now called *dental plaque,* which he found teeming with bacteria. He also mentions that plaque forms in greater abundance when oral hygiene is suspended, and he relates observations with regard to his own teeth. The following is part of a letter sent in 1683[10]:

> 'Tis my wont of a morning to rub my teeth with salt, and then swill my mouth out with water; and often, after eating, to clean my back teeth with a toothpick, as well as rubbing them hard with a cloth; wherefore my teeth, back and front, remain as clean and white as falleth to the lot of few men of my years, and my gums (no matter how hard the salt be that I rub them with) never start bleeding. Yet notwithstanding, my teeth are not so clean thereby, but what there sticketh or groweth between some of my front ones and my grinders (whenever I inspect them with a magnifying mirror), a little white matter, which is as thick as if 'twere batter. On examining this, I judged (albeit I could discern nought a-moving in it) that there were yet living animalcules therein. I have therefore mixed it, at divers times, with clean rain-water (in which there are no animalcules), and also with spittle, that I took out of my mouth, after ridding it of air-bubbles (lest the bubbles should make any motion in the spittle); and I then most always saw, with great wonder, that in the said matter there were many little living animalcules, very prettily a-moving.

Leeuwenhoek includes in this letter a drawing of the animalcules, in which cocci, rods, and spirochetes are easily identified (Fig 12). He also mentions that the animalcules are present in very large amounts in the mouths of men and women, young and old, and says, "[T]here are more animals living in the scum on the teeth in a man's mouth, than there are men in the whole kingdom." He mentions his surprise at the movement of the animalcules and has the following to add:

*Clifford Dobell has carefully analyzed these letters, including the Dutch original, the English version, and, when available, other translations. The interested reader is referred to the excellent and exhaustive study by Dobell[2] for further information on Leeuwenhoek's historic descriptions of protozoa and bacteria.

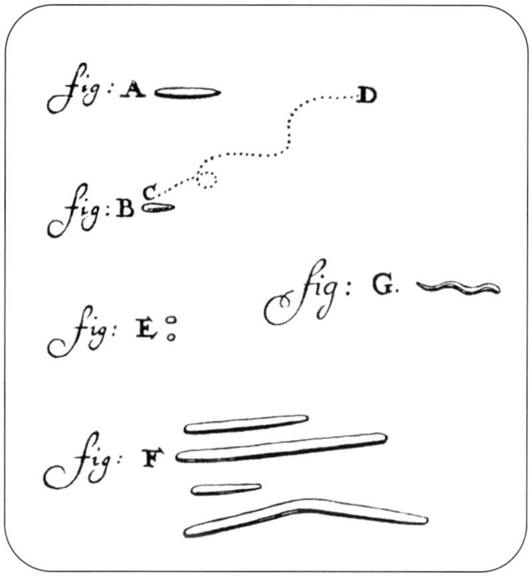


**Fig 12** Leeuwenhoek's drawing of bacteria from the human mouth, as appeared in letter No. 39, dated September 17, 1683.

> But we must be still more amazed when we consider how these animalcules can move, and shift 'emselves about, in stuff as thick as this when it is lodged upon and betwixt the teeth; and how hard and slow it must be for them to get about in such stuff. But when, on the other hand, the said stuff is mixed up with spittle, and by this mixing the animalcules find themselves in a fluid material, many of them feel released, as it were, and never stop moving, so far as the eye can see.

Several years later (1692) he revisited oral microorganisms, noting that at times he does not find living animalculae in his mouth, which is cause for speculation:

> The reason is, I most or pretty near always of a morning drink coffee, as hot as I can, so hot that it puts me into a sweat. ... Now the animalcules that are in the white matter on the front teeth, and on the foremost of the back-teeth, being unable to bear the hotness of the coffee, are thereby killed; like I've often shown that the animalcules which are in water are made to die by slight heating.

He later performed what can be considered the first anti-plaque experiment in history, as follows:

> Furthermore, I put some strong wine-vinegar in my own mouth, and then set my teeth, and let the vinegar run betwixt 'em after time; and after doing so, I rinsed my mouth thrice with fair water. Afterwards I once more fetched out some of the foresaid stuff from between my front teeth, as well as between my grinders; and I mixed it divers times both with spittle and with clear rain-water; and most always I discovered in it an unbelievable number of living animalcules, though most of 'em were in the matter I got from between my back teeth.

Then he performed an in vitro experiment:

> I have also put a little wine-vinegar to this stuff mixed with spittle, or with water; whereupon the animalcules fell dead forthwith.

He compares the in vivo findings with the in vitro experiment and explains the difference as follows:

> And from this I drew the conclusion that the vinegar, when I filled my mouth with it, didn't penetrate through all the matter that is firmly lodged between the front teeth, or the grinders, and killed only those animalcules that were in the outermost part of the white matter.

Five years later, in 1697, he relates that one of the back teeth in his mouth became loose and bothered him when chewing, and he pushed it with his thumb and removed it. He found that the molar in question had a huge cavity, from which he obtained a sample and found to his surprise that it contained so many animalculae that it appeared "to be alive." With respect to the size of the little animals he says that it "would take a thousand million of 'em to make up the bulk of a coarse sand-grain."

Finally in a letter dated June 29, 1708 he relates the following:

> At the latter end of the month of April, 1708, I was again seized with a high fever, which stayed with me for four days, rising higher each night; and as my tongue was again coated with a thick whitish matter, I oft-times removed some of it, which seemed stuck very tight to the parts of the tongue, with a small pen-knife or with a silver tongue-scraper; and viewing it many times through the magnifying glass, I could see nought else but what I have described in my previous discoveries.

He further took some of "the foresaid stuff from my tongue" and put it in a small clean china coffee cup, poured boiling rain water over it and let it stand "for a good half hour" to separate the particles.

> After a fortnight I saw that the water was well-nigh evaporated away, so I poured again a little rain water, which had stood some days in a clean phial in my closet, into the boiled water aforesaid. And five or six days afterwards ... I saw an inconceivable number of exceedingly small animalcules, and these of divers sorts.

Leeuwenhoek never associated bacteria to disease, probably because he had found bacteria in healthy mouths.

*Histologic observations.* Leeuwenhoek also studied the blood and blood vessels. William Harvey (1578–1657) had described in 1628 the circulation of blood in arteries and veins, with force provided by contractions of the heart. He could not determine, however, how the blood passed from the arteries to the veins. This was clarified in 1661 by Marcello Malpighi, who described the capillary network.

In 1665 Malpighi discovered the erythrocytes, which he incorrectly identified as fat globules.[8,11,14] Leeuwenhoek did not know of Malpighi's findings and rediscovered the red blood cells in 1674. In 1683, while investigating the embryonic development of the frog in vivo, Leeuwenhoek observed, in the capillaries, the rapid stream of erythrocytes, which he later found in other animals. Leeuwenhoek described the arterioles branching into innumerable capillaries, with red blood cells running in their interior and then reuniting in larger vessels (venules). He postulated that the smallest blood vessels have a wall, just as the arteries and veins, and that

> though each of the smallest blood vessels is provided with a wall, this said wall is so thin, open or spongy, that the thin watery liquid in the blood can get through it easily as water on a sieve.

Leeuwenhoek also made original observations on the structure of nerves and muscles: he described the optic nerve, other nerves, and the spinal cord as composed of little bundles of fibers, running parallel to each other, thus contradicting for the first time Galen's second-century theory that nerves are hollow and carry "animal spirits." He perceived that the muscular fiber had striations and studied the eyes of insects and of vertebrates (oxen and cows), describing the crystalline lens.[11,14]

In 1674 he described dentin, in teeth of humans and of other species, as composed of minute transparent tubes, and suggested that 600 or 700 of these would not excede the thickness of a hair. Leeuwenhoek did not distinguish bone from dentin, but observed in calf bone that the tubes formed a circumference, in the center of which was a larger tube: he was undoubtedly referring to a haversian system. He also showed, in a drawing, osteocytic lacunae.[17]

*Other observations.* The topics that most interested Leeuwenhoek were not oral microorganisms or blood circulation. His principal scientific interest centered on sexual reproduction,[13,17] which led him to refute the theory of spontaneous generation two centuries before this theory was finally laid to rest by Louis Pasteur.

Leeuwenhoek believed that microorganisms had male or female sex and reproduced by copulation and formation of the new organism inside the female body. This concept was accepted until the eighteenth century when Abraham Trembley, of England, and, later, Lazzaro Spallanzani, of Italy, described binary fission.

Leeuwenhoek, in 1677, observed the existence of motile cells in human sperm and postulated that these were normal components of human semen; in the following years he made similar observations in numerous species of mammals, birds, fish, and other phyla. Then, in 1683, he was the first to state that spermatozoa penetrated the ovum and fertilized it.

Leeuwenhoek carried out many studies of insects and lower animals, made discoveries in the area of anatomy of plants and the transport of nutrients within them, and investigated crystallography. He described plankton in salt water and fresh water and microorganisms in soil.

In addition to his concern for microscopy, Leeuwenhoek was interested in mathematics, especially geometry. His observations of blood in capillary tubes led him to advance a theory of capillary action. He performed experiments in chemistry to determine the specific gravity of various substances, and the "air expansion," produced by the combustion of gunpowder, as well as barometric and astronomic experiments.

Leeuwenhoek's work was recognized during his lifetime, and in his old age he was admired and venerated, appointed Fellow of the Royal Society, and received honors from the Academy of Sciences of Paris and the University of Louvain. When his discoveries made him famous, he was continuously disturbed by visitors eager to see his discoveries. Celebrities and nobility, as well as fellows of the Royal Society, numbered among his callers. Leeuwenhoek died on August 26, 1723, two months before his ninety-first birthday. He was buried in the Old Church of Delft.

Marcello Malpighi[8,11,19] was born in Bologna in 1628. He studied medicine and philosophy at the University of Bologna and then spent three years at the University of Pisa, where he was a student of the mathematician Giovanni Borelli. Malpighi taught at different times at the universities of Bologna, Pisa, and Messina and was the chief physician to Pope Innocent XII. From 1667 until his death in Rome in 1694, he maintained correspondence with the Royal Society of London, which supervised his publications.

Malpighi made fundamental anatomic and microscopic discoveries in many organs, and described numerous structures of basic interest to periodontology. He used instruments of different magnifying powers and made observations with both reflected and transmitted light.[8] Malpighi studied the structure of the lung, describing the pulmonary alveoli, and the missing link in Harvey's theory of blood circulation, the capillary network that connects arterioles and venules. Malpighi was the first to observe the erythrocytes and to study the "heart polyps," already described in patients who had died of heart disease, and to consider them intravascular coagulation of blood. He described the dental tissues (enamel and dentin), the tongue papillae (differentiating the horny outer layer of the tongue from the reticular mucous layer now called the *Malpighian layer*), and isolated the taste buds (determining their function as organs of taste). He also described the papillae of the skin, the organs of touch, and the secretory mechanisms of the salivary and other glands, as well as the now-called *Malpighian corpuscles of the kidneys.*[8]

Antony van Leeuwenhoek and Marcello Malpighi are two key figures in the development of sciences that later would become fundamental to periodontology. Leeuwenhoek's observations of oral flora, and of dental plaque and its suppression by external agents, are of particular interest since he explores a field that would require centuries to grow to primary importance for dentists and periodontists. Malpighi, too, broke new ground. He performed the initial microscopic studies of tissues, organs, and oral structures important to the discipline.

## References


1. Bulloch W. The History of Bacteriology. London: Oxford University Press, 1960.
2. Dobell C. Antony Leeuwenhoek and His "Little Animals." New York: Dover Publications, 1960.
3. Durant W, Durant A. The Story of Civilization. Vol 8: The Age of Louis XIV. New York: Simon & Schuster, 1963.
4. 'Espinasse M. Robert Hooke. Berkeley: University of California Press, 1956.
5. Harris H. The Birth of the Cell. New Haven: Yale University Press, 1999.
6. Henniger J. Leeuwenhoek, Antony van. In: Gillispie CC (ed). Dictionary of Scientific Biography. New York: Charles Scribner's Sons, 1973.
7. Hoffmann-Axthelm W. History of Dentistry. Chicago: Quintessence, 1981.
8. Huart P, Imbault-Huart MJ. Malpighi, Marcello. In: Gillispie CC (ed). Dictionary of Scientific Biography. New York: Charles Scribner's Sons, 1973.
9. Margotta R. The History of Medicine. New York: Reed International, 1996.
10. Leeuwenhoek A. The Collected Letters of Antony van Leeuwenhoek, vol I–XV. (Edited, illustrated, and annotated by a committee of Dutch scientists.) Amsterdam: Swets and Zeitlinger, 1952–1999.
11. Major RH. A History of Medicine. Springfield, IL: Charles C. Thomas, 1954.
12. McNeil WH. Plagues and Peoples. New York: Anchor Books, Doubleday, 1976.
13. Palm L, Snelders H. Antony van Leeuwenhoek 1632–1723. Rodopi BV (ed). Amsterdam: Swets and Zeitlinger, 1982.
14. Porter R. The Greatest Benefit to Mankind. New York: W.W. Norton, 1997.
15. Ring ME. Dentistry: An Illustrated History. St Louis: Mosby-Year Book, 1985. Reprinted, New York: Harry N. Abrams, 1992.
16. Ruestow EG. The Microscope in the Dutch Republic: The Shaping of Discovery. Cambridge: Cambridge University Press, 1996.
17. Rooseboom M. Leeuwenhoek's life in the Republic of the United Netherlands. In: Schierbeek A (ed). Measuring the Invisible World: The Life and Works of Antony van Leeuwenhoek, FRS. London: Abelard-Schuman, 1959.
18. Shklar G. Leeuwenhoek and Vermeer, an association of genius. J Hist Dent 1998;46:53–57.
19. Wilson C. The Invisible World: Early Modern Philosophy and the Invention of the Microscope. Princeton: University Press, 1995.

# 10

# The Eighteenth Century

After the years of French supremacy in the seventeenth century under Louis XIV, the eighteenth century saw the decline of France's political influence following a series of military defeats, and the rise of England's hegemony with the accession to the throne of the House of Hanover under George I, II, and III. The century ended with two important revolutions: the American Revolution in 1776, which brought democracy to the modern world, and the French Revolution in 1789, which ended the absolutist French monarchy but produced a period of chaos that gave rise to Napoleon's turbulent years.

The great political upheaval of the eighteenth century influenced all fields of thought, reducing the influence of academic dogmatism. Direct observation of phenomena and reproducible experiments gradually gained acceptance and became the basis of scientific research, following initial opposition that slowly gave way to the explosion of knowledge that would mark the following century.

The eighteenth century was the era of Voltaire (1694–1778), Diderot (1713–1784), Montesquieu (1689–1755), and Rousseau (1712–1788), in France; of John Wesley (1703–1791), and David Hume (1711–1746), in England; of Johann Sebastian Bach (1685–1750) in Germany; and Wolfgang Amadeus Mozart (1756–1791) in Austria.[5]

In medicine, a "spiritual doctrine" was a reaction against Descartes' idea of the body as machine. German Georg Ernst Stahl (1660–1734) advocated the existence of a "soul" that regulated health, while another German, Friedrich Hoffmann (1660–1742), claimed that the body functions through vital spirits that come from the brain and circulate in the blood and the nerves. Several other equally esoteric theories were advanced and to some extent delayed real scientific progress.[14,15]

In the eighteenth century, however, the first scientific studies that would end the theory of the humors proposed by Hippocrates and Galen two millennia earlier were presented by Morgagni and Bichat.

Giovanni Battista Morgagni[2,16,17] was born in Forli, a small town near Bologna, Italy, in 1682, and obtained a degree in philosophy and medicine from the University of Bologna in 1701. He studied under the noted anatomist Antonio Maria Valsalva, who had been a student of Marcello Malpighi. Morgagni became a professor at the University of Padua, where he occupied the position previously held by Vesalius, Fallopius, and Fabricius. He remained at Padua until he died.

Several scientists, including Francis Bacon, Vesalius, and Harvey had hinted at the possible correlation of clinical symptoms and autopsy findings, but none pursued the concept beyond rhetorical explanations. In 1679, Teophilus Bonetus, of Geneva, Switzerland, published a book entitled *Sepulchretum Sive Anatomica Practica*, in which he presented 3,000 clinical histories and autopsy findings. However, with many errors, poor organization, and no index, it was practically useless to physicians. René Laennec a century later called it an "undigested and incoherent compilation."[16]

Morgagni saw the deficiencies in Bonetus' work and sought to correct these errors, but in so doing he prepared a completely new work based on his own clinical observations and autopsies and those of his predecessors Valsalva, Albertini, and Malpighi. Entitled *De Sedibus et Causis Morborum per Anatomen Indagatis* (*On the Location and Causes of Diseases Researched Anatomically*), this work was presented in the form of seventy letters, written to an unidentified young physician. It contained about 700 cases and was organized in five books devoted to diseases of the head, thorax, abdomen, surgical and universal disorders, and an elaborate index.

Morgagni's descriptions clearly distinguished the important findings from the insignificant details, presenting the clinical signs and symptoms, the treatment performed, and the autopsy findings with an interpretation of their relationship to the clinical picture. It included the historical background and references on each topic and cited experiments conducted to clarify some points. Morgagni's work localized the diseases to the organs and gradually changed the emphasis from humors and general conditions to changes in the organs. Morgagni was a perfectionist, attending to every detail. He continued collecting cases and fine-tuning their presentation for decades, finally publishing the book when he was 79 years old. Considered the founder of modern pathology, Morgagni died in Padua ten years later, on December 5, 1771.

Marie-François-Xavier Bichat[12] was born in Thoirette in the Department of Jura, France, in 1771, less than one month before Morgagni's death. He studied medicine at Montpellier and Lyons and graduated from the University of Paris, where he was a student of Pierre Joseph Desault, a well-known surgeon. Bichat was appointed physician at the Hotel Dieu Hospital in Paris and devoted his time feverishly to the study of pathology, performing thousands of autopsies and publishing several important books early in his life, as if he knew he had little time. He died in 1802, at 31 years of age, apparently of tuberculous meningitis.

Bichat's contribution was to extend Morgagni's concept of organ pathology to the organ constituents, namely the tissues. He distinguished twenty-one tissues on the basis of their structure, texture, and properties. Bichat investigated the composition of organs by dissection and by different chemical and physical treatments such as heat, water, acids, desiccation, and maceration. Even without the use of a microscope Bichat discovered that organs are made out of tissues and that the tissues are the origin of pathologic changes. This revelation led to specific diagnoses such as pericarditis, myocarditis, and endocarditis, rather than the general "inflammation of the heart." Further development in this area would continue six decades later with Virchow's cellular pathology (see Chapter 16).

The eighteenth century produced many other key physicians such as Herman Boerhaave (1688–1738) of Holland, who envisioned health and sickness in terms of physical variables such as forces, weights, and hydrostatic pressure, distinguishing diseases of solids and diseases of "blood and humors"; Leopold Auenbrugger (1722–1809) of Italy, who founded the science of physical diagnosis and developed percussion as a diagnostic method; Lazzaro Spallanzani (1729–1799), also of Italy and a student of Morgagni, who made important discoveries of digestion, circulation, and reproduction; and Edward Jenner (1749–1823) of England, who developed the smallpox vaccine after observing that dairy maids who contracted cowpox were immune to the disease.[14,15,17]

In chemistry, it was the century of Antoine-Laurent Lavoisier (1743–1794), in France, who discovered oxygen and made important studies of respiration. He is considered the father of modern chemistry and was also an eminent physiologist. An aristocrat and a tax collector, Lavoisier died on the guillotine, sentenced by the French revolutionists as an "enemy of the people." It was also the century of Joseph Priestley (1733–1804), English theologian, politician, and scholar, who also discovered oxygen, probably before Lavoisier, but linked it to the phlogiston theory. Priestley was persecuted in England for his sympathies with the French Revolution, and emigrated to America where he died.[14]

At the end of the seventeenth century steps were taken to recognize and regulate dentistry, initially in Berlin, and then in Paris. In 1699 a decree of Louis XIV established that the hernia-operators, oculists, dentists, bone-resetters, and others had to pass a theoretical and practical examination to practice in Paris and its suburbs. Dentistry in general and periodontics in particular, especially because of Pierre Fauchard and John Hunter, went through a period of great progress in this century.

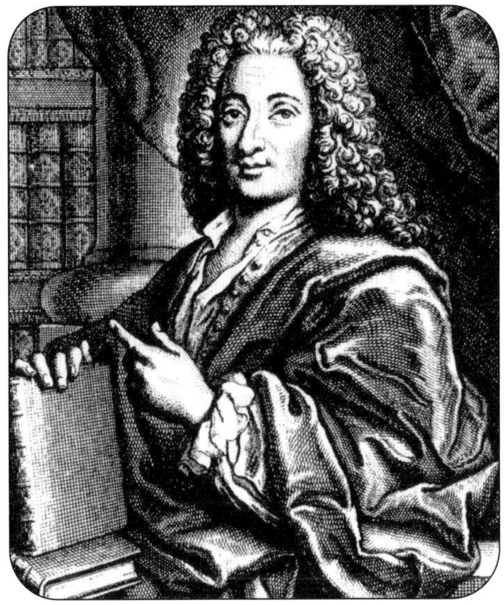

**Fig 13** Pierre Fauchard in the frontispiece of his book *Le Chirurgien Dentiste,* 1746.

## Pierre Fauchard

Pierre Fauchard (Fig 13) was born in Brittany in 1678. Little is known about his childhood and family. He received his training as a surgeon in the French Royal Navy, spending three years on a warship. The severe mouth diseases that sailors suffered, particularly scurvy, may have induced him to specialize in the treatment of diseases of the mouth. Furthermore, the surgeon-major of the Navy, under whom Fauchard served, was Alexander Poteleret, an expert in mouth diseases.

In 1696, after his military service, he opened his practice in Angers, at the time a university town. Dental extractions were performed by barbers, who also practiced bleeding through application of leeches. Fauchard was from the outset considered a "surgeon-dentist," and was probably the first to receive this title. His practice largely involved filling carious teeth and removing calculus and benign oral tumors. Prostheses were then practically nonexistent, except for ligating clumsy imitations of human teeth made out of bone or ivory to the remaining teeth.[20] Fauchard also traveled frequently to neighboring localities to see patients in order to increase his income.[20]

Although he enjoyed a good reputation in western France and patients came from distant places to see him, in 1718 Fauchard moved to Paris where he remained for the rest of his life. His practice at first was at Rue de la Comédie Française and, after 1747, at Rue des Grand Cordelier.[9,19,20] Fauchard quickly became well-known in Paris. His practice included various notables, and the best physicians and surgeons referred patients to him.[20]

In 1729 he married Mlle. Elisabeth Guillemette Chemin, whose father was a high-ranking dignitary. In 1734 Pierre Fauchard acquired the castle of Grand Mesnil, becoming a seigneur and a magistrate. Pierre and Elisabeth had only one son, Jean Baptiste Fauchard, who became an advocate in Parliament and counsellor to the French Admiralty, and later, after some political strife, went into exile in Belgium and became an actor and comedian.[20]

Fauchard was of the opinion that the examining commission set up by the edict of 1699 "lacked a skillful and experienced dentist," and therefore suggested that such a person be appointed to the commission, but his advice was ignored. Perhaps attempting to remedy this omission, Fauchard wrote a treatise of dentistry that offered candidates an authoritative source of information for their examination and subsequent practice.[9,19,20]

In 1723 Fauchard completed his manuscript, entitled *Le Chirurgien Dentiste, ou, Traité des Dents (The Surgeon Dentist, or, Treatise on the Teeth).* The text was published five years later, in 1728, and immediately became the foremost book on dentistry. It would remain so for more than a century. Indeed, many of his ideas remain valid. A second edition, considerably amplified and improved, was published in 1746. A third edition was published in 1786, after Fauchard's death.

Fauchard first had his friend, and probably mentor, Jean Devaux (1649–1729), critique the manuscript. Devaux was a prominent physician, considerably older than Fauchard, and some scholars assume that he collaborated with Fauchard, contributing experience and knowledge.[21,24]

A German translation of the first edition was published in 1733 and it greatly influenced the progress of dentistry in German-speaking countries. Unfortunately an English version did not appear until 1946. Of course, this late translation, by the British dental historian Lilian Lindsay, serves only a historical purpose.

Fauchard gained renown during his lifetime, to such an extent that in France and other countries periodontal disease was known for more than a century as *la maladie de Fauchard* (Fauchard's disease). He died in Paris on March 21, 1761.

Fauchard's *Le Chirurgien Dentiste* was published in two volumes of small format, with 39 chapters (494 pages) in the first volume and 26 chapters (425 pages) in the second. It reflects not only the methodical accumulation of data derived from his own observations, but also great respect for his predecessors, to whom he gives due credit. Fauchard's style is clear and concise, providing practical information as well as explanations of mechanisms and reasons for the phenomena described or the techniques proposed. The following comments refer to the 1746 edition of this text. All quotations are taken from the Lindsay translation.[6]

The first volume is largely devoted to the anatomy and pathology of teeth, gums, and tongue. Chapter 11 defines tartar as

> a substance that accumulates on the surface of the teeth and which becomes, when left there, a stony crust of more or less considerable volume. The most common cause is the negligence of those people who do not clean their teeth when they might, and that they perceive the lodgment of this foreign substance which produces disease of the gums.

He goes on to describe the causes of tartar, assigning primary importance to "the saliva when it is vitiated, as a result of some depravity of the lymph, and being charged with salts and much earthy matter, deposits them on the teeth."

In Chapter 16, titled "Of the structure, connection and use of the gums," Fauchard delineates the gingiva as follows:

> The tissue which composes the gums is firm and sufficiently hard. It is rather more glandulous than fibrous. It is contained and enveloped between the skin which lines the mouth, and the periosteum. This same tissue is penetrated and bathed by many different sorts of vessels, arteries, veins, nerves and lymphatic vessels almost all divided and multiplied into so many capillaries formed by the continuation of vessels supplying the neighboring parts of the gums.

The chapter goes on to detail gingival anatomy. The following chapter then deals with periodontal diseases, those being "the ones which destroy the teeth most frequently and cause them an infinity of troublesome accidents." The description that follows refers mainly to gingival enlargements, epulis, and abscesses. He depicts accumulations of calculus sometimes reaching monstrous proportions, and changes in the gingiva, such as swelling, bleeding, pain, and looseness of the teeth. He recommends the removal of calculus and the excision of the excessive gum tissue with straight or curved scissors.

Chapter 18 deals with epulis, of which he discerns a soft, white, nonpainful kind and a hard, red, painful variety. He details probing and removing the lesions surgically and includes postoperative management using various remedies. Gingival abscesses, including their treatment, are described in Chapter 19, ulcers in Chapter 20, and fistulae in Chapter 21.

Chapter 22 looks at "The ill effects of scurvy on the teeth, gums and bones of the jaws and the operation needed to treat them." The nutritional etiology of scurvy was not known at the time. The experiment of Admiral James Lind, of the British Navy, on the use of citric fruits to prevent the disease, took place in 1747. Lind's findings[13] were published in 1753 but his conclusions were generally rejected until 1782, when another British naval officer, known only as Mr. Young, corroborated Lind's findings.

Fauchard describes two kinds of scurvy. One appears to be real scurvy (vitamin C deficiency) causing the swelling, discoloration, ulcers, putrid exudation, bleeding, and, finally, gangrene and necrosis. He notes that the disease occurs on ships, seaports, and similar places, and is not so common in Paris and other inland cities. The other type is probably periodontitis. He says:

> [it] attacks the gums, alveoli and teeth. The complaint is recognized by a whitish, slightly glutinous pus which can be expressed from the gums by application of finger pressing pretty hard from below upwards in the lower jaw and from above downwards in the upper jaw.



Further along in the same chapter he remarks,

> What is singular, and which I have observed, is that those who have been treated for this complaint by internal remedies ... have not been cured, which makes me believe that there is no internal source or general cause, but that it has an accidental origin occasioned by the teeth. The better to understand this I have noticed that when the teeth have been lost as a result of this, their alveoli and their gums are so well joined, cicatrized and consolidated that there is no longer any appearance of purulent matter.

This statement indicates his belief in the local etiology of periodontitis, as opposed to the contemporary theory of a systemic causation. Based on this belief, he asserts the following:

> This loss can be avoided by the following means, that is to keep the teeth very clean, deplete the gums when they need it, by rubbing them vigorously every day with the end of the fingers dipped in one or other of the two dessicative, astringent and anti-scorbutic waters of which I have given the prescription in Chapter 5 of this first volume. Care must also be taken to wash the mouth after meals with a little wine and water and to observe each time to press the finger firmly on the gums when rubbing them in order to expel the pus which without that will consume and corrode the alveoli so that the teeth will become loose and finally fall out for want of support.

The remaining chapters focus largely on case reports of various dental and oral conditions.

Volume Two consists of twenty-six chapters mainly concerned with operative dentistry, prosthetics, and tooth extractions. The second and third chapters describe periodontal instruments and their uses. In Chapter 2, "Description of instruments appropriate for the removal of tartar of the teeth," Fauchard defines his five instruments—his own innovations—calling them the rabbet chisel, parrot's bill, graver with three facets, hook like a Z, and a knife (Fig 14). Then, in Chapter 3, "Manner of operating methodically in cleaning a mouth in detaching, removing and taking away the tartar without involving the enamel of the teeth," he details their use, including sharpening the instruments, positions of operator and patient, sequence of instruments to use, placement of the instrument in the mouth, separation of soft tissues, fulcrum, areas to be scaled with each instrument, including interdental surfaces, and so on.

Fauchard's *Le Chirurgien Dentiste* was for 150 years the most important source for learning and understanding the disease processes of the mouth and teeth and the methods for their treatment. It was not until the end of the nineteenth century that John Riggs and his followers improved on the clinical teachings of the French master, and N. N. Znamensky, with greatly improved methods of observation and based on the pioneering work of Virchow, Cohnheim, and others, improved the understanding of the tissue changes in periodontitis (see Chapter 12).

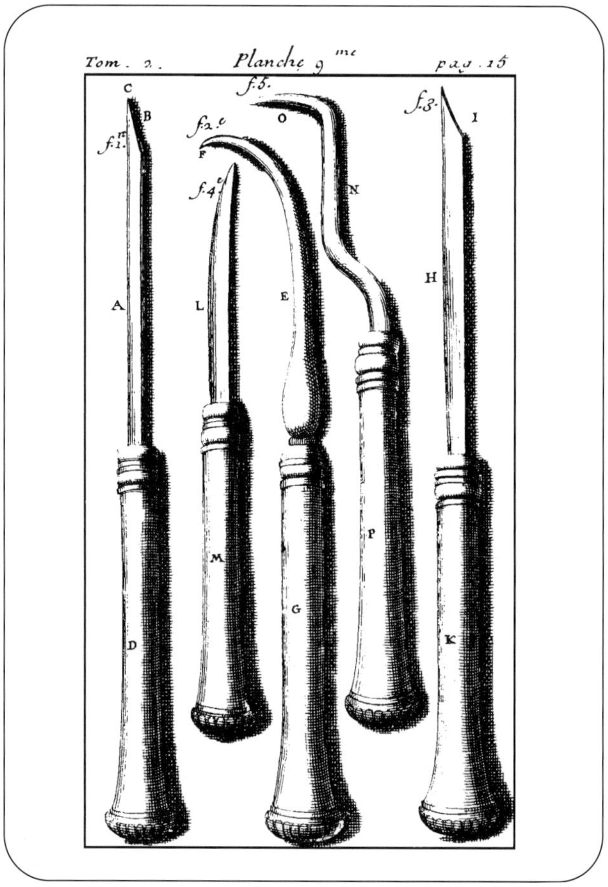


**Fig 14** Fauchard's set of scaling instruments.

Pierre Fauchard had many followers in France and also in Germany. Etienne Bourdet (1722–1789), from southern France, became the king's dentist in 1760. In 1757 he published *Recherches et observations sur touts les parties de l'art du dentist*, in which he quotes Fauchard extensively. The book went through several editions and was translated into a number of languages. Bourdet details severe periodontitis and its treatment by cleansing and in severe cases cauterizing the gingiva, or, when this fails, by gingival resection.[7]

Bourdet's treatment varied depending on the amount of bone lost; he explains it as follows[7]:

> Prior to bone loss and the manifestation of suppuration, at the onset of swelling and inflammation, if one obtains the services of a competent dentist the problem can be easily resolved by repeated disgorgements of the gingiva effected by small internal and external scarifications of the gingiva. This treatment when followed by one or more bleedings, mild purgations, and the use of an excellent opiate or mouth rinse will result in a complete cure.

In cases with bone loss, he recommended the following:

> One takes a flat, supple cautery instrument, heats it to red-hot, and insinuates it to the bottom of the void between the gingiva and the root, reintroducing it two or three times, observing to thoroughly burn the gingiva all along the surface corresponding to the root.

If suppuration persisted after repeating this treatment, he proceeded to excise the gingiva with scissors and clean the root surfaces.

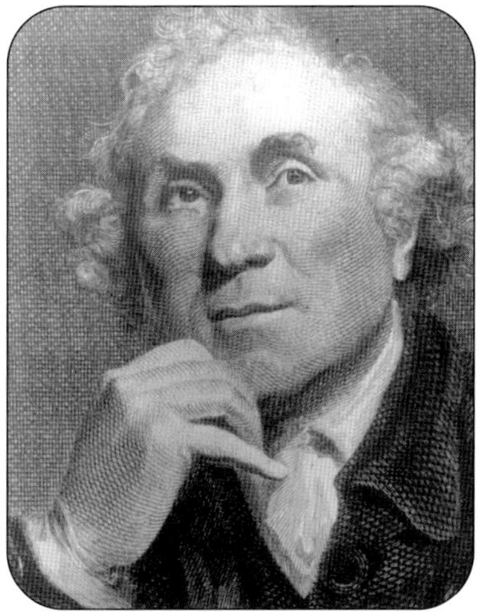

**Fig 15** John Hunter.

Another French author of the eighteenth century, Botot,[9] published *Observations sur la suppuration des gencives*, in which he differentiated three forms of periodontitis: suppuration of the gingiva, suppuration of the marginal bone, and suppuration of the socket itself. Botot thought of these diseases as infectious in nature. As a result, he rejects surgical treatment and recommends instead a treatment based on calculus removal, flushing, and rubbing with camphor oil.[9]

In Germany, Philipp Pfaff (1713–1766) of Berlin, was a military surgeon, and later court dentist, who in 1756 published *Abhandlung von den Zähnen des menschlichen Körpers un deren Krankheitn (Treatise on the Teeth of the Human Body and Their Diseases).*[9] Pfaff followed Fauchard's teachings and thus devotes a good part of the text to periodontal disease, recommending careful removal of calculus as its treatment. He suggests the use of mercury for the treatment of venereal diseases as one cause of gingival problems and, interestingly, mentions that smoking tobacco not only damages the teeth through biting on the pipe but also that smoke irritates the gums. Pfaff was the first to recommend taking an impression (with wax) to make a plaster model for denture construction.[9]

A Vienna surgeon, Joseph Jacob Plenk (1738–1807), published a book on diseases of teeth and gums, first in Latin in 1778, then in German in 1779, and in Italian in 1786 and 1790. This text reviews the literature and presents case reports, ordering the signs and symptoms of disease.[9]

August Gottlieb Richter (1742–1812), of Göttingen, Germany, published a text in 1798 that generally follows Fauchard's teachings.[8,9] Richter observes that calculus surrounds the gum and grows apically until the tooth falls off. He advocates calculus removal and says that this stimulates an inflammation in the detached parts of the gum, effecting its new adhesion to the tooth. This has been interpreted as an initial hint to reattachment.[8]

## John Hunter

John Hunter (Fig 15) was the youngest of ten children born to John Hunter and Agnes Paul. Two of the boys, John and William, would become leading physicians and teachers in Great Britain. John was born in 1728 in Scotland. William, ten years older than John, studied medicine at the University of Edinburgh and became a teacher of anatomy in London. John joined him in 1748 to study and research the field of anatomy. In 1761 John joined the army as a surgeon and participated in the Seven Years War against France. Upon returning to London, he opened what would become a successful private practice and continued his research and teaching of anatomy

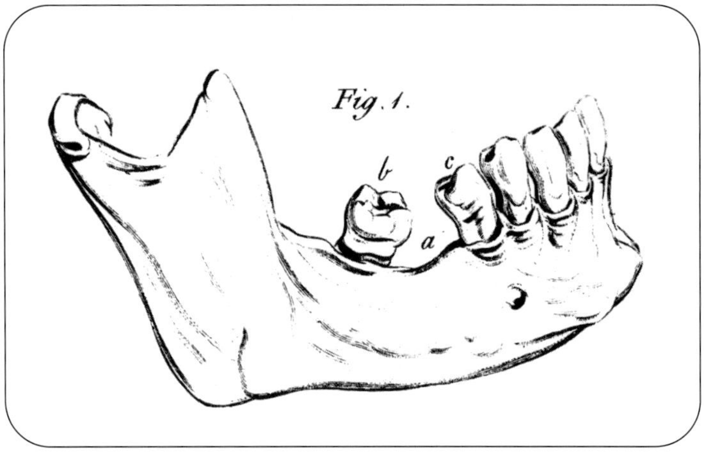


**Fig 16** Illustration from Hunter's book *The Natural History of the Human Teeth* showing the mesial migration of a mandibular second molar after loss of the first molar.

in Covent Garden. During his lifetime Hunter collected more than 13,000 anatomical specimens, which are now on display at the Hunterian Museum of the Royal College of Surgeons, in London. Hunter became widely respected, was appointed surgeon-extraordinary to King George III, and received numerous awards and accolades. He died in London in 1793.[4,14]

John Hunter published extensively and on a large number of topics. His treatise *The Natural History of the Human Teeth*, published in 1771 and 1778, was translated into several languages. A second volume, *A Practical Treatise on the Diseases of the Teeth*, was added to the second edition.[10,11]

The first part is a detailed anatomy of human teeth and jaws, with beautiful drawings of bone structures of the face, including primary and permanent teeth, edentulous jaws, sections of teeth showing enamel and dentin (not yet differentiated from cementum), and the pulpal space. He describes transplantation of teeth and also disagrees with the theory of continuous eruption of the teeth. He portrays the displacement of teeth as a consequence of the loss of adjacent or opposing teeth (Fig 16).

As a surgeon, Hunter contends that all diseases of the bone and soft tissues of the mouth should be treated by surgeons, limiting the role of the dentist to diseases of the teeth. Hunter traces the progress of dental caries, referring to initial white opaque spots that change, although not in all cases, to a dark brown speck before destroying the enamel and resulting in a carious lesion. Then he charts the destruction of a tooth by the carious process, the painful symptoms it produces, and abscess formation (gum boils).

The chapter "Diseases of the alveolar processes" refers to periodontal diseases.[11] Hunter describes pocket formation and bone loss as:

> a wasting of the alveolar processes, which are in many people gradually absorbed, and taken into the system. This wasting begins at the edge of the socket, and gradually goes on to the root or bottom.
>
> The gum, which is supported by the alveolar process, loses its connection, and recedes from the body of the tooth, in proportion as the socket is lost; in consequence of which, first the neck, and then more or less of the fang itself, becomes exposed. The tooth of course, becomes extremely loose, and at last drops out.

Hunter differentiates scurvy from other gum diseases, including necrotizing ulcerative gingivitis, which he describes as follows[11]:

> When the gums first begin to have a tenderness, we may observe it first on their edges: the common smooth skin of the gum is not continued to its very edge, but becomes at

> the edge a little rough like a border, and somewhat thickened. The part of the gum, between two teeth swells, and often pushes out like luxuriant flesh, which is frequently very tender.
>
> The inflammation is often carried so far as to make the gums ulcerate; so that the gums in many cases have a common ulcer upon them; by which process, a part of the teeth are denuded. This is often on one part only, often only on one jaw; while in some cases it is on the whole gums on both jaws.

Hunter describes another type of disease that usually occurs with the first type and consists of "a filling up of the socket at the bottom, whereby the tooth is gradually pushed out."[11] Hunter probably refers here to extrusion and exfoliation of the tooth, as may occur in aggressive periodontitis. He goes on:

> These diseases arise often from visible causes. Any thing that occasions a considerable and long continued inflammation in those parts, such particularly as salivation, will produce the same effect. The scurvy also, when carried to a great height, attacks the gums, and the alveolar processes, which becomes a cause of the dissolution of those parts. This is most remarkable in the scurvy at sea.

Hunter recommends a surgical treatment eliminating the gums "where they become luxuriant." Then he focuses several sections on tooth extraction, transplantation of teeth, which was a common treatment at that time, and problems arising from tooth eruption in children.

John Hunter's significant contributions to anatomy raised the scientific standards of dentistry. Other contributors to the development of periodontics in England include Thomas Berdmore, Bartholomew Ruspini, and Joseph Fox.

Thomas Berdmore (1740–1785) was a British dentist who held the title of Dentist to His Majesty, King George III. In 1768 Berdmore published *A Treatise on the Disorders and Deformities of the Teeth and Gums*,[3] in which he claims to base his conclusions on his personal experiences, having "purposely avoided quotations. … I could have quoted a few French authors, *who have written to make their names known*, and one or two English, who have translated very injudiciously."

These words written by Berdmore in the preface to his book reveal him as probably selfish and vain, contemptuous or jealous of foreigners (he probably refers mainly to Fauchard). Berdmore also despised his colleagues, of whom he further says that his book was "originally designed for artists, *who are not much given to reading*."

The book consists of 267 pages and is divided in three parts. The first, briefest part is concerned with anatomy and physiology of the teeth. The second, longest section describes diseases of teeth and gums and their treatment. The last part considers prevention, and several of its chapters focus on periodontal problems.

In Chapter 7, "On tartar of the teeth, and the recess of the gums and tooth-ache occasioned by the tartarous concretions long neglected," he has the following to say:

> For there are several sorts of Tartar differing remarkably in colour, thickness, hardness, and adhesion, from the soft slough that gathers overnight, or in sickly people, to the large and stony substance which often envelopes in one uniform crust all the Teeth of either jaw, together with a considerable part of the gums. …
>
> That soft matter that gathers on the Teeth overnight, is easily removed by brushing and washing them frequently, and freeing them carefully at night from the scraps of food that are apt to lodge after supper.
>
> … The crumbling of the hard scaly Tartar is to be removed by means of particular instruments, which the Surgeon-Dentists use, beginning at the gums and raising it off in layers from the Teeth.

> … The inflammation of the gums occasioned by Tartar is often very violent, and requires to be treated with emollients.

Berdmore also used surgery when necessary to remove hyperplastic gingival tissue once the tartar has been removed, "for without this, the gums will not closely embrace a tooth which has been made smaller at the collar by the removal of its tartar."

Berdmore stresses prevention and suggests methods for whitening the teeth. He also spells out splinting of loose teeth "by means of gold wire or silk ligature," and recommends the use of ligatures to correct irregularities of the teeth, but only in children:

> In advanced age it is well known, that the Teeth are so deeply and firmly fixed in the substance of the jaw-bone, that it requires a considerable power to force them out of their places, and that none of the bones at this period will yield to slight continued pressure, in the manner that the tender, growing bones of children will do.

## American Dentistry

American dentistry, which started to develop in the second half of the eighteenth century, arose from two different groups. The first was made up of individuals who had varying degrees of medical education and incorporated the care of teeth and mouth diseases into their practices. The second group consisted of barbers or craftsmen who were engaged in the manufacture of wood or metal instruments or utensils.[22]

The first qualified American dentists were trained in England or France. Robert Woffendale (1742–1828) was born in England and trained in London with Thomas Berdmore. Woffendale wrote one of the early dental books in America and was the first dentist to practice in the colonies, in New York City, from 1766 to 1768. In an advertisement in the *New York Weekly Journal* in 1766, he "begs Leave to inform the Public that he performs all Operations upon the Teeth, Gums, Sockets and Palate."

Similar advertisements were placed by other contemporary dentists. John Baker (1732–1796) was a dentist to George Washington and had a successful career. Baker imparted his dental knowledge to Paul Revere, Isaac Greenwood, and Josiah Flagg. In an advertisement in the *New York Weekly Journal* in 1768,[22] Baker tells the public that he

> cures the scurvy in the gums, be it ever so bad; first cleans and scales teeth from that corrosive tartarous gritty substance, which hinders the gums from growing, infects the breath and is one of the principle causes of scurvy, and, if not timely prevented, eats away the gums so that many people's teeth fall out fresh. … His dentifrice with proper directions for preserving the teeth and gums is to be had at his lodgings.

## References

1. Bellagarda G, Bellagarda M. Storia Illustrata dell'Arte Dentaria. Torino, Italy: Medica Minerva, 1987.
2. Belloni L. Morgagni, Giovanni Battista. In: Gillispie CC (ed). Dictionary of Scientific Biography. New York: Charles Scribner's Sons, 1973.
3. Berdmore TA. Treatise on the Disorders and Deformities of the Teeth and Gums. Birmingham, AL: Classics of Dentistry, 1981.
4. Dobson J. Hunter, John. In: Gillispie CC (ed). Dictionary of Scientific Biography. New York: Charles Scribner's Sons, 1973.
5. Durant W, Durant A. The Story of Civilization. Vol 9: The Age of Voltaire. New York: Simon and Schuster, 1965.

# Part IV

# The Nineteenth Century

# 11

# The Century in Perspective

Economic and ideological changes affected daily life in the nineteenth century more than at any previous time.[1–5] The economic changes encompassing what is called the Industrial Revolution started in Great Britain during the last decades of the eighteenth century when the United States and France were experiencing political and social transformation.

In the realm of economics, changes occurred in the production of wealth, in manufacturing techniques, exploitation of natural resources, formation of capital, and distribution of products to consumers. In the domain of sociopolitical philosophy, thinkers recognized that social hierarchies were not God's will, and concepts of individual independence and government by popular consent gained ground.

The ideological revolution stemmed from the French encyclopédie and gained momentum through two violent revolutions and the events surrounding them. First was the American struggle for independence, in 1776, followed by the drafting of the American Constitution, which proclaimed persons' equality before God and the law and instituted an elective, not hereditary, government. Second was the French Revolution, in 1789, which marked the end of the absolutist monarchy but led to a period of turmoil that ended with Napoleon's defeat at Waterloo and the return to power of the Bourbon dynasty, this time was a constitutional monarchy.

After mid-century, the problems created by industrialization with the new proletarian class and the rapid, uncontrolled urbanization led to the surge of new ideas such as communism, nationalism, and imperialism.

Ordinary people in the early nineteenth-century Western world continued to live as their ancestors had in preceding centuries: life was marked by scarcity, fear of pestilence, and insecurity with respect to the future, both near and distant. Work was manual, with few tools, moved by muscle power of man or beast, and sometimes aided by energy from rivers or wind.

As the century progressed other sources of power were developed, such as steam machines, electricity, and gas combustion. Agriculture progressed, with innovations such as fertilizers and new tools. Factories started to appear, initially for the production of fabrics, and new mining techniques improved the extraction of coal and iron. The steam machine, originally invented to pump water out of carbon mines, was found to have numerous uses, particularly in locomotives and steam ships. Inventions such as the sewing machine, Portland cement, the typewriter, electricity and incandescent light, the telegraph, telephone, and electric tramways, improved living conditions.

There were also great innovations in the work of engineers and architects, who applied technological advances to introduce greater comfort and hygiene to daily life. These innovations, together with the work of medical and basic scientists, were part of an important revolution that improved and prolonged people's lives.

## Medical Sciences

The French revolutionaries, in their efforts to destroy all aristocratic and oligarchic traditions, abolished the old universities and academies and founded, in 1794, the *Ecole de Santé*, which was free of the restrictions that tradition imposed on the old institutions and allowed scientific research to be conducted in the large public hospitals. Thus, Paris gradually became the most important medical center, with a new type of medicine based on the findings of physical examination and autopsy.

Prominent physicians included Jean Nicolas Corvisart (1755–1821), Napoleon's physician, who popularized and perfected the percussion technique first described by the Viennese Leopold Auerbrugger (1722–1809); René T. H. Laennec (1781–1826), who developed the stethoscope; and Pierre C. A. Louis (1787–1882), who used numerical methods to demonstrate the benefit, or lack, of therapeutic methods.[9,10,11,14]

Vienna was another important medical center, with pathologist Carl Rokitanski (1804–1878), Joseph Skoda (1805–1881), who furthered physical diagnosis, and Ferdinand von Hebra (1816–1880), who pioneered scientific dermatology. London, too, was a principal city, with Thomas Hodgkin (1798–1866), Thomas Addison (1793–1860), and Robert Graves (1796–1853).

In the second half of the century German medicine came to the fore, with an emphasis on laboratory diagnosis and microscopic studies. Chemist Justus von Liebig (1803–1873) and Johannes Müller (1801–1858), renowned teacher and researcher in anatomy, physiology, and pathology, along with his eminent disciples Rudolf Virchow (1821–1902), Jacob Henle (1809–1896), and Herman von Helmholtz (1821–1894), among others, shine in this period.

Microbiology and immunology emerged as serious scientific disciplines in the second half of the century, with the French chemist Louis Pasteur (1822–1895), German physician Robert Koch (1843–1910), and a host of disciples. Their studies led to the development of pharmacology as a discipline, pioneered by Paul Ehrlich (1854–1915), and other investigators.

Surgery started to gain stature with the discovery of anesthesia by Horace Wells and William Morton (see Chapter 12), along with Joseph Lister's (1827–1912) application of Pasteur's concepts to medicine, which introduced the era of antisepsis. Later two Germans, Ernst von Bergmann (1836–1907) and Theodor Billroth (1829–1894), developed aseptic techniques in surgery.

## Dentistry

The eighteenth century saw the birth of dentistry as a profession, and the work of Pierre Fauchard and John Hunter consolidated its scientific base. In the nineteenth century, medical advances and technological developments further established the foundations of dentistry, expanding its diagnostic and treatment techniques. American scientists' contribution to this expansion and consolidation gained momentum in the second half of the century but concentrated mainly on the practical and technical aspects of dentistry.

*Clinical dentistry.* Dental practice continued slowly to shift away from the territory of traveling tooth extractors, barbers, and even blacksmiths—itinerant dentists who were generally self taught or had apprenticed with other practitioners, and, undoubtedly, filled a public need when there were no trained dentists or physicians.[13] In the cities first and in smaller towns later, these early dentists were replaced by physicians or others who had trained under practitioners, so gradually, toward the end of the century, the newer generation of dentists could boast a university education.

Porcelain dentures had been introduced in the late eighteenth century, and industrial production of porcelain teeth started in Philadelphia in 1825. Use of vulcanized hard rubber for denture bases started by mid-nineteenth century, and use of gold clasps for partial dentures and

6. Fauchard P. Le Chirurgien Dentiste ou Traité des Dents. Lindsay L (trans). Birmingham, AL: Classics of Dentistry, 1980.
7. Garant PR. The contributions of Etienne Bourdet (1722–1789) to the diagnosis and treatment of periodontal disease. Bull Hist Dent 1993;41:69–72.
8. Held A-J. Periodontology. From Its Origins up to 1980: A Survey. Basel, Switzerland: Birkhäuser, 1989.
9. Hoffmann-Axthelm W. History of Dentistry. Koehler HM (trans). Chicago: Quintessence, 1981.
10. Hunter J. The Natural History of the Human Teeth, vol 1 (ed 2). London: Johnson, 1778.
11. Hunter J. The Natural History of the Teeth. Vol 2: A Practical Treatise on the Diseases of the Teeth (ed 2). London: Johnson, 1778.
12. Kopal Z. Bichat, Marie-François-Xavier. In: Gillispie CC (ed). Dictionary of Scientific Biography. New York: Charles Scribner's Sons, 1973.
13. Lind J. A Treatise on the Scurvy (ed 3). Birmingham, AL: Classics of Dentistry, 1981.
14. Major RH. A History of Medicine. Springfield, IL: Charles C. Thomas, 1954.
15. Margotta R. The History of Medicine. London: Reed International Books, 1996.
16. Nuland SB. Doctors. The Biography of Medicine. New York: Vintage Books, 1995.
17. Porter R. The Greatest Benefit to Mankind. New York: W.W. Norton & Co, 1997.
18. Prinz H. Pierre Fauchard and his works. Dent Cosmos 1923;65:827.
19. Ring ME. Dentistry: An Illustrated History. St Louis: Mosby-Year Book, 1985. Reprinted, New York: Harry N. Abrams, 1992.
20. Viau G. The life of Pierre Fauchard (1678–1761). Dent Cosmos 1923;65:797.
21. Viau G. The manuscript of Fauchard. Dent Cosmos 1923;65:823.
22. Waite FC. The background of modern American dentistry. J Dent Educ 1936;1:91.
23. Walsh JJ. Fauchard, the father of modern dentistry. Dent Cosmos 1923;65:809.
24. Weinberger BW. An Introduction to the History of Dentistry, 2 vols. St Louis: Mosby, 1948.

suction to replace springs in full dentures started in the last decades of the century. In 1820, in Paris, Christophe François Delabarre (1784–1862) published the first book on prosthetics.[6]

Improvements in crown-and-bridge prostheses also took place in this century, with development of cement in the 1860s, improvements in gold crowns, dowel crowns, and many others. Restorative dentistry went through the "amalgam war" between the proponents of the new technique (amalgam) and those fanatically defending the gold foil. The contributions of G. V. Black established rational technical bases for operative dentistry procedures.[12]

*Basic sciences in dentistry.* Germany led the world in the second half of the nineteenth century in biomedical sciences, mostly due to the importance given to basic sciences research in medical training.[7] This scientific research philosophy included dentistry, and dental training stressed basic science training and not just the formation of skillful operators.[8] Numerous Americans emigrated to Germany to practice dentistry. At the time American dentistry was practical and technically oriented, while German dentistry had a more solid scientific background. The different philosophies of the American and the German approaches to dentistry in the nineteenth century is reflected in the comment of American dentist Dr. William Bonwill after he visited W. D. Miller, who had emigrated to Germany to practice dentistry in Berlin (see Chapter 13).

> I have found no inducement to change my own simple ways of treatment, which for 45 years have been satisfactory, notwithstanding all that has been said on the germ theory. … Antiseptic treatment has done a wonderful work, and all praise to the agitators! But let us not lose sight of the fact that all our operators in the various branches of our art would be not worth a farthing without mechanical engineering details being carried out faithfully.[7]

The divergent approaches to dental science and art were clearly reflected in the curricula of the schools or institutes of dentistry that appeared in America and later in Europe in the nineteenth century (see Chapter 28).

The difference may also have had an important business component. In America many devices and materials could be patented, therefore becoming highly profitable. In addition, most American dental journals were published by dental supply companies, and this literature greatly influenced dentistry.[7] The relationship between dentistry and commercial companies started to wane in the beginning of the twentieth century, and by the 1930s and 1940s the United States was at the forefront of basic research as well as dental technology.

## References

1. Briggs A (ed). The Nineteenth Century. New York: Bonanza Books, 1985.
2. Carranza FA. Revolucionarios de la Ciencia. Buenos Aires: Vergara, 1998.
3. Hobsbawm E. The Age of Revolution: 1789–1848. New York: Vintage Books, 1962.
4. Hobsbawm E. The Age of Capital: 1848–1875. New York: Vintage Books, 1975.
5. Hobsbawm E. The Age of Empire: 1875–1914. New York: Vintage Books, 1989.
6. Hoffmann-Axthelm W. History of Dentistry. Chicago: Quintessence, 1981.
7. Huff DE. A comparison of American and German dentistry, 1850–1900. Bull Hist Dent 1985;33:47.
8. Jenkins NS. Modern dentistry in Germany. Dent Cosmos 1912;54:1225.
9. Major RH. A History of Medicine. Springfield, IL: Charles C. Thomas, 1954.
10. Margotta R. The History of Medicine. New York: Smithmark, 1996.
11. Porter R. The Greatest Benefit to Mankind. London: W. W. Norton, 1997.
12. Ring ME. Dentistry: An Illustrated History. St Louis: Mosby-Year Book, 1985. Reprinted, New York: Harry N. Abrams, 1992.
13. Ring ME. Quackery in dentistry. Past and present. J Calif Dent Assoc 1998;26:818–826.
14. Shryock RH. The Development of Modern Medicine: An Interpretation of the Social and Scientific Factors Involved. Madison, WI: University of Wisconsin Press, 1947.

# 12

# Anesthesia

In the second half of the nineteenth century, three major developments in medical science had a particular impact on periodontics. They were the discovery of anesthesia, the development of germ theory of disease, and the discovery of X rays. Each of these three findings merits a chapter.

First came the discovery of anesthesia. Until the middle of the nineteenth century, surgery was torture and patients were reluctant to submit to it because of the terrible pain and the uncertainty of the results. The best surgeons were those who could operate fastest, for example, amputating a leg in 90 seconds. And of course the patient had to be held immobile by several strong assistants and in many cases received, prior to the procedure, a hefty dose of alcohol.

Yet for many centuries there had been some knowledge about suppression of pain during surgical procedures. Soporific agents from plants such as hyoscyamus and mandragora, and administration of alcohol had been used for thousands of years.[7] In one manuscript found in the Benedictine monastery at Monte Cassino, near the city of Salerno, Italy, and dated in the eleventh century, are instructions from Hippocrates and Galen on how to prepare a soporific sponge, as follows[7]:

> Hypnotic Aid, that is the soporific suitable for those who are treated by surgery, so that asleep, they do not feel the pain of cutting. Rx, opium one half ounce, mandragora the juice from the leaves eight ounces, the juice of fresh hemlock, hyoscyamus three ounces of the juice together with sufficient water so that it forms a liquor, and then absorb in a fresh dry sponge and dry it carefully. And when thou wouldst employ this sponge, dip it in warm water, place it over the nose and cause the patient to breathe deeply until he sleeps. And when thou wouldst wake him up, apply to his nose another sponge well soaked in vinegar and thou wilst end the sleep.

This formula was later included in the *Antidotarium*, used as a textbook in Salerno. Another document from the School of Salerno, called the *Antidotaria Parva*, dated at the beginning of the twelfth century, contains the following passage:

> And it is noted that opium, hyoscyamus and mandragora produce a deep slumber, because of its great humidity, if you make a cataplasm from these and it is placed on the spot on which an incision or an operation will be performed, they abolish sensation completely so that pain in any form is not felt.[7]

All this knowledge about general and local anesthesia was lost for almost a milennium. In the eighteenth century, "mesmerism" (hypnotism) had been attempted to induce anesthesia prior to operations, but the medical profession did not find this method effective.[8] It was only toward the middle of the nineteenth century that an American dentist discovered a method to induce general anesthesia. Half a century later a Viennese ophthalmologist found a method to induce local anesthesia.

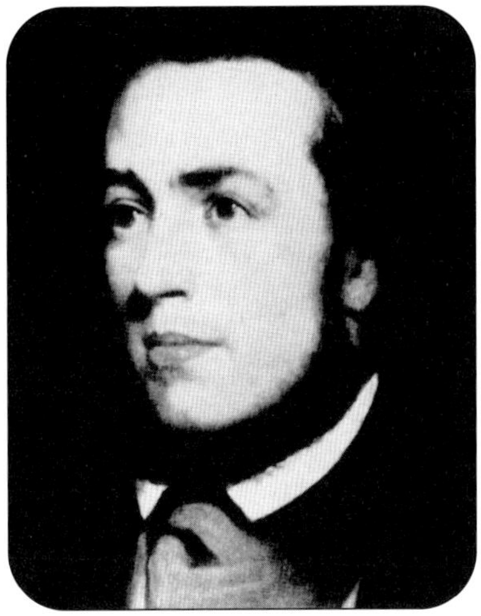

**Fig 17** Horace Wells (anonymous painting, Hunt Memorial Medical Society, Hartford, Connecticut).

## The Discovery of General Anesthesia

There is a certain amount of disagreement on who discovered anesthesia[2]: Crawford Long (1815–1878), a physician from Jefferson, Georgia; Horace Wells (1815–1848), a dentist from Hartford, Connecticut; or William Morton (1819–1868), a dentist from Boston, Massachusetts. Long may indeed have been the first to use inhalation anesthesia in 1842, in the privacy of his office in a rural area of Georgia. However, he never communicated his experiences, nor did he perform demonstrations to the medical community or to the public. Long published a paper in 1849, relating experiments he had performed seven years earlier, but his claim to priority for the year 1842 is weak because his procedures were not made public and did not benefit people outside his small circle of patients.

Wells and Morton did in fact discover the anesthetic effects of nitrous oxide and ether, respectively, and made definite attempts, unsuccessful for Wells but successful for Morton, to generalize the use of inhalation anesthesia.

Horace Wells (Fig 17) was a successful dentist in Hartford, Connecticut. Born in Vermont in 1815, to a well-to-do family, he received a solid general education and obtained his dental training under a preceptor in Boston. On December 10, 1844, Wells and his wife attended a show in a local theater, presented by a Mr. Gardner Q. Colton, who called himself a professor and chemist. Colton sought to amuse the public by administering to volunteers from the audience the so-called laughing gas (nitrous oxide)* which causes a loss of inhibition, a state of euphoria and excitement, and loud, unprovoked laughter (Fig 18). While leaving the stage, one of the volunteers tripped and fell, injuring his leg. He sat next to Wells, who inquired about his injury, and the man replied that he had not felt any pain. Impressed by this, Wells immediately conceived the idea of using the gas to anesthetize patients prior to surgery.

Wells contacted Colton and told him to bring the gas next day to his office. Wells also contacted his friend and student, John Riggs, and both planned the experiment to be performed the next day. On December 11, 1844, John Riggs extracted a molar from Dr. Wells—the first painless extraction of the modern era of medicine.

* Prior to the stage of sedation and loss of consciousness, nitrous oxide produces a state of excitement and relaxation. Numerous theater performances used nitrous oxide to entertain the public. Students in universities and medical schools also used it for this purpose not knowing that it caused loss of consciousness and insensitivity to pain.

The British chemist Joseph Priestley (1733–1804) discovered the "laughing gas" in 1787, and Humphry Davy (1778–1829) and Michael Faraday (1791–1867) suggested its use in surgery. However, surgeons and physicians did not adopt this method.

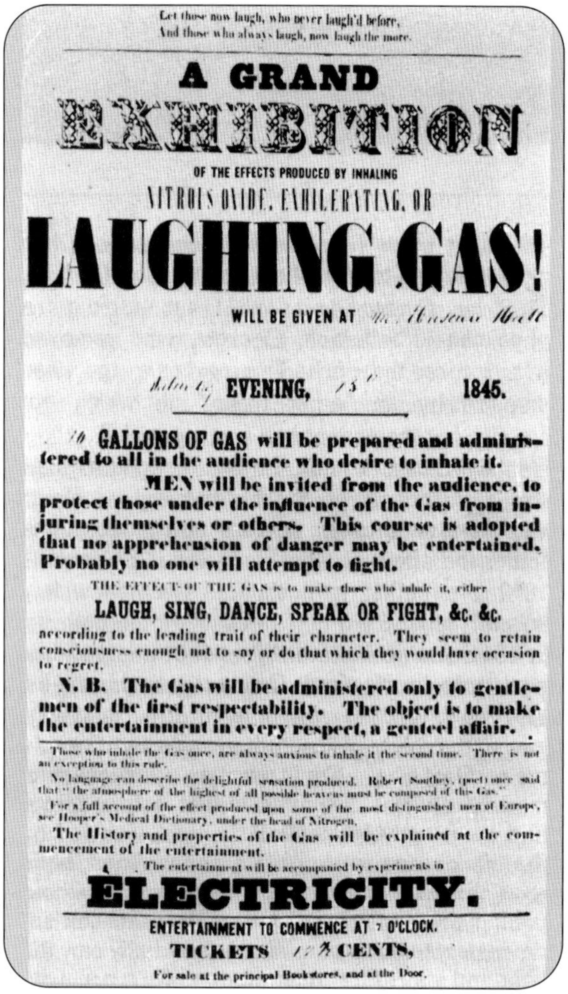


**Fig 18** Announcement of a laughing gas party, 1845.

Horace Wells attempted immediately to communicate his findings to the medical world. He contacted Massachusetts General Hospital, in Boston, where Professor of Surgery John Collins Warren agreed with some reluctance to have Wells demonstrate his technique. On January 20, 1845, Wells was nervous as he attempted to extract a student's tooth in front of an audience of incredulous students and staff. His demonstration failed when the patient screamed and later said he had felt pain. Wells returned to Hartford humiliated and discredited and had a nervous breakdown that forced him to leave his practice for several months.

More than a year later, William Morton (Fig 19) became interested in the problem. Born in 1819, Morton had been one of the first students at the Baltimore College of Dentistry, but left before graduation to complete his training with Horace Wells as his preceptor. Morton had helped Wells in his failed demonstration and in 1846 consulted with Charles Jackson, professor of chemistry, about other drugs that could have an effect similar to nitrous oxide. Jackson suggested ether.

On September 30, 1846, Morton extracted a patient's tooth in a painless procedure, and on October 16, performed a successful demonstration at Massachusetts General Hospital (Fig 20), in which Warren removed a tumor from the neck of a patient.

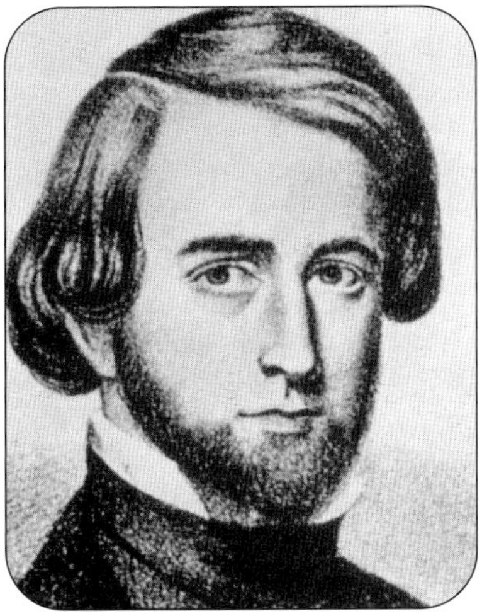

**Fig 19** William G. T. Morton.

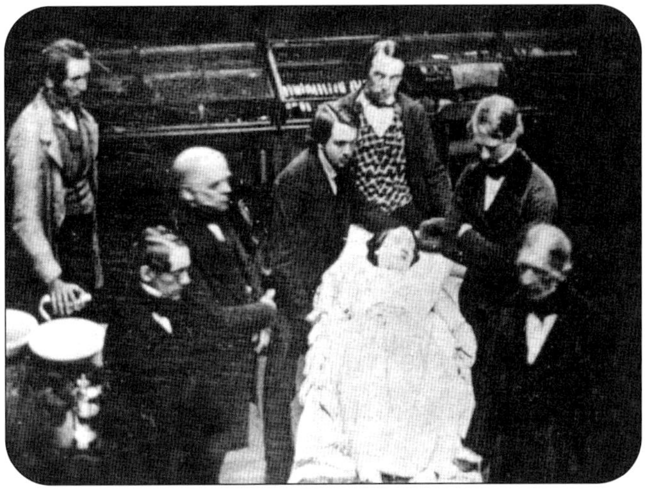

**Fig 20** Daguerrotype of the second operation performed under ether anesthesia, at the Massachusetts General Hospital in Boston, October 17, 1846. The man behind the patient, with checkered vest, is William Morton. The surgeon, John Collins Warren, is at the bottom right.

After Wells' demonstration on the anesthetic effect of nitrous oxide and Morton's on ether, the use of both gases rapidly became generalized in Europe and other parts of the world. In 1847, Dr. James Young Simpson, professor of obstetrics at the University of Edinburgh, was the first to use ether to eliminate pain during childbirth.* A few months later Simpson discovered the anesthetic effects of chloroform. For several decades ether and chloroform were the preferred anesthetics for childbirth and for surgery.

A bitter contest arose between Wells, Morton, and Jackson for priority in the discovery of general anesthesia, and soon after Dr. Crawford Long joined the dispute, adding his name to the candidates for the honor, which included an award of $100,000, voted by the U.S. Congress as reward to the discoverer.[9]

In January 1848, Horace Wells moved to New York, where he began experimenting with chloroform. After an unfortunate incident, he landed in jail where he committed suicide on January 24, by severing his femoral artery under the influence of the drug. He was 33 years old. Shortly after his death, news arrived in New York that the Medical Society of Paris had honored him as the discoverer of anesthesia. In 1864 the American Dental Association, and in 1872 the American Medical Association, recognized Wells as the discoverer of anesthesia.

After Wells' death, the conflict continued between Morton and Jackson, but neither of them was successful in his endeavor. Morton died of a heart attack in 1868, in mental and physical ruin, impoverished by years of bitter controversy. Jackson continued to pursue the congressional award after Morton's death but became mentally deranged and was institutionalized for years. He died in 1880.

The use of nitrous oxide and other general anesthetics for extractions of teeth was later developed commercially by the same person who, in 1844, conducted theatrical shows on the effects of the laughing gas: Gardner Quincy Colton. He and his associates claimed to have administered anesthesia to more than 100,000 persons between 1864 and 1897, with no fatalities.

The contributions of Wells and Morton are exceptional landmarks in the progress of surgery, and the operating room and dental office gradually ceased to be a last resort, dreadful and terrifying, and became a real health service.

---

*Initially the use of an anesthetic during childbirth was rejected for religious reasons, adducing that a painful childbirth was God's will. This idea was rejected only after Queen Victoria gave birth to Prince Leopold in 1857 under ether anesthesia administered by Dr. John Snow.

## The Discovery of Local Anesthesia

Since the sixteenth century, when Francisco Pizarro conquered Perú for Spain, Europeans knew of a plant, *Erythroxylon coca*, that, when chewed, produced remarkable physical strength and endurance. The active ingredient of this plant was isolated in 1860 by the German chemist Albert Niemann (1834–1861), who gave it the name *cocaine.*

In the early 1880s Sigmund Freud (1856–1939), before starting his psychoanalytic work, became interested in a German military experiment, which consisted of providing cocaine to soldiers during maneuvers to help them overcome the hardships of military campaigns. He noted in himself that the drug induced a euphoric stage that lifted him out of his periods of depression. In 1884 he published a paper on the effects of this drug, noting, too, that cocaine, when placed on the tongue, induced localized numbness. He related this finding to his friend and collaborator, ophthalmologist Carl Koller (1857–1944), and gave him a small amount of the alkaloid.

Carl Koller was born in Bohemia in 1857 and received his medical degree from the University of Vienna in 1882. Freud and Koller had collaborated in the research on cocaine, but Freud was more interested in the systemic effects of the drug while Koller, who had already investigated other drugs for their anesthetic effects, was interested in this property of cocaine. Koller initially induced anesthesia to the eye with drops of a cocaine solution, and in 1884 presented his findings at the German Ophthalmologic Congress in Heidelberg. In 1888, Koller, a Jew, perceiving a growing anti-Semitic sentiment in Austrian academic circles, emigrated to America where he practiced ophthalmology in New York City, until his death in 1944.

Use of cocaine as a local anesthetic spread rapidly, especially in the United States, where, in 1884, techniques were developed to anesthetize the nose, mouth, larynx, trachea, rectum, and urethra. Toward the end of the same year, New York surgeon William Stewart Halstead (1852–1922) described techniques for regional anesthesia by injection, using 4% cocaine. Experimenting with the drug, Halstead became addicted and underwent months of treatment. He later became professor of pathology at Johns Hopkins University and had a successful career.*

Richard Hall, surgeon at New York's Roosevelt Hospital, introduced local anesthesia to oral surgery, by performing a block anesthesia of the mandibular nerve. On November 26, 1884, dentist Charles Nash anesthetized Hall, injecting cocaine at the infraorbital foramen, for the treatment of a carious incisor. This was probably the first operative dentistry procedure performed under anesthesia.[5]

Local anesthesia by injection was made possible by the syringe. Hoffmann-Axthelm[5] attributes this invention to the orthopedic surgeon Charles-Gabriel Pravaz (1791–1853), of Lyon, France, in 1852. The syringe was known as the *Pravaz syringe* and later as the *Luer syringe*, after its manufacturer.

According to Glenner and Pick,[3] Pravaz's invention did not have a needle but a screw-piston rod and allowed only for administration of very small amounts of fluid. Glenner and Pick point to Daniel Ferguson, a surgical instrument maker of London, as the first to develop a true hypodermic syringe, later modified by Alexander Wood, of Edinburgh, Scotland. The first trial, in November 1853, involved injecting opiates into painful areas.

Anesthesia by cocaine was not satisfactory and, furthermore, it carried the danger of addiction. Chemists Alfred Einhorn (1857–1917) and Richard Willstätter (1872–1942), in the Hoechst plant in Munich, developed procaine in 1905, which received the commercial name of *Novocaine.* The addition of epinephrine, isolated a few years earlier by Japanese researcher

*Halstead introduced rubber gloves for surgeons and nurses, although not to prevent infections but to avoid the skin irritation caused by disinfectants. Rubber gloves had been developed years before (in 1840) by Charles Goodyear (1800–1860), for use in dissections.

Jokichi Takamine (1854–1922) and American investigator Thomas Bell Aldrich (1861–1938), both working independently in the United States, resulted in the most widely used anesthetic solution of the twentieth century.[5]

With the progress in general and local anesthesia, development of periodontal surgical techniques gradually became more and more complex and sophisticated, directed not only to solve disease problems but also to treat esthetic and functional derangements.

## References


1. Atkinson RS, Boulton TB (eds). The History of Anesthesia. Park Ridge, NJ: Parthenon, 1989.
2. Caverley RK. Anesthesia as a specialty: past, present and future. In: Barash PG, Cullen BF, Staelling RK (eds). Clinical Anesthesia. Philadelphia: J.B. Lippincott, 1989.
3. Glenner RA, Pick RM. A history of local anesthesia armamentarium. Bull Hist Dent 1986;34:1.
4. Herschfeld JJ. Carl Koller and the discovery of local anesthesia. Bull Hist Dent 1986;34:122.
5. Hoffmann-Axthelm W. History of Dentistry. Chicago: Quintessence, 1981.
6. Keys TE. The History of Surgical Anesthesia. New York: Dover, 1963.
7. Major RH. A History of Medicine. Springfield, IL: Charles C. Thomas, 1954.
8. Margotta R. The History of Medicine. New York: Smithmark, 1996.
9. Miller AH. Two notable controversies over the invention of the electric telegraph and the discovery of surgical anesthesia. Ann Med Hist 1934;6NS:110.

# 13

# Microbiology

The transmission of disease by contact was suspected in antiquity but it was assumed to be caused by supernatural forces. Many centuries later this idea was replaced by a belief in cosmotelluric phenomena such as eclipses, earthquakes, comets, floods, atmospheric changes, heat, cold, humidity, dryness, winds, and air changes known as *miasmas*, a term probably similar to *pollution* today.[6,24]

With the great epidemics of the Middle Ages, the concept of contagion began to emerge, and quarantines were imposed on persons traveling from suspicious sites. Boccaccio's *Decameron* describes people's reactions to the bubonic plague of the fourteenth century, as they attempted to isolate themselves in rural areas, away from the dead and dying in the cities.

Girolamo Fracastoro (1478–1553), a typical Italian Renaissance poet, physician, astronomer, mathematician, and geologist, in a 1546 publication conceives contagion as the product of seeds or germs (*seminaria*) of disease, thus creating the theory of *animated contagium.* Fracastoro describes contagium as occurring by direct contact, by touching clothing, linen, and other items he calls *fomites*, and at a distance.[8]

Fracastoro's theory would not be confirmed until the discovery of the microscope in the seventeenth century. Dutch microscopist Antony van Leeuwenhoek discovered the invisible world of microscopic living creatures (see Chapter 9), but neither he nor his contemporaries linked these animalcules to disease.

In 1720, Benjamin Marten, an obscure London physician, published *A New Theory of Consumptions: More Especially of a Phthisis or Consumption of the Lungs*, in which he clearly opines that the cause of consumption (tuberculosis) may be certain species of animalculae.[10] Marten's assertion, however, did not alter current medical thinking.

A Viennese physician, Marcus Anton von Plenciz (1705–1786) also presented, in 1762, a theory about the bacterial causes of disease. And in the first half of the nineteenth century, Italian researcher Agostino Bassi (1773–1856) and German scientist Jacob Henle (1809–1885) looked at animalculae as causes of contagious diseases.

## The Germ Theory of Disease

Until the 1860s, however, the causes of most human diseases were unknown. The big breakthrough came when French chemist Louis Pasteur and German physician Robert Koch, established beyond any doubt the concept of bacteria-caused disease, and English surgeon Joseph Lister carried Pasteur's concepts to medical and surgical practice.

Louis Pasteur (Fig 21)[7,11,13,33] was born in the town of Dole, in the Franche-Comté region of France, near the Swiss border, on December 27, 1822. Soon after, his family moved to the nearby town of Arbois where he grew up. He attended school in Besançon and studied chemistry in Paris where he obtained his doctorate in 1846.

Pasteur's first scientific interest was crystallography, to which he made important contributions. He was assistant professor of chemistry at the University of Strasbourg, then professor and dean of sciences at the University of Lille, and finally he accepted the position of chief ad-

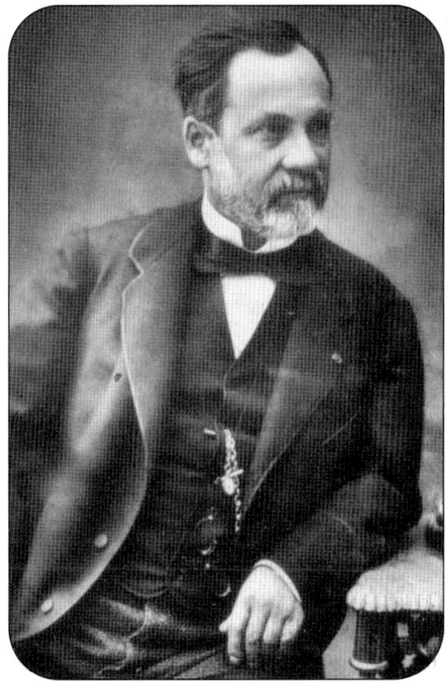

**Fig 21** Louis Pasteur, 1875.

ministrator and scientific director at Paris' *Ecole Normal*, where he remained until 1867, when he became professor of chemistry at the Sorbonne. At the *Ecole Normal* he began his investigations on fermentation, and in a series of careful studies demonstrated that bacteria involved in putrefaction and fermentation come from the air and do not generate spontaneously. He rediscovered the existence of anaerobic bacteria, not knowing that they had been described one century earlier by the Italian Lazzaro Spallanzani.

In 1865, at the request of the Emperor Napoleon III, Pasteur investigated diseases in the silk worm that were devastating the French silk industry, and found that they were caused by a protozoan, thus demonstrating for the first time that a microorganism can cause disease.

After the Franco-Prussian War of 1870–1871, Pasteur, already highly respected, investigated fermentation procedures for wine and beer, creating the process known as *pasteurization*, to sterilize these drinks and, later, milk and others, by heating to 55°C and maintaining the temperature for a given time.

Eventually Pasteur turned his attention to developing vaccines for various diseases. Edward Jenner's discovery of the smallpox vaccine eight decades earlier had resulted from the application of the common knowledge that milkmaids infected with cowpox did not contract smallpox. Pasteur went further, to analyze scientifically the problem of vaccination and immunology, thus formulating vaccines against chicken cholera, the cattle disease anthrax, and finally rabies.

In 1886 the Pasteur Institute was created with worldwide donations for the study of rabies and other microbiological problems. Pasteur and his disciples discovered the causal agents for several diseases—including puerperal fever, foruncles, and bone infections—and pioneered the sterilization of surgical instruments. Pasteur died in Paris on September 28, 1895.

Robert Koch (Fig 22)[5,7,25] was born in the mining town of Clausthal, near Hanover, Germany, on December 11, 1843, and received his medical degree from the University of Groningen in 1866.

In 1872 he became district medical officer in the small town of Wollstein, now part of Poland, halfway between Berlin and Breslau (now Wroclaw). At the time, medical experts were divided on the possible microbial origin of diseases. Prestigious scholars such as Rudolf Virchow were skeptical, while others, such as Edwin Klebs, favored the idea. It was Klebs who originally

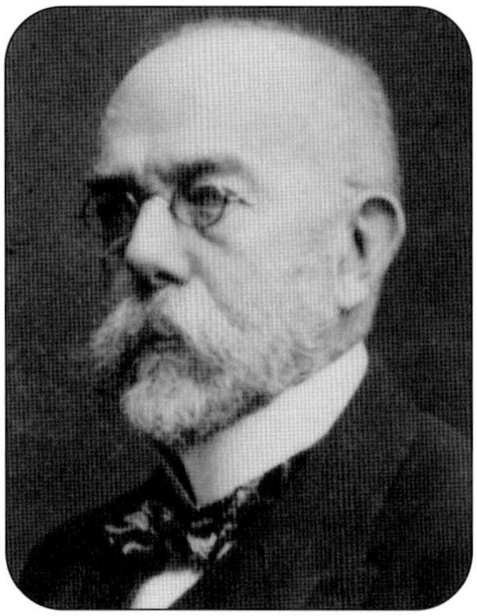

**Fig 22** Robert Koch, 1907.

developed the postulates, later modified by Koch and known as *Koch's postulates,* regarding the conditions required to certify the microbial origin of a disease.

In Wollstein, Koch started to investigate the cattle disease anthrax, discovering the causal microorganism, including its life cycle and the formation of spores. Koch's studies on anthrax are astonishing, particularly considering that he worked alone, and in addition to his public health work and his private medical practice. He later developed methods to stain bacteria, started microphotography to document his findings, and studied the microbiology of wound infections.

As a consequence of his work, he was offered and accepted a position in Breslau, and shortly thereafter, at the Imperial Health Office in Berlin. Here he led a group that developed many of the classic bacteriological techniques, including cultivation of bacteria in solid media, such as agar in Petri dishes, bacteria staining techniques, microphotographic techniques, and so on. Technical improvements in the microscope, such as the use of condensers and oil-immersion lenses, pioneered by Ernst Abbe (1840–1905) of the University of Jena, and manufactured by the Carl Zeiss Microscope Company, were a valuable help to Koch's work.

Koch's interest turned to tuberculosis, and after a series of brilliant investigations, he discovered the bacterial etiology of the disease. He then looked at cholera, epidemics of which were devastating areas in Southeast Asia, China, Persia, and Egypt, and reaching Europe and North America. He traveled to Egypt and Asia and discovered the microbial agent responsible for this disease, the *Vibrio cholera.*

Koch became an internationally recognized researcher, and the University of Berlin created an institute, later called the Koch Institute, for his research group, which included other renowned microbiologists. Together they discovered the microbial causes of serious diseases that included gonorrhea, typhoid fever, diphtheria, dysentery, and pneumonia.

Koch received the Nobel Prize in 1905. He died April 27, 1910.

Until the 1860s surgery was performed without any regard to cleanliness or hygiene. Physicians used the same bloody apron for every operation, over their street clothes. The same instruments were used over and over again with only a brief wash or none at all. Physicians were offended at the idea of washing their hands before operating, since their social status prohibited them from admitting to dirty hands.

In the 1840s two visionaries, Oliver Wendell Holmes (1809–1894), in Boston, and Ignaz Semmelweis (1818–1865), in Vienna, mentioned lack of hygiene as the cause of puerperal fever. Oliver Wendell Holmes[3,7] was a prominent physician, who, after obtaining his medical degree

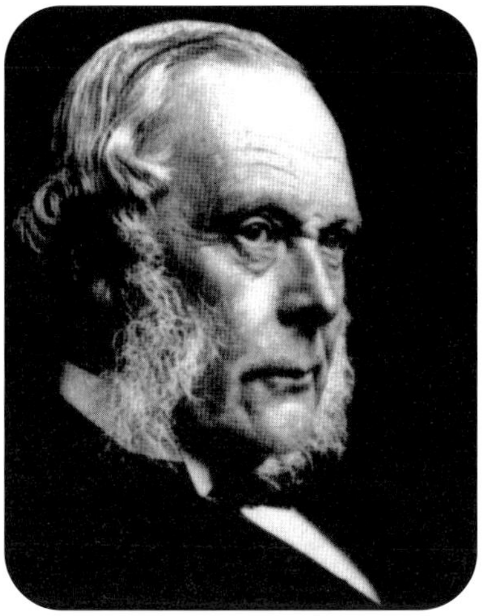

Fig 23 Joseph Lister.

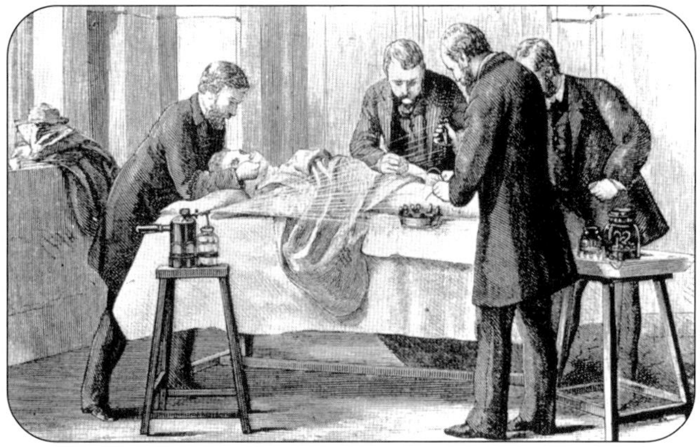

Fig 24 Surgical operation performed in 1882 using the carbolic acid spray recommended by Lister to eliminate bacteria from the air. (Note that the surgeons wear street clothes.)

at Harvard, studied in Paris under Pierre-Charles Louis. Holmes became professor of anatomy and dean of the Harvard Medical School, and was an eloquent speaker, gifted writer, and poet. He was the father of the Supreme Court justice Oliver Wendell Holmes, Jr.

Ignaz Semmelweis[18] was born in Budapest, Hungary, and studied medicine in Vienna. After graduation he entered the Department of Obstetrics of the University of Vienna where he carefully recorded deaths by puerperal fever at the two clinics, one teaching medical students and the other, midwives. The medical students also performed autopsies of the deceased patients, and their clinic had a much higher percentage of deaths due to puerperal fever than did the midwives' clinic.

Both Holmes in Boston, in 1843, and Semmelweis in Vienna, in 1847, realized that the high incidence of puerperal fever, usually a fatal disease, stemmed from the transmission of "poisonous substances" carried by doctors and nurses from patient to patient. They did not know that living beings of microscopic size were the agents that carried the infections. Holmes and Semmelweis recommended cleanliness and hygiene—carefully washing the hands with chlorinated water—before delivering a baby, to avoid transmission of disease. Their warning would not be heeded.

Joseph Lister (Fig 23)[12,14] was born in the small town of Upton, outside London, in 1827, and obtained his medical degree from the University College Hospital in 1850 and his certification as a surgeon in 1852. In 1865 Lister was professor of surgery at the University of Glasgow and later at King's College in London. Impressed by Pasteur's work, Lister thought that wound infections, the greatest scourge of surgery, could be prevented by antimicrobial agents, so he started to protect the surgical wounds with carbolic acid. (*Carbolic acid* was the name used to designate phenol, a compound obtained by distillation of coal tar; it is closely related to creosote.)

During a symposium in Dublin on August 9, 1867, Lister read his findings, which were published in *The Lancet* the same year:

> [when it was shown] by the researches of Pasteur that the septic property of the atmosphere depended not on the oxygen or any gaseous constituent, but on minute organisms suspended in it, which owed their energy to their vitality, it occurred to me that decomposition in the injured part might be avoided without excluding the air, by applying as a dressing some material capable of destroying the life of the floating particles. … The material which I have employed is carbolic or phenic acid, a volatile organic compound which appears to exercise a peculiarly destructive influence upon low forms of life, and hence the most powerful antiseptic with which we are at present acquainted.[22]

To clean wounds, Lister applied cloths soaked in carbolic acid. Following Pasteur's discovery of bacteria in the air, Lister developed a machine to spray an aerosol form of the acid over the wound during an operation (Fig 24).

His results were astonishing, and although it took some time, his methods prevailed, and the era of antisepsis in surgery was born. The search for other antiseptic agents continued uninterrupted, and Lister made many other improvements to surgical techniques, including the use of catgut ligatures. He received the recognition of his country and the world and died in London in 1912.

Two German surgeons, Theodor Billroth (1829–1894) and Ernst von Bergmann (1836–1907), developed the aseptic technique.[24] Billroth, who obtained his medical degree at the University of Berlin and later became professor of surgery in Vienna, was a gastrointestinal surgeon with extensive training in pathology and bacteriology. He refined Lister's antiseptic methods and developed numerous surgical techniques, and was also a pioneer in monitoring patient temperatures, a method discovered by Carl Wunderlich (1815–1877).

Von Bergmann graduated in Berlin, served as an army surgeon, taught at Würzburg as well as his alma mater, and was a leading surgeon of his era. He was an early follower of Lister's methods, but carbolic acid irritated his skin. He developed steam sterilization of instruments as well as methods to clean the operating room, the patient, and the surgeon.

Lister's antiseptic technique was introduced in France by Just Lucas Championnière (1843–1913) and in the United States by William Halsted (1852–1922).[29]

*Sterility in dental offices.* The pioneering studies of Pasteur, Koch, and Lister, and W. D. Miller's book published in 1890 (see below) were important factors in bringing sterility to dental offices.[16] By the end of the century dentists started washing their hands more scrupulously, sometimes with antiseptic solutions, and sterilizing instruments with boiling water, antiseptics such as carbolic acid, formaldehyde gas, or steam under pressure.[16] These methods remained common until midtwentieth century. The use of sterile disposable needles started in the early 1960s.

## Periodontal Microbiology

German physician Robert Ficinus (1809–1852) of Dresden is credited by Hoffmann-Axthelm[20] as the first to describe a microbial etiology of periodontal disease. In his 1847 publication "Über das Ausfallen der Zahne" ("Concerning the loss of teeth"), Ficinus mentioned that "these animals force their way into the fibers between the gingiva and the cement, loosen the former and here form the tooth-loosening calculus."[20]

In the 1880s the germ theory of disease, recently proven by Pasteur and Koch, and the identification of a bacterial cause of many diseases, suggested to scientists and clinicians that periodontal disease was also caused by germs. The proof of this causation, however, would be difficult and would take almost a century to determine conclusively.

In 1881 German physician Adolf Witzel (1847–1906) (Fig 25), of Essen, mentioned microorganisms as the cause of periodontal disease. Witzel was a renowned dentist who made important contributions to the amalgam problem and to the treatment of pulp diseases, including the antiseptic method of therapy.[20]

In a paper presented on August 1, 1881, at the annual meeting of the Dental Association of Germany, Witzel presented the clinical manifestations of periodontal disease (which he called *infectious alveolitis*), describing gingival recession, pocket formation, calculus deposits, and suppuration.[37] He mentioned that the roots of diseased extracted teeth

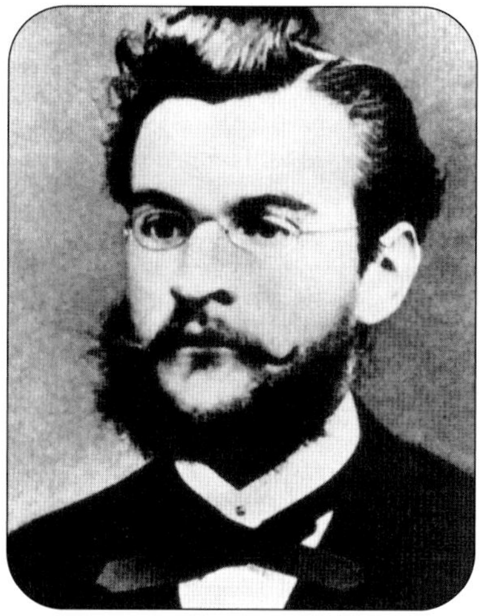

**Fig 25** Adolph Witzel.

are velvet-like and loosened, and present a brilliant vascular injection increasing towards the root, and associated with small nodules and lobular granulations. I have not yet examined these growths for nests of micrococci, but I have no doubt that they are to be found, not only in the granulations, but also in the medullary tissue of the interalveolar partition. In the pus which may be obtained from the affected alveoli by pressing the gum we observe under the microscope a countless number of micrococci and bacteria, which doubtless find in the pockets of gum tissue *the most favorable conditions for their continuous development.*

He further differentiated bone loss caused by "senile atrophy of the alveoli" as follows:

[Senile atrophy of the alveoli] occurs more frequently in strong and healthy persons in middle life, and, according to my observations, seldom, I might almost say never, attacks carious teeth with diseased pulps. Senile atrophy consists of the steady disappearance of the socket, by means of which the fangs of the teeth are gradually laid bare; there is no necrosis of the alveolar margin, and the gum remains firmly attached to the latter and to the periosteum of the jaw. In alveolar pyorrhœa, on the other hand, there is, as already mentioned, a loosening of the gum from the outer border of the alveolus, by means of which the periosteum of the latter becomes exposed and destroyed by colonies of micrococci, while the margin of bone, thus robbed of its covering, is infected and finally becomes softened by caries.

Witzel then described his treatment for alveolar pyorrhea, recommending extraction of all teeth that have lost more than half their osseous support and of molars with furcation involvement. Extractions should not be delayed, and he explained why:

I have dwelt on this comparison with the view of showing that in alveolar pyorrhœa there is a certain something cooperating, either a *predisposition* on the part of the alveoli, or, as to me appears more probable, a virus, of the nature of which we are as yet ignorant. It is true that I have not hitherto made any attempts to convey the affection from one individual to another by transferring the pus from a diseased alveolus to a healthy one. The fact, however, that it usually begins in the neighbourhood of one tooth and never attacks a whole row of teeth at once, and that its extension is best prevented either by treating the diseased alveolus antiseptically as soon as possible or by extracting the tooth, proves that we have to deal with a *local contagium.*

After the extractions of teeth with more than half the bone lost, he proceeded to "cleanse the remainder from all concretions situated below the gums." For this he recommended Riggs' instruments and the excavators. Then he disinfected the diseased areas, using a small glass syringe with a fine gold cannula, which he described in detail, adding,

> For it is only by using such an instrument that we can bring the solution of carbolic acid and chloride of zinc which I recommend in this treatment into immediate contact with the pockets of gum and diseased portions of the alveoli.

The disinfectant that Witzel used was carbolic acid, probably following Lister's use of the same substance for treatment of wounds. Witzel recommended the following prescription:

| | | |
|---|---|---|
| Rx Acid. Carbolic. 5.0 | Aq. Menthæ Pip. 100.0 | Ol. Cinnamon. Acut. 0.5 |
| Spir. Vini Rectif. 400.0 | Ol. Anisi 1.0 | |

He mentioned that this treatment should be carried out three times during the first week and that it is not painful. For the few cases in which it is painful, he suggested first injecting into the pocket a few drops of tincture of iodine and aconite, before applying the carbolic acid.[37]

In an 1882 paper, George Cunningham, of Cambridge, Massachusetts, also recommended careful and complete scaling followed by an application, into the pockets, of "deliquesced carbolic acid, dental tincture of iodine, or a combination of both."[9]

A paper by A. O. Rawls, of Lexington, Kentucky, read before the Southern Dental Association, in New Orleans on March 31, 1885, summarizes the contemporary knowledge of the etiology of periodontal disease[30]:

> If I am not misinformed, Dr. Riggs claims that salivary calculus is the immediate cause, and his treatment, so far as I have been able to learn, is certainly consistent with such view, besides being, in my estimation, far superior to the local treatment of other theorists. Dr. Ingersoll, of Iowa, advocates the theory of sanguinary calculus as a cause, stating that often when no salivary deposits were present the sanguinary calculus would be found far up the roots of the teeth,– which I think correct, but would prefer the term serumal calculus. Dr. Black, of Illinois, presents the latest local-origin theory, in support of which, and confirmatory of his microscopic findings, he has the results of similar research by Dr. Witzel, of Essen, Germany, whose article bearing upon the subject was somewhat earlier than that of Dr. Black's. This is one of the numerous germ theories, and is founded upon the fact of the presence in these cases of little hot-beds of peculiar organisms of fungi, which, according to supporters of the theory, cause a melting away of the pericemental membrane – by what means is not definitely understood, but presumably by the "digestive fluids of the fungous growth causing a remolecularization of tissues exposed to their action."

Rawls described the clinical features of the disease, surprisingly mentioning that the disease progresses more slowly in tobacco chewers,

> possibly [because] the narcotic properties of tobacco may to some degree lessen the intensity of the trouble, but I apprehend the differences apparent are due more to the mechanical effects in exercising and cleaning the teeth of food, rather than any therapeutic action of the tobacco *per se.*

His opinion on treatment is interesting. Rawls believed that in addition to "the most thorough removal of all deposits of a foreign nature," antiseptic agents and surgery are needed. The following excerpts from his paper give an idea of his treatment, which is "to incise or split the gum slightly over or in the vicinity of the parts to be operated upon. …"

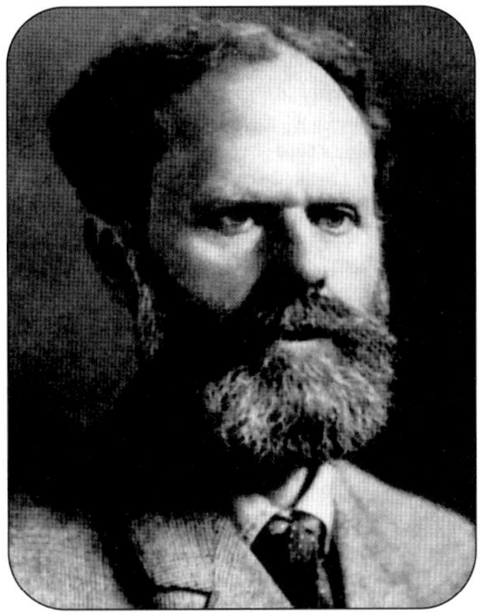

**Fig 26** Willoughby D. Miller.

> During this operation it is well from time to time to syringe well the parts with tepid salt water, mixed with which may be any one of the many good antiseptics now in common use. About as good a preparation as you will find for this purpose is Listerine, which combines the qualities of an antiseptic with that of a stimulant and does not perceptibly coagulate.
>
> When reasonably assured that the teeth are well cleansed, your attention should then be directed to the removal of all disintegrating and lifeless bone. How easy to say and yet seldom accomplished! Indeed this is often a very difficult and painful operation, not only to perform but doubly to ascertain when it is complete. ...
>
> Following this operation, an antiseptic in solution with tepid water may be thoroughly used about the teeth; but as far as strong escharotics, caustics, and such like preparations, especially on pledgets of lint or cotton to be left in the pockets for hours at a time, I think it entirely contrary to our best conceptions of the laws governing the reproduction of tissue. ...
>
> The patient ... should be instructed to keep the teeth scrupulously free of food, to gently manipulate the parts by rubbing or pressing the gums with thumb and finger.[30]

Witzel, Cunningham, and Rawls all were clinicians, with no training in bacteriology, who applied some of the recent findings of Pasteur, Koch, and others to the treatment of periodontal disease. They believed that microbes were involved in the etiology of the disease and used antimicrobials to combat them.

The first oral microbiologist with formal training was Willoughby D. Miller, and his book *The Microorganisms of the Human Mouth*[26] constituted a seminal contribution to dentistry and to microbiology.

Miller[17,21] was born on a farm in Alexandria, Ohio, on August 1, 1853 (Fig 26). His parents were German immigrants, and he spoke German fluently. Miller spent his youth on the farm and at 18 years old enrolled in the University of Michigan, where he majored in mathematics and physics, graduating with honors in 1875.

To complete his training he traveled to Scotland, but had financial difficulties and accepted a job as translator and teacher to the wife and daughter of an American dentist, Dr. Frank Abbot, in Berlin. Miller and Abbot's daughter soon fell in love; Miller also became interested in his future father-in-law's profession. Dr. Abbot supported Miller's dental studies at the University of Pennsylvania, where he graduated in 1879. Back in Berlin he practiced dentistry with his father-in-law and continued his interest in basic sciences, at a time when Robert Koch was the leading figure in microbiology.

Between 1871 and 1907, Miller published 164 papers on various dental science problems, and in 1889 the first edition of his classic book, *The Microorganisms of the Human Mouth*, appeared in German; the English translation was published in the United States the following year. His greatest accomplishments were in caries research, where he developed the chemoparasitic theory of caries.

Miller described the features of periodontal disease and considered the role of predisposing factors, irritational factors, and bacteria in the etiology of pyorrhea alveolaris. He believed that the disease was not caused by a specific bacterium but by a complex array of bacteria normally present in the oral cavity. This theory came to be known as the *nonspecific plaque hypothesis*, and it went unchallenged for seven decades.

Part I of Miller's book is devoted to general bacteriology and the etiology of dental caries. Part II covers "The pathogenic mouth bacteria and the diseases which they produce." In this second part Miller describes the tissue invasion of pathogenic bacteria following mechanical injuries, gangrenous tooth pulps as centers of infection, lung diseases caused by aspiration of oral bacteria, and so on.

He describes pyorrhea alveolaris as "a disease of probably parasitic nature," and he offers detailed bacteriologic analysis of thirty-nine cases of human periodontal disease as well as six cases of the disease in dogs. He was, however, unable to cultivate a single responsible bacterium, and concludes that

> pyorrhœa alveolaris is not caused by any specific bacterium, which occurs in every case (like the tubercle-bacillus in tuberculosis), but various bacteria may participate in it, just as in suppurative processes. ... Besides, as far as we know, there is no bacterium which, inoculated under the gums, is able to provoke the disease in healthy persons.

Miller contends that the normal oral flora proliferated when tissue resistance was reduced:

> As regards the participation of bacteria in pyorrhœa alveolaris, our present knowledge of suppurative inflammations compels us to consider the former as the cause of the suppurations incident to this disease. Micro-organisms which possess pyogenic properties temporarily or permanently inhabit every mouth. If, therefore, the power of resistance of the peridental tissue be impaired by any of the above-mentioned local or constitutional causes in such a manner as to furnish a suitable culture medium for the bacteria, they will, of course, begin their ravages, and the usual symptoms will follow.[26]

In 1891, Miller published a long paper entitled "The Human Mouth as a Focus of Infection,"[27] in which he calls attention to

> the human mouth as a gathering-place and incubator of diverse pathogenic germs, performs a significant rôle in the production of various disorders of the body, and that if many disorders whose origin is enveloped in mystery could be traced to their source, they would be found to have originated in the oral cavity.

Miller details numerous oral and systemic diseases supposedly caused by oral bacteria, then the microbiologic features of the bacteria themselves, and finally the antiseptics that can be used in conjunction with oral hygiene (brushing and flossing) to combat these bacteria.

W. D. Miller was appointed professor at the University of Berlin, and, in 1892, head of the Department of Dentistry. By then he was widely esteemed, the recipient of many awards and honors. In 1906, unhappy because of scarce official funds for his department, he accepted an offer from the University of Michigan and returned to America. But before reaching Ann Arbor, he stopped to visit his sister in Alexandria, Ohio, where he suffered an attack of appendicitis and died on July 27, 1907.

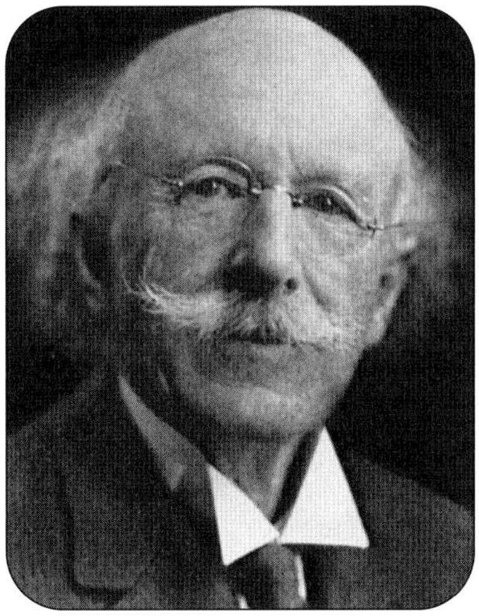
**Fig 27** James Leon Williams.

Miller did not recognize the existence of dental plaque, which was described for the first time by James Leon Williams (Fig 27). Williams was born on a farm in Maine, in 1852, apprenticed with Dr. E. J. Roberts and was a self-taught dental histologist. His field of interest was the study of dental caries, and for his important contributions on this topic, the Baltimore College of Dental Surgery bestowed upon him the DDS degree in 1883. In 1887 Williams moved to London where he conducted a successful practice and died in 1932.[31]

In a paper published in 1897, dealing with pathology of enamel in relation to dental caries,[36] Williams demonstrates that

> Lining the cavities or covering the surface where decay has commenced there is always to be seen a thick felt-like mass of acid-forming organisms. This mass of fungi is so dense and adhesive as to make it highly improbable that the enamel is affected, except in rare and special instances, by any acid other than that which is being excreted by the bacteria at the very point where they are attached to the enamel. The thick glutinous-like mass of fungi also prevents the excreted acid from being washed away, so it exerts its full chemical power upon the calcific tissue.

This description is accompanied by a photomicrograph of human enamel (ground section) covered by a "gelatinous accumulation of bacteria, attached to the tooth surface and related to the development of dental caries."[36]

In 1899, Greene Vardiman Black coined the term *gelatinous microbial plaque*,[4] although for many years it was known as *plaque of Leon Williams*. The actual relationship of the microbial plaque to gingival inflammation was not recognized until several decades later.

Other European investigators, such as Emile Magitot (1834–1897), Louis Charles Malassez (1862–1910), V. Galippe (1847–1922), and J. Arkövy (1851–1932), investigated the etiology of periodontal disease, which they considered of parasitic nature. Galippe made the most extensive investigations, injecting purulent material from pockets into guinea pigs and other experimental animals, and finding they developed abscesses. This theory was not supported by Miller.[26]

*Necrotizing ulcerative gingivitis (NUG).* Acute necrotizing ulcerative gingivitis was apparently recognized early in history, but in many descriptions it is difficult to differentiate between NUG and scurvy (or NUG occurring in cases of scurvy). The lack of systemic symptoms in the descriptions may point to cases of NUG with no underlying nutritional deficiency.

As far back as the fourth century BC, the Greek general and writer Xenophon noted that his soldiers were affected with sore mouth and foul-smelling breath, and since other systemic symptoms were not mentioned, it is believed not to have been scurvy.[19] The Roman medical literature records cases of noma (Celsus, first century AD), and cases of what is possibly so-called trench mouth are mentioned by Aellius Gallus in Arabia and Pliny of the troops under Germanicus.[19]

In 1778, John Hunter (see Chapter 9) described the clinical features of this disease and differentiated it from scurvy and chronic periodontitis. NUG struck in epidemic form in Napoleon's army during the Italian campaign of 1793–1794, and later was mentioned numerous times as occurring among soldiers, as well as in debilitated children.[19] In 1859, E. J. Bergeron stated that the condition, whether found in soldiers or in children, is the same disease.[2,19] In 1886, the German pathologist A. Hirsch discussed some of the features associated with the disease, such as enlarged lymph nodes, fever, malaise, and increased salivation.[19] In 1906, T. L. Gilmer described the interdental papilla as being ulcerated.[19]

In 1893, V. Babes[1,17] described a gingival ulcerative condition in soldiers, associated microscopically with streptococci and fusiform bacilli in close relation to leukocytes. He assumed, however, that the organisms were weakly pathogenic and attributed the disease to the low systemic resistance of the soldiers.[17] The first clear mention of fusiform bacilli and spirochetes as etiologic agents appears to have been made by German researcher F. Früwald in 1889.[17]

In the same year (1896), Hyacinthe Jean Vincent (1862–1950), a French physician working at the Pasteur Institute in Paris, and Hugo Carl Plaut (1858–1928), in Germany, described the spirillum and fusiform bacilli associated with what later became known as *Vincent's angina*.[28,34] J. Bernheim in 1898 and Vincent in 1904 described these organisms as *ulceronecrotic gingivitis*.[19,35]

## References


1. Babes V. Über einen die Gingivitis und Hemmörrhagieen verursachenden Bacillus bei Skorbut. Dtsche Medizin Wochenschr 1893;19:1035.
2. Bergeron AJ. De la stomatite ulcéreuse des soldats et de son identité avec le stomatite des enfants, dites conneuse diphtherique ulcéromembraneuse. Paris: Labé, 1859.
3. Beruti JA. Vida y Obra de Oliver Wendell Holmes. Un Gran Médico y un Gran Literato. Buenos Aires: El Ateneo, 1939.
4. Black GV. A Work on Special Dental Pathology Devoted to the Diseases and Treatment of the Investing Tissues of the Teeth and the Dental Pulp. Chicago: Medico-Dental, 1915.
5. Brock TD. Robert Koch: A Life in Medicine and Bacteriology. Washington: ASM Press, 1999.
6. Bulloch W. The History of Bacteriology. London: Oxford University Press, 1938.
7. Carranza F. Revolucionarios de la Ciencia. Buenos Aires: Vergara, 1998.
8. Clendening L (ed). Source Book of Medical History. New York: Dover Publications, 1960.
9. Cunningham G. Gum treatment. Br J Dent Sci 1882;25:472,523.
10. Daniel TM. Captain of Death: The Story of Tuberculosis. Rochester, NY: University Press, 1997.
11. Debré P. Louis Pasteur. Foster E (trans). Baltimore: Johns Hopkins University Press, 1998.
12. Dolman CE. Lister, Joseph. In: Gillispie CC (ed). Dictionary of Scientific Biography. New York: Charles Scribner's Sons, 1973.
13. Dubos RJ. Louis Pasteur, Free Lance of Science. Boston: Little, Brown & Co, 1950.
14. Gaw JL. A Time to Heal: The Diffusion of Listerism in Victorian Britain. Philadelphia: American Philosophical Society, 1999.
15. Geison GL. The Private Science of Louis Pasteur. Princeton, NJ: University Press, 1995.
16. Glenner R. Sterility in dentistry. Bull Hist Dent 1990;38:33.
17. Gold SI. Periodontics. The Past. Part III. Microbiology. J Clin Periodontol 1985;12:257–269.
18. Gortvay G, Zoltan I. Semmelweis: His Life and Works. Budapest: Akadémiai Kiadó, 1968.

19. Hirschfeld I, Beube F, Siegel EH. The history of Vincent's infection. J Periodontol 1940;11:89.
20. Hoffmann-Axthelm W. History of Dentistry. Chicago: Quintessence, 1981.
21. König KG. W. D. Miller and his contributions to dental science. In: Miller WD (ed). The Microorganisms of the Human Mouth (reprinted edition). Basel: S. Karger, 1973.
22. Lister J. On the antiseptic principle in the practice of surgery. Lancet 1867;2:353.
23. Loesche WJ. Chemotherapy of dental plaque infections. Oral Sci Rev 1976;9:65.
24. Major RH. A History of Medicine, 2 vols. Springfield, IL: Charles C. Thomas, 1954.
25. Metchnikoff E. The Founders of Modern Medicine: Pasteur, Koch, Lister. New York: Walden, 1939.
26. Miller WD. The Microorganisms of the Human Mouth. Philadelphia: S. S. White, 1890.
27. Miller WD. The human mouth as a focus of infection. Dent Cosmos 1891;33:689,789,913.
28. Plaut HC. Studien zur bakteriellen Diagnostik der Diphtherie und der Anginen. Dtsche Medizin Wochenschr 1894;20:920.
29. Porter R. The Greatest Benefit to Mankind. New York: W. W. Norton, 1997.
30. Rawls AO. Pyorrhea alveolaris. Dent Cosmos 1885;27:265.
31. Ring ME. The contributions of Dr. J. Leon Williams, pioneer dental histologist and prosthodontist—and his London practice, as recorded in his day books. J Hist Dent 1995;43:59–65.
32. Shklar G, Carranza FA. The historical background of periodontology. In: Newman MG, Takei HH, Carranza FA. Carranza's Clinical Periodontology, ed 9. Philadelphia: W.B. Saunders, 2002.
33. Vallery-Radot M. Pasteur. Paris: Perrin, 1994.
34. Vincent HJ. Sur l'etiologie et sur les lesions anatomopathologiques de la pourriture d'hopital. Ann l'Inst Pasteur 1896;10:448.
35. Vincent HJ. Recherches sur l'etiologie de la stomatite ulceromembraneuse primitive. Arch Internat Laryngolog 1904;17:355.
36. Williams JL. A contribution to the study of pathology of enamel. Dent Cosmos 1897;39:169,269,353.
37. Witzel A. The treatment of pyorrhœa alveolaris, or infectious alveolitis. Br J Dent Sci 1882;25:153,209,257.

# 14

# The Discovery of X rays

The discovery of X rays by Wilhelm Röntgen in 1895, started as a purely basic science finding, but it revolutionized medicine, dentistry, and periodontics. Wilhelm Conrad Röntgen (Fig 28) was born in 1845 in the small town of Lennep, in Prussia, and grew up in Apeldoorn, Holland. He graduated with a degree in physics from the University of Zurich and in 1888 was appointed professor and director of the Institute of Physics at the University of Würzburg.[3,11,19]

Toward the end of the century invisible rays, such as ultraviolet, infrared, and Hertzian, were recognized. The English chemist William Crookes (1832–1919) had already designed the tube that bears his name, which consists of two metal plates, known as *anode* and *cathode*, at each end of a tube, from which most of the air can be pumped out. When electricity is applied to the plates, the tube glows as cathode rays (electrons) move through it, escaping through a small aluminum window, and the wall opposite the cathode turns green.

On November 8, 1895, Röntgen was experimenting with the penetrating power of cathodic rays, using a Crookes tube covered with light-tight black cardboard. By chance he had left a barium platinocyanide screen a few feet from the tube. To his amazement a strange fluorescence appeared on the screen when the power was on (he could not see that the fluorescence was green because he was color-blind). He repeated the experiment countless times, over a period of weeks, with the same result. He found that the strange rays could go across a sheet of paper, then a book, a piece of wood or rubber or tin foil, and even a thin aluminum plate, but was stopped by a lead plate. Then he tried holding a lead ring with his fingers and was amazed to find that he could see not only the ring and his fingers but also the bone within them. He doubted what he was seeing, but knowing that the cathodic rays could impress a photographic plate, and trusting this image more than his eyes, he proceeded to take the first-ever radiograph. On December 22, Röntgen took a radiograph of his wife's hand (Fig 29). Thus radiology was born.[3,11,19,20]

Röntgen wrote a paper relating his experiences with these strange invisible rays that he called *X rays* (and were soon called *Röntgen rays* by his colleagues). The paper was immediately published by the local physics society (on December 28, 1895). Within just a few days he sent reprints of his paper to the more important physicists in the world, and his amazing discovery attained worldwide acclaim. In less than a week the news had appeared in important newspapers around the world; on January 12, Röntgen was decorated by Kaiser Wilhelm II. Throughout his life he earned multiple awards and prizes, including the 1901 Nobel Prize in physics. Röntgen died in 1923.

For Röntgen the discovery was only of basic science interest, and after two more papers on X rays, published in March 1896 and March 1897, he returned to his other basic science investigations. For the medical and dental professions, however, the discovery of the X ray not only was a ground-breaking finding for basic science, but also had extraordinary diagnostic potential. The discovery triggered unprecedented interest, and researchers throughout the Western world began to investigate the use of X rays, developing its indications and improving the equipment. As early as February 1896, papers started to appear in England on the use of X rays for bone fractures. In 1896 alone, more than 1,000 papers and 48 books appeared on the use

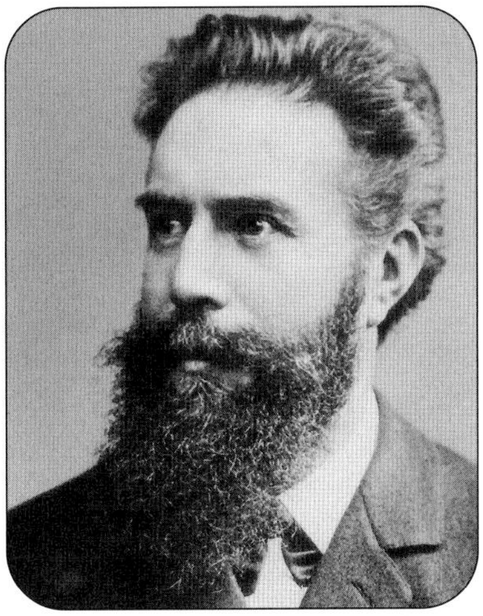

**Fig 28** Wilhelm Conrad Röntgen, by Dittmar, Kgl. Hofphotograph, Munich, 1900.

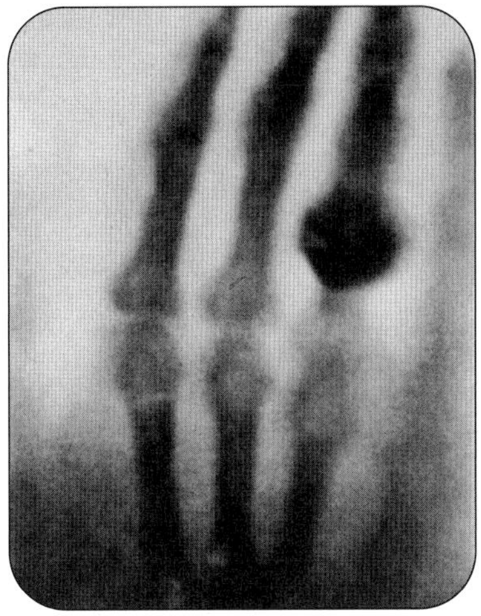

**Fig 29** Radiograph of Bertha Röntgen's hand, taken on December 22, 1895.

of X rays. That same year radiographs were accepted as evidence in a criminal case in Canada and in a civil case in the United States.[3,11]

In the first two months after Röntgen's discovery, three individuals reported taking dental radiographs.[1,4,5,7,9] In mid-January 1896, German dentist Otto Walkhoff (1860–1934), of Braunschweig, an 1881 graduate of the University of Berlin, took an intraoral radiograph of his own jaw, using a glass photographic plate wrapped in black paper and covered with rubber dam, with an exposure time of 25 minutes (Fig 30). Otto Walkhoff was one of the most highly esteemed dentists of his time. A renaissance man of dentistry, Walkhoff excelled in anatomy, physiology, histology, pathology, anthropology, pharmacology, microphotography, and metallurgy. He was professor at the University of Berlin before moving to Munich and finally to Würzburg. Author of many books and research papers, his seminal work on endodontics introduced chlorophenol combined with camphor for the treatment of diseased pulp. This treatment, known as *Walkhoff's paste*, was introduced in the United States by Hermann Prinz and used around the world.[16]

Even as Röntgen's conclusions were being published, in February 1896, another German, Walter König (1859–1936), of Frankfurt, took a series of fourteen dental radiographs. Likewise, in England, Frank Harrison, of Sheffield, reported taking dental radiographs in January 1896.[1,4,5,7,9]

In an article published in *Dental Cosmos* in March 1896, William J. Morton, wrote:

> The application of X ray will, I believe, greatly aid the art of dental surgery. ... Radiographs ... open out a wondrous field of investigation and study and diagnosis. Each errant fang is distinctly placed; teeth before their eruption stand forth in plain view; an unsuspected exostosis is revealed; a pocket of necrosis, of suppuration, or of TB revealed. Extent and area of metallic filling are sharply delineated. Most interesting is the fact that the pulp chamber is beautifully outlined.[14]

Morton was a physician and the son of the discoverer of ether anesthesia. The younger Morton demonstrated the use of X rays before the New York Odontological Society, taking intraoral radiographs of a skull.[9]

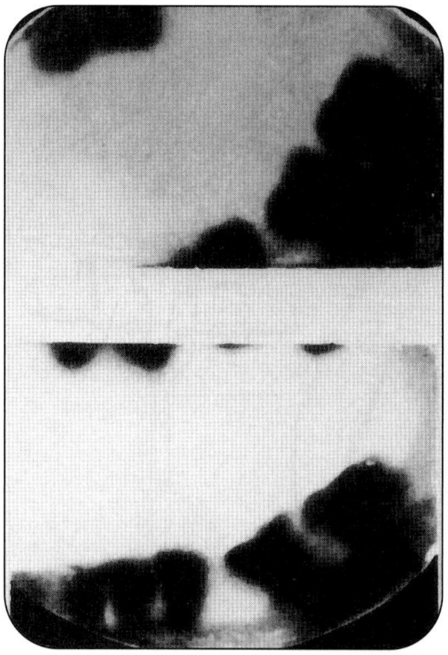

**Fig 30** Radiograph taken by Otto Walkhoff of his own mouth two weeks after Röntgen's discovery.

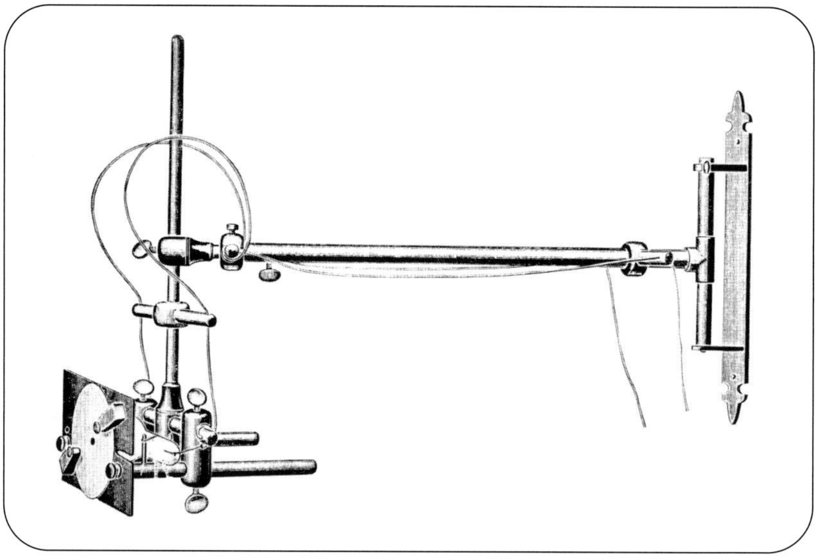

**Fig 31** First commercially manufactured dental X-ray machine (Reinger-Gebbert and Schall, Germany, 1905).

In July 1896, William H. Rollins invented an intraoral cassette and intraoral fluoroscope, and later that same year, an X-ray tube arm and bracket for use in the dental office (Fig 31).[6] This equipment was described in the literature but never manufactured.[6] (See also Chapter 20).

In Europe, Julius Albrecht, of Frankfurt,[1] stated the following four indications for "X-ray photographs":

1. It is possible to determine the position of an emerging third molar and, as required, remove it.
2. It can be determined if there is any damage in the case of persistent milk teeth, and in general, to clarify the situation of the permanent teeth and their location at an early point in time.
3. Possible denticles can be detected and root anomalies or fractures can be identified.
4. Possible bone fragments with persistent pus secretions can be detected.

In July 1896, Dr. C(harles) Edmund Kells was the first American dentist to use X rays. Kells was born in New Orleans on October 21, 1856. His father was also a dentist and Edmund practiced with him in New Orleans after obtaining his dental degree from the New York College of Dentistry in 1878. He was a skilled clinician, with great expertise in dental prosthetics and exodontia, and a defender of root-canal therapy when the focal infection theory demanded extraction of all pulpless teeth.[21] He was also a talented inventor, whose innovations went beyond dentistry to include a thermostat, an electromagnetic clutch and engine, an automobile jack, and an elevator starter and brake.[21] The first in the United States to use commercially produced electricity in his dental office, he invented an electric dental engine and pump to clear the operating field by aspirating fluids. He also built his own X-ray machine immediately after learning of Röntgen's discovery.[5,7,9,17]

Dr. Kells was a prolific writer, having published more than 200 articles on all aspects of dentistry. He was also a remarkable speaker and an able debater, defending his beliefs with energy and conviction.[12]

Practitioners quickly began to detect the dangers of X-ray exposure. Hair loss and skin blistering and peeling were seen after the long exposures required at the time. Reports on these dangers started to appear in 1897, and the cumulative effect of the damage was recognized years later.[13]

Kells, who held the film to take radiographs of his patients, developed a carcinoma in his right hand. He had a number of operations in the next twenty years, attempting unsuccessfully to stop the progress of the cancer. His hand and then his entire arm and shoulder had to be amputated. When he learned that he had lung metastasis, he committed suicide on May 7, 1928.

Development of dental radiology in the twentieth century is discussed in Chapter 20.

## References


1. Bober-Moken I, Perez RS. Historic insights on dental radiography. Bull Hist Dent 1986;34:13.
2. Franke OC. Wilhelm Conrad Roentgen and other X-ray pioneers. Bull Hist Dent 1983;31:11.
3. Glasser O. W. C. Röntgen, ed 2. Springfield, IL: Charles C. Thomas, 1972.
4. Gardiner JF. C. Edmund Kells: New Orleans' gift to dentistry. Bull Hist Dent 1981;29:2.
5. Glenner RA. 80 years of dental radiography. J Am Dent Assoc 1975;90:549.
6. Glenner RA. The Dental Office: Pictorial History. Missoula, Montana: Pictorial Histories, 1984.
7. Gold SI. Diagnostic techniques in periodontology: A historical review. Periodontol 2000 1995;7:9.
8. Hoffmann-Axthelm W. History of Dentistry. Chicago: Quintessence, 1981.
9. Jacobsohn PH, Fedran RJ. Making darkness visible: The discovery of X ray and its introduction to dentistry. J Am Dent Assoc 1995;126:1359.
10. Kells CE. Thirty years' experience in the field of radiography. J Am Dent Assoc 1926;13:693.
11. Kevles BH. Naked to the Bone. New Brunswick, NJ: Rutgers University Press, 1997.
12. Langland OE, Fortier AP. The contributions of Dr. C. Edmund Kells: A bibliography. Bull Hist Dent 1971;19:34.
13. Mazzola PV. Early reports of X-ray dangers. Bull Hist Dent 1974;22:31.
14. Morton WJ. The X ray and its application to dentistry. Dent Cosmos 1896;38:478.
15. Obituary, Dr. C. Edmund Kells. Dent Cosmos 1928;70:747.
16. Rezai RF. Otto Walkhoff—Renaissance man of dentistry. Bull Hist Dent 1986;34:115.
17. Ring ME. Dentistry: An Illustrated History. St Louis: Mosby-Year Book, 1985. Reprinted, New York: Harry N. Abrams, 1992.
18. Rollins W. Radiography in pyorrhea alveolaris. Int Dent J 1897;18:140.
19. Röntgen Rays Centennial. Würzburg University, 1995.
20. Sarton G. The discovery of X rays. Isis 1937;26:349.
21. Varnado MB. Dr. C. Edmund Kells: As I remember him. Bull Hist Dent 1971;19:27.

# 15

# Clinical Periodontology

In the eighteenth century, France and England were leaders in the development of dentistry, represented principally by Pierre Fauchard and John Hunter. In the following century, particularly in its latter half, the leadership was shared by Germany, in the area of scientific research, and the United States, in the area of technology and clinical methods.

One European dentist who moved to America was Leonard Koecker; he advanced innovative ideas on periodontal disease and its treatment. Koecker (Fig 32) was born in Bremen, Germany, in 1785, and, after apprenticing with an itinerant dentist in his native town, moved to Baltimore as a financial agent. When his business failed, he turned to his old interest in dentistry and began what would become a successful practice in Baltimore; later, in 1812, he would practice for a short while in Lancaster, Pennsylvania, until he took up residence in Philadelphia. In 1822 Koecker moved to London, for health reasons, where he also had a successful practice until his death in 1850.

In a paper in 1821, in the *Philadelphia Journal of Medicine and Physical Sciences*, he describes as follows the inflammatory changes in the gingiva and the presence of calculus on teeth, leading to their looseness and exfoliation[15]:

> The gums are, for the most part, much swelled and inflamed, attended by a thin pus-like discharge from between them and the roots of the teeth, occasioning an offensive smell. These parts sometimes exhibit a pretty healthy appearance, though never, as far as my experience extends, perfectly free of inflammation, as Hunter and Fox have stated.
>
> As already intimated, this disease frequently in the beginning, proceeds very slowly, and often affects only certain parts of the gums for many years. When once, however, it becomes general, it goes on with such rapidity, that while one tooth is dropping out, others are so loose, that the slightest pressure almost, will make them fall from their sockets.

After mentioning a number of "remote causes of the disease," he recognizes the role of local causes[15]:

> scorbutic or scrofulous habit affecting the gums, the frequent and inordinate use of mercury, great irregularities in the position of the teeth, neglect of cleanliness, smoking and chewing of tobacco, operations of different kinds injudiciously performed, such, for example, as the filing of the teeth. ...
>
> By the above causes, a collection of tartar, without which I have never seen the disease, is deposited upon particular parts of the teeth, and this becomes the immediate or exciting cause of the disease.

Koecker goes on to prescribe treatment that should follow extraction of hopeless teeth. He mentions the careful removal of tartar and the need for oral hygiene by the patient, which he recommends be performed in the morning and after every meal, using an astringent powder and a toothbrush, placing "the bristles ... into the spaces of the teeth." He discourages splinting on the grounds that it loosens firm teeth; he recommends that treatment of caries be postponed until after gingival treatment is completed and that placement of artificial teeth be avoided.

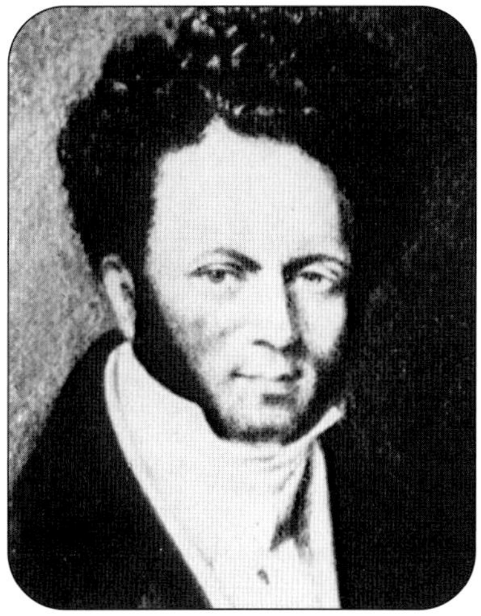

**Fig 32** Leonard Koecker.

In 1826 Koecker published *Principles of Dental Surgery*,[16] in which he describes periodontal disease as in the 1821 article, details recommended treatment, and recounts cases he treated.

Koecker was an early advocate of the odontogenic focal infection theory and recommended the extraction of all severely involved teeth and roots, including all unopposed molars, to prevent systemic infections. Koecker also made important contributions to endodontics (pulp capping) and operative dentistry (gold foil). Indeed, evidence proves that Koecker was ahead of his time. But the dental profession did not give his work the attention it deserved, and his contributions went unnoticed.[17]

Levi Spear Parmly (1790–1859), a New Orleans dentist, is considered the father of oral hygiene and the inventor of dental floss.[7] In a book published in 1819 he states that dental caries can be controlled by brushing and by using

> a waxen silken thread ... which is to be passed through the interstices of the teeth, between their necks and the arches of the gum, to dislodge that irritating matter which no brush can remove and which is the real source of distress.[7]

Johann Jacob Joseph Serre[13] (1759–1830) was born in Belgium but carried out his professional activities mostly in Vienna and Berlin. He wrote several books, the most important of which was a 564-page treatise, published in 1803, and entitled *Praktische Darstellung aller Operationen der Zahnheilkunst* (*Practical Presentation of All the Operations of the Art of Dentistry*). In two previous publications, one devoted to "toothache of the prettier sex during their pregnancies," Serre emphasized the importance of oral hygiene.[12]

The term *pyorrhea alveolaris* was used for the first time by Alphonse Toirac (1791–1863) in 1823, although some scholars dispute this.[13] The term was introduced in the United States at a meeting of the American Dental Association in Chicago in 1877 by Frederick Henry Rehwinkel (1825–1889), a German physician who emigrated to the United States, attended the Baltimore College of Dental Surgery, and practiced in Chilicotte, Ohio.[12,21]

Chapin Harris was born in Pompey, New York, on May 6, 1806, and after training with his older brother, became an itinerant dentist throughout the South, finally settling in Fredericksburg, Virginia, then in Baltimore in 1835.[2,13]

Harris was a man of culture who befriended prominent writers and artists, and had a vast personal library. Harris was one of the founders (with Horace H. Hayden), and the first dean and professor of practical dentistry, of the Baltimore College of Dental Surgery. In addition, he was the founder (with Eleazar Parmly) and editor of the first dental journal in the world, the *American Journal of Dental Science*, as well as a founder of the American Society of Dental Surgeons.[2,13,19]

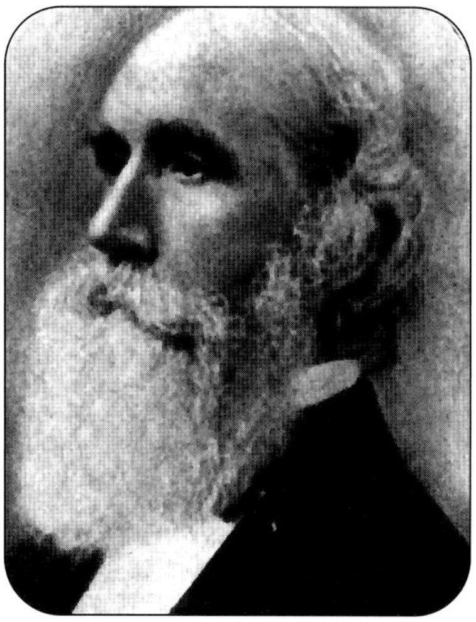

**Fig 33** John Riggs.

In 1839 he published the book *The Dental Art, Practical Treatise on Dental Surgery*,[10] which had numerous editions and translations into the beginning of the next century. This book deals with all aspects of dental practice and includes chapters on diagnosis and treatment of periodontal diseases. In his book Harris recognizes that

> The gums and alveolar processes, from apparently the same cause, frequently assume morbid conditions. Every unhealthy action in one, is almost certainly to be followed by some disorder in the other. The most common form of disease, to which these parts are subject is usually, though very imperfectly, denominated scurvy, from its being supposed to resemble *scorbutus*. ... To this disease, however, it bears no resemblance ...

Harris mentions that, according to Thomas Bell, there are two types of disease, one resulting from local irritation and the other from constitutional causes. He further recognizes, again following Bell, that

> were it not for local irritation, the constitutional tendencies to disease, in these parts, would rarely manifest themselves; and, on the other hand, were it not for constitutional tendencies, the effects of local irritation would seldom be of a serious character.

As far as treatment is concerned, Harris followed the recommendations of Leonard Koecker and credited John Hunter, Joseph Fox, and Thomas Bell.

In his final conclusions Harris insisted that the proper sequence of treatment should be first to extract the teeth that cannot be treated, then treat the gingiva, and finally supply the patient with artificial teeth as needed. Chapin Harris died in 1860.

The leading authority on periodontal disease and its treatment in the United States in the mid-nineteenth century was John M. Riggs (Fig 33). Born October 25, 1811, on a farm in Seymour, Connecticut, Riggs had a natural mechanical ability and worked as a youth in a blacksmith shop making farm tools of his own invention. Following his family's wishes, he later enrolled at Trinity College in Hartford with the idea of entering the Episcopal ministry. But after graduating in 1837, he changed his mind and began to teach school, and later enrolled at Jefferson Medical College in Philadelphia. After one year he became interested in dentistry and apprenticed with Dr. Horace Wells, in Hartford. He later practiced in Hartford, as Wells' associate, and in 1844 performed the first surgical operation under anesthesia, extracting a tooth of Dr. Wells' under nitrous oxide (see Chapter 12). When Wells retired following his failed demonstration of nitrous oxide anesthesia, he referred his clientele to Riggs, who practiced in Hartford for the rest of his life. Riggs, in turn, was a strong supporter of Wells and later of Wells' widow in their unsuccessful attempt to have the U.S. Senate recognize Wells as the originator of general anesthesia.

Very early in his career Riggs became interested in gingival diseases and devised treatments for curing them. Because he was successful and decided to limit his practice to the diagnosis and treatment of periodontal disease, Riggs can be considered the first periodontist in history.[12,21]

Riggs described his treatment of periodontal disease to an audience at the Connecticut Valley Dental Society at Northampton, Massachusetts, in June 1867, mentioning that in twenty-five years the majority of the treatments had been successful.[20] A year later the society honored Riggs for his accomplishments.

Riggs presented his ideas and treatment methods to numerous audiences in the United States and abroad. His publications, however, were few.[27,28] In an 1876 paper[27] he says,

> This disease is called by many the disease of old age, as formerly it was more particularly noticed in persons of advanced age, but at the present we find the middle-aged and even the young affected by it. Many of the textbooks consider it hereditary, or constitutional, or bone disease. The result from whatever cause is most disastrous to the teeth, and in many cases to the health of the patient, for one by one the teeth become loose because of loss of bony support, and are plucked out as an intolerable annoyance. If the inflammatory action be great and involve most or all of the gum embracing the teeth, pus tinged with blood exudes from around the necks of the teeth on the slightest pressure of lips or tongue or in mastication.

Riggs describes periodontal disease as occurring in four stages:

> As the disease exists in a less annoying and less dangerous form for several years previous to the above aggravated symptoms covering from 10 to 20 years before it culminates in its miserable characteristic—the loss of teeth—I have thought it best to tabulate its progress by treating it under four heads or divisions:
>
> *First:* Where the margins of the gums showed decided inflammatory action with some absorption of its substance and bleeding at the slightest touch of the brush.
> *Second:* Where the inflammation extends over the thinner alveolar border causing absorption of the bone as well as of gum tissue, forming small pockets beneath the gums filled with pus.
> *Third:* Where the disease action takes deeper hold involving thicker portions of the process absorbing it most rapidly near the tooth.
> *Fourth:* Where the disease has swept away all of the alveola and much of the gum.

This description of the different stages of the disease, from marginal gingivitis to periodontitis to tooth loss, could scarcely be improved today.

As a preventive measure, Riggs strongly advocated cleanliness of the mouth, as he points out, "[T]he teeth themselves, with their accumulated accretions and roughened surfaces ... are the exciting cause of the disease."[27]

He strongly opposed surgery, which at the time consisted of resection of the gums. He thought this type of surgery barbaric, and instead advocated deep subgingival curettage reaching the bone margin (also quite gory). For this he devised six small curettes, for instrumentation in left and right sides (see also Chapter 21). Riggs performed his treatment under chloroform anesthesia.

Arthur Merritt (1870–1961), a prominent periodontist and historian, mentions that he contacted a former associate of Riggs, Dr. Levi C. Taylor, who told him in a personal letter: "Dr. Riggs was very rough and seemingly harsh but for all of that, he produced the best results I have ever seen and especially in bad cases. He would place his patients in some instances under chloroform far enough to do his work satisfactorily. The results were always good."[20]

Riggs was part of a committee that attempted unsuccessfully to establish a dental school at Yale University, but in 1867 Harvard University approved the project, creating such a school, and Riggs was appointed clinical instructor.[12,21] Gradually his views and ideas on periodontal therapy attained wide acceptance, he was recognized as the leading authority in the field, and the disease became known as *Riggs' disease.* Some of his contemporaries criticized Riggs for having allowed the disease to bear his name, but he responded that he had not proposed it; some of his disciples had, and he had never used it himself.[20] This appears to be the case judging from the literature of the era.

His merits were recognized by the Baltimore College of Dental Surgery, which conferred upon him the honorary degree of Doctor of Dental Surgery.[12,21] Riggs' ideas were supported by the *Missouri Dental Journal*, whose editor, Dr. H. S. Chase, published several articles describing his techniques.[11,12]

An interesting anecdote: Dr. Sheldon Baumrind, of Berkeley, California, discovered among the Mark Twain papers in the Library of the University of California, Berkeley, an incomplete and unpublished manuscript entitled "Happy Memories of the Dental Chair," in which the famed author relates his visits to Dr. Riggs' office. As Baumrind relates,[3] sometime in the early 1870s, Mark Twain was referred by a friend to Riggs to be treated for "Riggs' disease." Twain describes Riggs as "gray and venerable, and humane of aspect; but he had the calm, possessed, surgical look of a man who could endure pain in another person." He relates his first impressions of Riggs' office as follows[3]:

> I got into the chair and looked about me, noting the cuspidor at my left elbow, the convenient glass of water; the table at my right covered with long steel bodkins laid out in rows on a white napkin; then laid my head back in the rest, feeling pale and nervous, for this thing was all new to me; new and hellish, if I may use such a word without offense. The doctor bent over me, I spread my mouth and he put a mirror the size of a nickel into it, and inspected it all around. And began to talk. Not swiftly, not excitedly; but evenly, smoothly, tranquilly.

After relating Riggs' description of Twain's oral condition, Twain gives an account of the clinical procedures:

> He put his tools into my mouth, rooted it under a gum and began to carve. He seemed to fetch away chips of bone the size of my hand. In truth what he removed could hardly have been seen without a microscope, I suppose—but my imagination is a microscope. If I had been honest enough to speak my mind I would have said, 'Ow!' to every dig; but I was ashamed to do that, and so only said 'Um,' in a low voice, and kept back the exclamation point. The doctor worked fast and with a hand that was as sure as it was vigorous. ...

Riggs offered Twain the option of chloroform analgesia which "made everything comfortable and pleasant." Finally Twain summarizes his experiences, saying,

> I was in the chair a good part of two days—nine hours the first day and five the next—and came out of it with my 32 teeth as polished and ship-shape and raw as if they had been taken out of their sockets and filed. It was a good job, and quickly and skillfully done; but if I opened my mouth and drew in a cold breath it woke up my attention like pouring ice water down my back. ... But after that they became as tough as iron, and a thorough comfort.

In 1881 Riggs attended the 7th International Dental Congress in London, chaired by Sir James Paget and counting among the attendants Louis Pasteur, Robert Koch, and Joseph Lister.

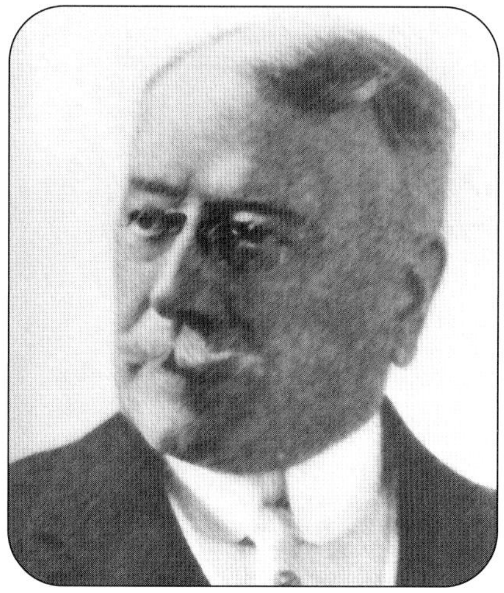

**Fig 34** William Younger.

Riggs was received in London with great respect and met and discussed his method of treatment with Emile Magitot, Joseph Arkövy, and Sir John Tomes.[20,21]

Riggs was a modest, unassuming man, who attended meetings infrequently and seldom spoke. He never married. On November 11, 1885, Riggs died of pneumonia, in Hartford, Connecticut.

Riggs and his disciples had great influence on the dental profession. They were proponents of the so-called conservative approach to periodontal therapy, developing the concept of oral prophylaxis and prevention. Among Riggs' followers were W. J. Younger, R. B. Adair, D. D. Smith, and L. Taylor.[12] Many papers by followers and contemporaries of Riggs described clinical features and treatment of periodontal disease, the latter based mostly on hygienic measures.[19,22]

William J. Younger (Fig 34) was born in 1839 in Santiago, Chile, where his British parents were missionaries. He grew up in San Francisco, where he obtained a medical degree from the University of the Pacific in 1862, and practiced medicine, but soon became interested in dentistry and made it his specialty. For many years he was chair of dental medicine in the medical department of the University of California.[25] In 1897 he moved to Chicago and in 1900 established himself in Paris, France, where he practiced for twenty years, becoming a respected professional.[21,25]

The periodontal treatment that Younger advocated was less aggressive than Riggs', in that he contended that bone curettage was not indispensable.[8] The scaling instruments designed by Younger in 1897, and later modified by his student, Dr. Robert Good, of Chicago, constituted the so-called Younger-Good set, widely used until well after World War II. Hans Sachs, in Germany, a student of Robert Good, also introduced some modifications to the original Younger design, and these instruments were widely used in Europe.[9] Younger's instrument design has been the basis for modern instruments used to this day. Information on the development of scaling instruments is given in Chapter 21.

Younger considered periodontal disease a local infection and was the first to discuss, in 1892, the possibility of reattachment:

> I am satisfied that attachment takes place in these cases, otherwise the teeth could not become so firm and the gums and tissues of the socket cling so to the tissues of the root. It is therefore an easy matter for direct union to be established between these healthy, living tissues when the partition of calculus is thoroughly removed from the root, and a granulating surface produced in the environment tissues of the gingivus.[sic][21]

Although Younger could not have established that new attachment had taken place, he had a clear idea that it was the ideal outcome of treatment, resulting in obliteration of the pocket rather than removal of its external wall.

In addition, after his careful root instrumentation, Younger used various medicaments, particularly 50% lactic acid and other organic and inorganic acids, to flush out debris and bacteria and to remove metabolic products that sealed cemental channels[8,9] and thus favor reattachment.

In 1902, Younger reported at a meeting of the American Dental Club of Paris, on a case[1] of root coverage using gingival grafts (see Chapter 21). His best-known paper was published in German in a Swiss dental journal in 1905.[33] Younger died in Paris on July 23, 1920.

Other followers of Riggs' concepts and methods were Dr. Robin B. Adair (1878–1929), who practiced in Atlanta, Georgia, for more than fifty years,[20] and was a pioneer in the oral hygiene movement, and Dr. David D. Smith (1839–1920), a graduate, and later professor and dean of the Philadelphia Dental College. He also obtained a medical degree from the Jefferson Medical College. Smith practiced in Germantown, Pennsylvania, and in the early part of the twentieth century, dentists who came to his office to observe his treatments formed a society that later became the American Academy of Periodontology[24] (see Chapter 26).

It is interesting to note that root resection techniques, including hemisections, were already practiced in the latter part of the nineteenth century. In 1884, J. N. Farrar of New York City, described the technique, which was intended mostly for the treatment of periapical abscesses but also was recommended in deep pocket formation resulting from "discharge of pus along the outside of the root of the tooth." Detailed drawings accompany the paper.[6]

In America, particularly under the influence of John Riggs and his followers, and probably also due to the early creation of dentistry as an independent discipline with recognized university status, the concept of a local origin of periodontal disease prevailed, and techniques for its local treatment were advanced. In Europe, on the other hand, and particularly in France, dentistry remained a specialty of medicine, and etiologic concepts and the treatment techniques derived from them remained in the realm of systemic and constitutional disorders.

French researcher Emile Magitot (1833–1897) (Fig 35) was a strong proponent of these ideas. Born in Paris, the son of a dentist, Magitot studied medicine. And although his life was devoted to research in areas related to dentistry, such as the development of tooth structures in man and in various animals, dental caries, and dental anomalies, he rejected the manual and mechanical part of dental therapy performed by dentists. He claimed to be a stomatologist and was instrumental in establishing the medical specialty of "stomatologie" in France.[23]

Magitot considered calculus an accidental factor rather than a causative one, although he recommended its removal. He assumed that the disease he called *alveolo-dental periostitis* started in the periodontal membrane and the cementum, evolving toward the apex and only secondarily affecting the gingiva. He thought the disease was caused by general nutritional deficiencies, gout, diabetes, rheumatism, and albuminuria.[9]

Hungarian physician Joseph Arkövy (1851–1922) was also a proponent of the systemic causation of periodontal disease. Arkövy thought the primary site of periodontal disease was the alveolar bone margin and that from there it proceeded to the periodontal ligament and the cementum.[13] Other European clinicians, however, followed the American lead and developed treatment techniques more in accordance with the concept of a local etiology.

L. Cruet, in France, in 1888, advocated the gingivectomy technique.[4,12]

Salomon Robicsek[31] (Fig 36) was born in Bajsa, Hungary, in 1845, grew up in Prague and attended the University of Vienna School of Medicine where he studied under such prominent teachers as Carl Rokitanski and Joseph Skoda. After graduation in 1868, he specialized in dentistry, and opened his practice in Vienna in the 1870s. Robicsek published several papers in German between 1877 and 1902. Robicsek died in Vienna in 1928.

Although his method of treatment of periodontal disease is not described in any of his papers, Robicsek presented it at various scientific meetings in 1883 and 1884, and Stern and others[31] obtained, in the 1960s, information from Robicsek's son Karl, who had practiced with his

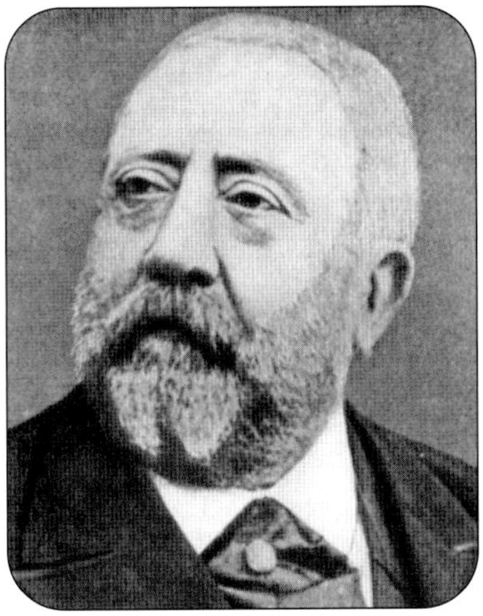

**Fig 35** Emile Magitot.

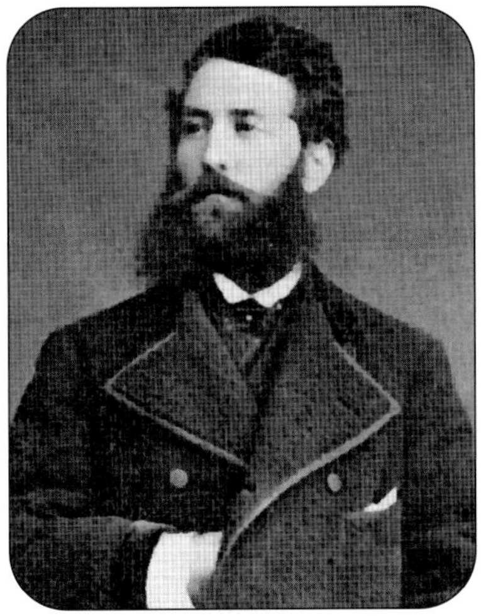

**Fig 36** Salomon Robicsek.

father. The Robicsek technique consisted of a straight-line gingivectomy, exposing and scraping the osseous margin, using burs. The area was then painted with iodine tincture and the patient was instructed to rinse with a disinfectant solution, preferably hydrogen peroxide.[31]

This historical account would not be complete without mention of dental quacks.[14,30,32] Charlatans have, on both sides of the Atlantic and throughout the centuries, performed dental work whenever trained dentists were unavailable or too expensive for the general population.

In the early years, there was no clear distinction between charlatans and trained practitioners, and many used strange concoctions with "magical properties" to treat medical and dental ailments. Flamboyant individuals, sometimes backed by an entire quasi-theatrical production, were the most successful. With the advent of formal university training in the latter part of the nineteenth century, charlatans gradually lost their appeal, but they persisted (and still do) when other methods were unavailable or unaffordable.

Itinerant charlatans performed extractions and treated all kinds of oral aches and pains, as well as headaches, earache, neuralgias, lumbago, and many other ailments. They used little understood forces such as electricity or magnetism, fumigation, and a variety of patent medicines. Ring mentions that an "electric" toothbrush was manufactured by a London company and imported into the United States; it was "charged" by rubbing its *wooden* handle with a special cloth.[30] Patent medicines containing secret ingredients were banned in the United States in 1906.

Mandel[18] mentions the faith healers who "depend on divine intervention and the placebo effect of their cures." The following excerpt from Mark Twain's autobiography, is transcribed from Mandel[18]:

> We had the "faith doctors," too, in those early days—a woman. Her specialty was toothache. She was a farmer's old wife and lived five miles from Hannibal. She would lay her hand on the patient's jaw and say, "believe," and the cure was prompt.

Every age has its quackery and some professionals find it quite lucrative, even in the dental field.[18] Currently, some types of "alternative medicine" advocate unproved methods of treatment and continue to find receptive minds in the uninformed or the disillusioned.

## References


1. American Dental Club of Paris. Meetings of December 1902 and January and March 1903. Dent Cosmos 1904;46:39.
2. Asbell MB. Chapin A. Harris and Horace H. Hayden: An historical review. Bull Hist Dent 1969;17:27.
3. Baumrind S. Mark Twain visits the dentist. J Calif Dent Assoc 1964;Dec. Reprinted in: Bull Hist Dent 1973;21:25.
4. Cruet L. Traitement chirurgicale de l'ostéopériostite alvéolodentaire. Revue Odont 1888;7:494.
5. Epstein HD. John Riggs and his disease. Bull Hist Dent 1969;17:1.
6. Farrar JN. Radical and heroic treatment of alveolar abscess by amputation of roots of teeth, with description and application of the cantilever crown. Dent Cosmos 1884;26:79, 135.
7. Fischman SL. The history of oral hygiene: How far have we come in 6000 years? Periodontol 2000 1997;15:7.
8. Gold SI. Hans Sachs: Pioneer periodontologist and dental historian. Bull Hist Dent 1986;34:28.
9. Gold SI. Periodontics. The past. Part II. The development of modern periodontics. J Clin Periodontol 1985;12:171.
10. Harris CA. The Dental Art: Practical Treatise on Dental Surgery. Baltimore: Armstrong and Berry, 1839.
11. Hartzell TB. The story of the origin and development of periodontoclasia. J Am Dent Assoc 1935;22:1899.
12. Held AJ. Periodontology. From Its Origins Up to 1980: A Survey. Boston: Birkhauser; 1989.
13. Hoffmann-Axthelm W. History of Dentistry. Chicago: Quintessence, 1981.
14. Jago JD. Early dental charlatans and quacks. Bull Hist Dent 1984;32:118.
15. Koecker L. An essay on the devastation of the gums and the alveolar processes. Philadelphia J Med Phys Sci 1821;2:282.
16. Koecker L. Of the devastation or absorption of the gums and sockets on the teeth. In: Principles of Dental Surgery. London: Underwood, 1826. Reprinted in: J Periodontol 1940;11:82.
17. Leonard HJ. Diagnosis and treatment of periodontoclasia. J Periodontol 1940;11:67.
18. Mandel I. Dental quackery: A retrospective view. J Am Dent Assoc 1994;125:153.
19. McManus C. The makers of dentistry. Dent Cosmos 1902;44:1105.
20. Merritt AH. A brief history of periodontology. J Dent Res 1921;3:149.
21. Merritt AH. Periodontal Diseases: Diagnosis and Treatment. New York: Macmillan, 1935.
22. Mills GA. Some of the phases of Riggs' disease (so-called). Dent Cosmos 1877;19:185,254,347.
23. Obituary, Dr. Emile Magitot. Dent Cosmos 1897;39:680.
24. Obituary, Dr. David D. Smith. Dent Cosmos 1920;62:911.
25. Obituary, Dr. William J. Younger. Dent Cosmos 1920;62:1365.
26. Rawls AO. Pyorrhea alveolaris. Dent Cosmos 1885;27:265.
27. Riggs JM. Suppurative inflammation of the gums and absorption of the gums and alveolar process. Pennsylvania J Dent Sci 1876;3:99. Taken from: Arch Clin Oral Path 1938;2:423.
28. Riggs JM. Pyorrhea alveolaris. Dent Cosmos 1892;24:524.
29. Ring ME. Dentistry: An Illustrated History. St Louis: Mosby-Year Book, 1985. Reprinted, New York: Harry N. Abrams, 1992.
30. Ring ME. Quackery in dentistry. Past and present. Calif Dent J 1998;26:819.
31. Stern IB, Everett FG, Robicsek K. Robicsek: A pioneer in the surgical treatment of periodontal disease. J Periodontol 1965;36:325.
32. Young JH. The long struggle against quackery in dentistry. Bull Hist Dent 1985;33:69.
33. Younger WJ. Pyorrhea alveolaris. Schweiz Vierteljähresscrift Zahnheilk 1905;15:87.

# 16

# Pathology

As seen in Chapter 10, the shift from seeing disease as a generalized problem, as indicated by the theory of humors of Hippocrates and Galen, to viewing it as a localized disorder started with clinical and autopsy studies of Giovanni Battista Morgagni (1682–1771), published in 1761, and subsequently those of the young French physician Marie-François-Xavier Bichat, (1771–1802), who concluded that the organs were composed of tissues and that these were the seat of disease.[14,18]

Carl Rokitanski (1804–1878), professor at the University of Vienna, performed tens of thousands of autopsies and expanded the knowledge of pathologic anatomy. But, in spite of the fact that the microscope had been used since the middle of the seventeenth century, neither Rokitanski nor any of his predecessors used it extensively. In the nineteenth century, as advances were made in the microscope, including achromatic lenses (developed by Joseph J. Lister, the father of Joseph Lister), researchers began to use it in more generalized ways, contributing greatly to the progress of anatomy and pathology.[6,18]

The cellular theory developed after the investigations of botanist Mathias Schleiden (1804–1881) and zoologist Theodore Schwann (1810–1882). Schleiden published, in 1838, a paper stating that all plants are made of cells, and in the following year Schwann extended these observations to animal tissues. Their discoveries are referred to as the *Schleiden-Schwann cell theory*. They still believed, however, that cells originated not from parent cells but instead from a so-called blastema, by a process comparable to the formation of crystals.

This was the general state of pathology when Rudolf Virchow entered the field. His contributions, more than 2,000 publications, established modern pathology. He became the leading force in the latter half of the nineteenth century, together with Robert Koch, to bring Germany to the forefront of medical research and clinical practice,[19,21,23] a position that would gradually be relinquished to the United States after World War I.

Virchow (Fig 37)[1,6,18,26] was born in 1821 in the rural town of Schivelbein, in Eastern Pomerania, Prussia. After completing his secondary education with high honors, he enrolled at the tuition-free Friedrich-Wilhelms Institut, a branch of the University of Berlin devoted to the training of military physicians. Here, he studied medicine under the tutelage of Johannes Peter Müller, well-known biologist, anatomist, and biochemist.

Toward the middle of the century Rokitanski was the most renowned pathologist in Europe, but he continued to believe that cells grew from an amorphous matter, the *blastema*, and that the fundamental pathologic changes occurred in the blood. In other words, he returned to the theory of humors. Virchow opposed this theory vigorously and essentially demolished it, in a paper published in 1846.

Virchow introduced the systematic use of the microscope to pathology and taught his students to "learn to see microscopically." For this purpose he developed a moving track that carried a series of microscopes from one student to the next so they could observe the microscopic fields prepared by the teacher.[19]

Virchow strongly supported the concept that life is a series of physicochemical phenomena that follow mechanical laws, and that scientific research should be based on clinical observations, physical and chemical tests, animal experimentation, necropsies, and microscopic analyses.

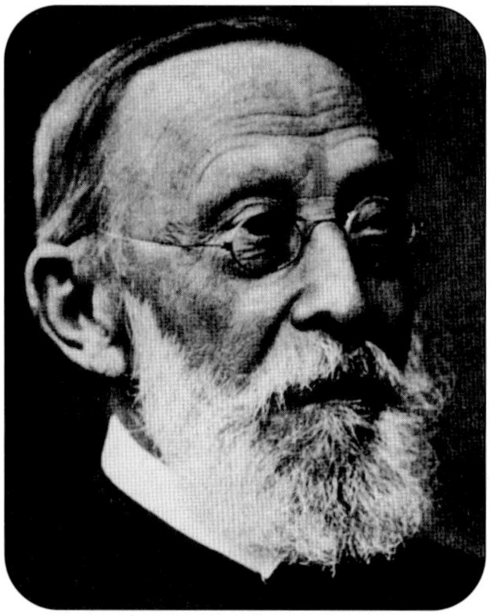

**Fig 37** Rudolf Virchow.

Virchow was the first to describe many diseases, such as leukemia, thrombosis and embolism, malignant tumors, syphilis, tuberculosis, inflammation, necrosis, and gangrene.[23] His observations resulted from refined microscopic and staining techniques.

Virchow founded and edited the *Archives for Pathological Anatomy and Physiology and for Clinical Medicine* and the *Yearbook of Accomplishments and Progress in Medicine*, known as *Virchow's Yearbook*, and edited both until his death. He also wrote the first volume and edited the remaining six volumes of *Handbook of Special Pathology and Therapeutics*, which was the first of many world-renowned, multiple-author German series.

During his tenure as professor at the University of Würzburg (1849–1856), he conceived his "cellular pathology," establishing his adage *omnia cellula a cellula* that cells originate in other cells. The Schleiden-Schwann cell theory presented in 1838–1839 continued the notion of blastema as the origin of the cells. Virchow's concept established that all pathologic processes were physicochemical disturbances of cellular activity leading to alterations in function, and that all cells come from parent cells.

In 1856 he was recruited by the University of Berlin, where he headed an Institute of Pathology, and founded a school that produced many esteemed pathologists such as Friedric von Recklinghausen, Julius Cohnheim, Theodor Klebs, and Paul Langerhans.

Virchow excelled in several fields other than pathology. He was an important politician, founder of the German Progressive Party, and for many years member of Parliament and head of the opposition to Chancellor Otto Bismarck. As a parliamentarian he frequently spoke against anti-Semitism and the expansion of colonialism.[26]

Virchow was also deeply interested in public health and epidemiological issues, proposing important sanitary measures in parliament. He was concerned with anthropology, and his studies on skulls and physical data of children disproved the concept of an Aryan race. In addition, he made important contributions to archeology. Virchow died in Berlin in 1902.

## Inflammation

The improved microscopic technology of the latter half of the nineteenth century allowed for more sophisticated and accurate analyses of the cellular and tissue changes involved in inflammation. Two principal researchers of this issue were Cohnheim and Metchnikoff.

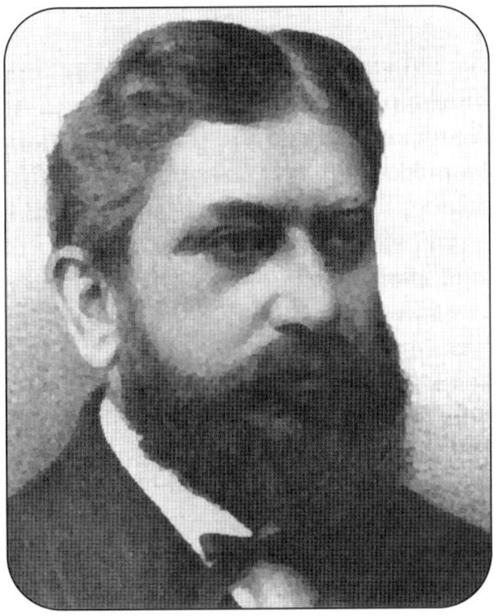

Fig 38 Julius Cohnheim.

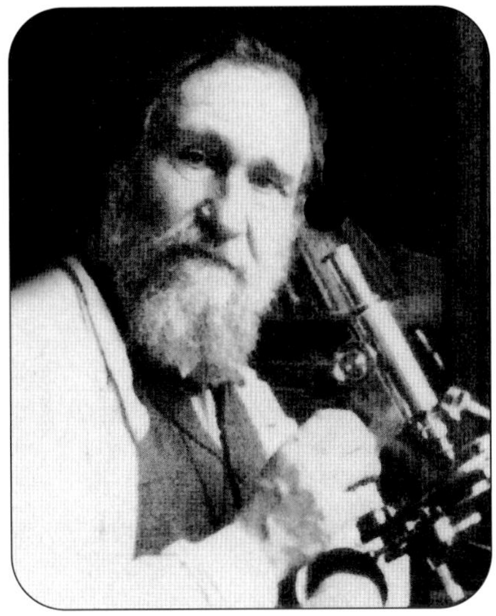

Fig 39 Elie Metchnikoff.

Julius Friedrich Cohnheim (1839–1884) (Fig 38) was born in Demmin, Pomerania, and received his medical degree at Berlin in 1861. After a short period in the army, he became assistant to Virchow, and subsequently professor of pathology at Kiel, Breslau, and Leipzig. Paul Ehrlich and Carl Weigert were among his disciples.[18]

He studied the essential features of inflammation induced in transparent tissues, such as the drawn out intestine of a curarized frog or tongue of a frog after removal of papillae. He showed the dilatation of blood vessels, a slowing down of the bloodstream, and the margination and emigration of leukocytes from the blood vessels (diapedesis). Moreover, he demonstrated the formation of pus from extravasated polymorphonuclear leukocytes. He assigned primary importance in inflammation to a lesion in the vessel wall.[7,8] Cohnheim's inflammation studies appeared in 1873 and 1882. He died from complications of gout at the age of 45.

Elie (Ilya) Metchnikoff (Fig 39)[5,18,25] was born in Russia, in the town of Ivanovska, Kharkov Province, in 1845, and obtained a doctorate in zoology at St. Petersburg. In 1888 Metchnikoff moved to Paris where he worked at the Pasteur Institute.

In 1882 while in Messina, Italy, Metchnikoff made his greatest scientific discovery: he recognized the role of phagocytes in the defense mechanisms of animals—the basis of his theory that phagocytosis was the chief protection of the animal body against bacterial invasion. These ideas triggered an enormous controversy between the defenders of Metchnikoff's theory of a cellular defense mechanism and opponents who believed in a humoral mechanism of defense. The first group was composed largely of French investigators, led by Pasteur, while the second was made up, principally, of German, and more specifically Prussian, followers of Koch. The rivalry between Pasteur and Koch was political as well as scientific, in the aftermath of the Franco-Prussian war.

A compromise between the two antagonistic positions came in 1903 when the English researchers Almroth E. Wright (1861–1947), later to be Alexander Fleming's mentor, and Stewart R. Douglas (1871–1936) discovered the opsonins, a humoral substance that helps leukocytes digest bacteria. The Swedish Academy of Sciences also found a middle ground when, in 1908, it awarded the Nobel Prize to Metchnikoff, the champion of the cellular theory, and Paul Ehrlich, strong proponent of the humoral theory.[18,24] Metchnikoff died in Paris in 1916.

## Periodontal Histopathology

Joseph Fox was born in 1776 and died in London in 1816. Little is known about his early years, except that he conducted in London an extensive and very successful dental practice. Early in the nineteenth century, Fox published two books that represent a seminal contribution to the knowledge on periodontal disease and its treatment: *The Natural History of the Human Teeth*, published in 1803, followed in 1806 by *The History and Treatment of the Diseases of the Teeth, the Gums and the Alveolar Processes.* The second volume has an extensive section dealing with periodontal diseases.

Fox distinguishes between periodontal disease caused by tooth diseases, by gum diseases, and by constitutional diseases. He notes that cases of periodontal disease often have no carious teeth and that calculus occurs in neglected mouths. Fox describes two types of periodontal disease:

> The most common disease is that which has been called scurvy in the gums, thus denominated from assuming an appearance similar to that which happens to persons afflicted with the sea-scurvy. This disease is generally marked by the gums becoming redder than ordinary and enlarged from a turgessence of the vessels, which are made to bleed by the slightest causes, such as the use of a toothbrush, the biting of a crust, or even by only sucking on them. ...
>
> The disease next proceeds to the alveolar processes, the substances of which are destroyed by absorption; at length the teeth become loose, and, in a few years, drop out, one after the other, at short intervals, until the person is rendered toothless.[9]

In another chapter Fox describes diseases of the alveolar bone: "The alveolar processes are always sympathetically affected by all the diseases of the teeth and gums."[9] But also:

> The alveolar processes have certain diseases peculiar to themselves, independent from affections arising from the teeth and gums. The most common disease to which they are subject, is a gradual absorption of their substance, whereby the teeth lose their support, become weak, and at length are so loosened as to drop out.[9]

Fox observes that the first disease occurs "at a very early period in life," while the second appears between 40 and 50 years of age. Fox's detailed drawings trace tooth anatomy, gingival disease, recession, bone loss, edentulous jaws, and calculus (Fig 40). With respect to calculus formation, Fox argues,

> Almost every person is subject to a formation of [tartar] in a greater or lesser degree; in some the deposit is so habitual or copious, that, without unremitted attention, their teeth cannot be preserved in a decent state; whereas, in others, it is so small in quantity that the least degree of care is sufficient to keep the teeth perfectly clean. ...
>
> In the formation of tartar about the teeth, it insinuates itself under the gums, and detaches them from the necks of the teeth; the gums are thus brought into a diseased state, are subject to inflammation and pain, and at last gradually recede from the teeth. This state of the gums soon causes the alveolar process to become affected, and absorption of them is induced. ...
>
> The tartar always accumulates in greater quantity about those teeth situated near to the openings of the salivary ducts.

Fox recommends oral hygiene with a toothbrush and water, and if this is not sufficient, a tooth-powder. When tartar has collected about the teeth "scaling is most useful and necessary for their preservation." Fox also presents a chemical analysis of calculus, which he sees as consisting of:

| | |
|---|---|
| Phosphate of lime—35 | Animal fat, or oil—3 |
| Fibrina, or cartilage—9 | Loss—3 |

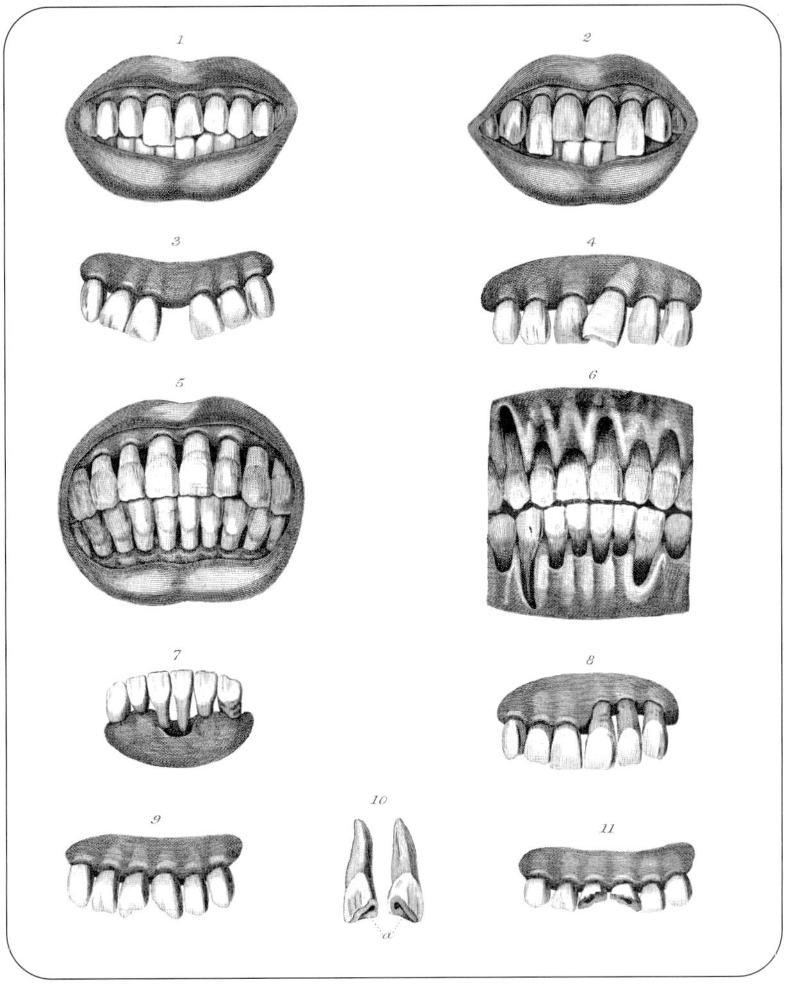


Fig 40 Illustration from John Fox's book[9] showing different periodontal pathologies.

Fox also recognizes that teeth loosen for various reasons—among them "absorption of the alveolar process,"—and recommends ligating with silk the loosened tooth or teeth to stronger teeth.

Joseph Linderer (1809–1878), the son of Callman Jacob Linderer, was an itinerant German dentist later recognized by the university, and author of a book on dentistry.[12] A student of Johannes Müller, Joseph Linderer published his research findings in his father's book. Linderer's 1851 publication describes a non-inflammatory form of periodontal disease, almost free of inflammation, in which the gingiva shrinks progressively so that the neck of the tooth is exposed; additionally, the study details gingival fibromatosis.[11,13] Further, he provides a careful description of the enamel organ.[13]

In 1841 English scientist William Lintott described two types of periodontitis, one of local origin and the other of systemic origin,[11] while French researcher E. Andrieu (1833–1889) in 1885, analyzed "alveolo-dental periostitis" as an inflammation of the gum leading to resorption and even necrosis of the bone.[11]

Sir John Tomes (1815–1865) (Fig 41), surgeon-dentist at the Middlesex Hospital School of Medicine, in London, published in 1848 his lectures on dental physiology and surgery.[27] He in-

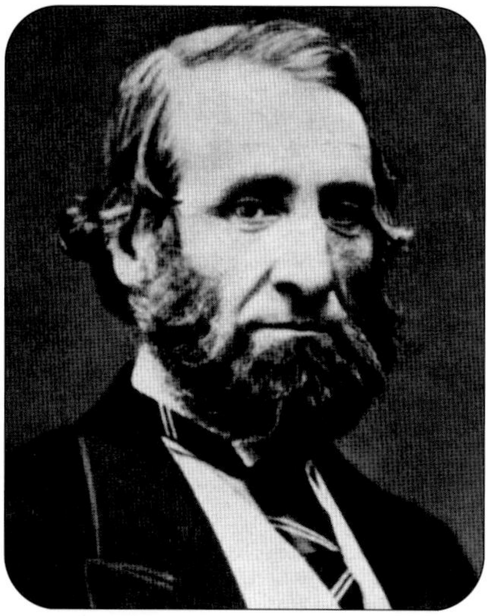

**Fig 41** Sir John Tomes.

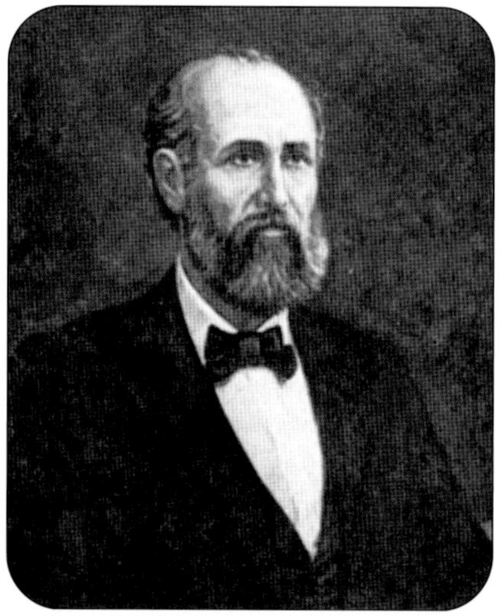

**Fig 42** G. V. Black.

vestigated, among other conditions, acute and chronic inflammation of the gums, the latter resulting in tooth loss, ulceration of the gums, and various tumors. His treatment of chronic inflammation consisted of scarifying the tissues with a lancet and applying astringents. Tomes identified the dentinal fibrils that still bear his name.

In the United States, Greene Vardiman Black (1836–1915) (Fig 42), known for his development of operative dentistry, also made important contributions to periodontology. In a book published in 1887, Black described two types of periodontal disease, one of local origin, caused by poor oral hygiene, which he called *calcic pericementitis*, and another called *phagedenic pericementitis*, caused by dietary deficiencies and constitutional imbalances.[11] In an 1899 paper on the periodontal membrane,[2] he outlines the fiber system and notes the presence of glands (probably epithelial rests of Malassez). Interestingly, in 1817 French investigator Etienne Reynaud Augustin Serres (1786–1868) had described glands in the gingiva and periodontal ligament of the newborn. These *glands of Serres*, as he called them, were thought to secrete calculus. In fact they were epithelial rests, later described by Malassez.[13]

As the nineteenth century progressed, improved histological techniques, as well as technological advances in the microscope, permitted several scientists to describe the dental and periodontal tissues. Their names are found today, in many of the structures they described. Among these scientists: Alexander Nasmyth (1789–1848), of London, distinguished the transparent pellicle that covers the enamel. Adolph Retzius (1796–1860), of Stockholm, detailed enamel and dentin histology and embryology. Rudolph Albert Kölliker (1817–1905), of Würzburg, colleague and friend of Virchow and Röntgen, made extensive studies in histology and embryology, identifying the osteoclast, and elucidating dental and oral tissues, including the fibrous systems of the gingiva.[12] Berlin anatomist Oscar Hertwig (1849–1922) recognized the root-forming epithelial sheath in tooth formation. Louis Charles Malassez (1862–1910), a Parisian surgeon and pathologist, refuted Magitot's theory of the origin of epithelium in cysts from an irritation of the pulp; Malassez discerned the periodontal ligament epithelial rests that bear his name. Wilhelm Waldeyer (1836–1921), of Strasbourg and Berlin, described the ring of lymphoid tissue of lingual, pharyngeal, and faucial tonsils.[11–13] Victor Ebner von Rofenstein (1842–1925), a histologist at the University of Vienna Medical School, developed methods for the study of the dental hard tissues, and made detailed studies of the salivary glands and other oral structures. His name is applied to structures, such as the glands of von Ebner in the posterior part of the tongue, and the incremental lines of Ebner in the dentin. Anatomist Julius Tandler (1869–1936), Harry Sicher's mentor, was interested in the oral tissues.

The nineteenth century saw new studies in a variety of related areas. In 1869, Moriz Heider (1816–1866) and Carl Wedl (1815–1891), a histopathologist, published an *Atlas of Pathology of the Teeth*, which proposes the theory of a bacterial etiology of dental caries.[17] Moriz Heider, at the University of Vienna, developed the philosophy that dentistry should be studied in connection with the entire organism and not as an independent science disconnected from medicine.[17]

Gingival and periodontal changes during pregnancy were recognized by J. Pitcairn in 1818,[22] and in 1877, A. Pinard published a case study on pregnancy gingivitis.[20]

The possibility of a relationship between forces exerted on the teeth, mainly occlusal forces, and pathological changes in the periodontium were suspected in the second half of the nineteenth century. William Gibson Arlington Bonwill (1833–1899), of Philadelphia, introduced a truly useful articulator, which he presented in 1864 at the meeting of the Delaware Dental Society. The articulator was based on "geometrical, mathematical and mechanical laws" and represented a notable advancement in prosthetics.[11,13] At the same time Bonwill considered that dental occlusion might play a role in the etiopathogenesis of periodontal disease.[11]

Moritz Karolyi (1865–1945) would describe grinding and clenching of the jaws early in the following century[11,13,16] (see Chapter 18).

## References


1. Ackerknecht EH. Rudolf Virchow. New York: Arno Press, 1981.
2. Black GV. The fibers and glands of the peridental membrane. Dent Cosmos 1899;41:101.
3. Bonwill WGA. Articulation and articulators. Transact Am Dent Assoc 1864;76.
4. Bonwill WGA. The scientific articulation of the human teeth as founded on geometrical, mathematical and mechanical laws. Dent Items 1899;21:617.
5. Brieger GH. Metchnikoff, Elie. In: Gillispie CC (ed). Dictionary of Scientific Biography. New York: Charles Scribner's Sons, 1973.
6. Carranza FA. Revolucionarios de la Ciencia. Buenos Aires: Vergara, 1998.
7. Cohnheim J. The Phenomena of Inflammation. In: Lectures on General Pathology, vol 1 (in German). London: The New Sydenheim Society, 1882. Translated and reprinted in: Clendening L. Source Book of Medical History. New York: Dover and Henry Schuman, 1942.
8. Florey HW. The history and scope of pathology. In: Florey L (ed). General Pathology. Philadelphia: WB Saunders, 1970.
9. Fox J. The History and Treatment of the Diseases of the Teeth, the Gums and the Alveolar Processes. Birmingham, AL: Classics of Dentistry Library, 1981.
10. Harris H. The Birth of the Cell. New Haven: Yale University Press, 1999.
11. Held A-J. Periodontology. From Its Origins Up to 1980: A Survey. Basel: Birkhäuser, 1989.
12. Hintzsche E. Koelliker, Rudolph Albert von. In: Gillispie CC (ed). Dictionary of Scientific Biography, vol 7. New York: Charles Scribner's Sons, 1973.
13. Hoffmann-Axthelm W. History of Dentistry. Chicago: Quintessence, 1981.
14. Hudson RP. Disease and Its Control. New York: Praeger, 1987.
15. Huff DW. A comparison of American and German dentistry 1850–1900. Bull Hist Dent 1985;33:47.
16. Karolyi M. Beobachtungen über Pyorrhoea alveolaris. Öst-ung Vjschr Zahnheilk 1901;17:279.
17. Kremenak NW, Squier CA. Pioneers in oral biology: The migrations of Gottlieb, Kronfeld, Orban, Weinmann, and Sicher from Vienna to America. Crit Rev Oral Biol Med 1997;8:108.
18. Major RH. A History of Medicine. Springfield, IL: Charles C. Thomas, 1954.
19. Nuland SB. Doctors. The Biography of Medicine. New York: Vintage Books, 1995.
20. Pinard A. Gingivitis in pregnancy. Dent Register 1877;31:258.

21. Plaut A. Rudolf Virchow and today's physicians and scientists. Bull Hist Med 1953;27:236.
22. Pitcairn J. A case of disease of the gums which occurred during pregnancy. Dubing Hosp Rep 1818;2:309.
23. Rather LJ. Rudolph Virchow's views on pathology, pathological anatomy and cellular pathology. Arch Path 1966;82:197.
24. Silverstein AM. A History of Immunology. New York: Academic Press, 1989.
25. Tauber AI, Chernyak L. Metchnikoff and the Origins of Immunology. New York: Oxford University Press, 1991.
26. Thomas R. Rudolf Virchow: Pathologist, public health physician, liberal politician, anthropologist, and opponent of anti-Semitism. J Med Biogr 1999;7:200.
27. Tomes J. A Course of Lectures on Dental Physiology and Surgery. London: John W. Parker, 1848.

# Part V

# The Twentieth Century

# 17

# The Century in Perspective

The twentieth century was marked in the West by accelerated, continuous technological and scientific progress and by three devastating wars that involved most of the western world. The Great War, later called the First World War (1914–1918) brought about new technologies, deadly gases, and attacks on civilian populations, and resulted in enormous human and material losses. The war ended with the fall of governments, the realignment of political systems, and revolutions that promoted ideologies of the left and the right. U. S. power grew in spite of the Great Depression of the 1930s, as British hegemony continued to wane.

The Second World War (1939–1945) involved not only a European but also a Pacific theater of operations. U. S. military and industrial power tilted the balance against the forces of the German empire and solidified American leadership of the free world. The end of the war revealed the terrible genocides performed by Hitler's Nazi regime and Stalin's communist regime. As with World War I, this war brought technological developments, most significant of which was the unleashing of nuclear power that would not only end the war in the Pacific, but inaugurate decades of fear of world destruction.

The Cold War (1948–1990), resulting from the political confrontation of the United States and the Soviet Union after World War II, did not reach a real conflagration because both sides feared nuclear annihilation and had a military equilibrium. The collapse of the Soviet Union resulted in relative peace, threatened only by terrorist attacks and localized conflicts. Differences in the degrees of development of different areas of the world persisted, however, and gaps among the various nations have widened probably due to the commercial and economic globalization. Democratic governments replaced former unstable regimes and dictatorships in Latin America and other less developed areas.

## Medical Sciences

Scientific progress has been incessant and tremendous throughout the century.[1] The following are just a few examples of twentieth-century breakthroughs that changed science and the world:

1. The new fields of endocrinology, nutrition, hematology, immunology, and other areas of medicine brought an understanding of the etiology of many noninfectious diseases and clinical solutions to problems.
2. Discovery of antibiotics solved many infectious diseases, although resistant strains of microbes created some as yet unsolved problems.
3. Invention of the electron microscope, toward the middle of the century, allowed larger magnifications and better resolution, permitting exploration of the unknown world of cells and viruses.
4. Discovery in 1953 of the double helix structure of the DNA molecule, by James Watson and Francis Crick, allowed geneticists to reach a new level, and the identification of the human genome in 2000 promised solutions to numerous biological and medical puzzles.

5. The use of statistics to analyze clinical and basic problems and application of computers to medical science allowed the organization and analysis of experimental data, and the collection of personal and collective data in centers. This led to improvements in diagnostic and therapeutic decisions and development of mathematical models to analyze the causes and evolution of disease and the spread of epidemics.
6. New diagnostic methodology combined the computer with radiographic images or magnetic resonance, the development of renal dialysis, the heart-lung machine, and the transplantation of organs.

Two devastating worldwide epidemics decimated many populations: the 1918 influenza epidemic and, beginning in the 1980s, AIDS.[4,8] Also environmental contamination with the increase in toxic substances used in pesticides, detergents, solvents, and other synthetic chemical products, increased the incidence of certain types of malignancies and some chronic degenerative disorders such as Alzheimer disease.

Medical practice changed drastically. Private general practice that had expanded in the nineteenth century with the growing middle class, started to subdivide into specialties and subspecialties. This greatly improved the degree of expertise and the success in treatment and prevention of many diseases, but gradually resulted in reduced personal contact between physicians and patients. In addition, modern treatment required the use of expensive analyses and complicated equipment that increased greatly the cost of medical care. Higher costs meant increased reliance on medical insurance, and gradually the insurance companies created an industry in which the patient was relegated to a secondary role and profits governed medical decisions—a dilemma that continues to defy resolution.

## Dentistry

Dental practice advanced in the late nineteenth and early twentieth centuries by virtue of two important changes.[7] First, the gradual introduction of technological advances. For example, the use of electricity led to the operating light that freed the dentist from daylight, and permitted the redesign of dental offices to include the ergonomic design of equipment and improved positioning of the patient. Moreover, the use of electrically driven rotary cutting instruments revolutionized operative dentistry; the use of local anesthesia (Chapter 12) made possible not only improved surgical techniques (Chapter 22), but also operative dentistry and prosthodontic methods; the discovery and development of radiology improved diagnosis and therapy (see Chapters 14 and 20).

Second, dentists realized that single-handed dentistry could be vastly improved by dental assistants. So early in the century practitioners began delegating some aspects of dental therapy, particularly those related to prevention, to trained assistants that became dental hygienists (see Chapter 29).

In the second half of the century, dental practice continued its incessant evolution, to some extent subdividing into multiple specialties (endodontics, oral surgery, orthodontics, pediatric dentistry, periodontics, and prosthodontics). The majority of practitioners, however, continued to be generalists.

Progress in dentistry was marked in the twentieth century by the discovery of the preventive effect of fluoride on dental caries and by researchers' and clinicians' efforts to unravel the intricacies of the periodontal disease problem, and develop methods for its solution and prevention. The preventive effect of fluoride on dental caries was hinted in Europe in the nineteenth century,[3] but it was the efforts of a group of American researchers that brought the caries problem to a satisfactory solution.

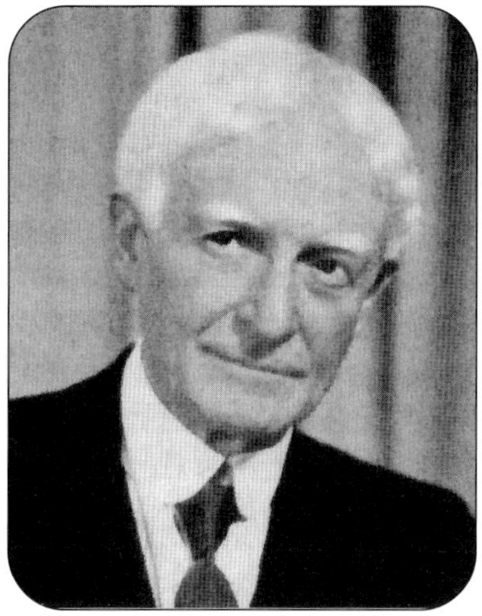

**Fig 43** William G. Gies.

In May of 1908, American scientist Frederick McKay (1874–1959), of Colorado Springs, first identified the relationship between mottled enamel, common in that region, and the presence of fluoride in drinking water. In 1925, McKay established that fluoride in drinking water not only produced mottled enamel, but also inhibited dental caries.

After a number of laboratory and epidemiologic studies, a team of researchers at the U.S. Department of Public Health, led by H. Trendley Dean (1893–1962), confirmed the caries-preventive effect of fluoride in drinking water. This led to the fluoridation of water supplies in many communities throughout the world, which, in addition to the incorporation of fluorides in dentifrices, and its preventive application in children, has resulted in the virtual elimination of dental caries in populations where these methods are applied.

The development of basic biomedical research in dentistry constituted the foundation for the sustained progress of periodontology in the twentieth century. One force in biomedical research was a scientist whose vision and leadership guided dental investigation at this time. William G. Gies (1872–1956) (Fig 43) was a biochemist at Columbia University, promoter of dental research and dental education, and an inspiration to many dentists to learn the basic sciences and follow a career in dental research. Gies was one of the founders of the *Journal of Dental Research* in 1919, and in 1920, the International Association of Dental Research.[6]

The dean of the Chicago College of Dentistry at Loyola University, William H. G. Logan (1873–1943), a man of vision and integrity, a scientist and a leader, created in 1927 an Institute of Dental Research at Loyola, following the lead of Bernhard Gottlieb's institute at the University of Vienna.[5] The creation in 1948 of the National Institute of Dental Research, as part of the National Institutes of Health, in Bethesda, Maryland, gave extraordinary impetus to dental and oral research, through research at the institute and grants awarded to investigators in other research facilities.

All these efforts resulted in a new generation of periodontal researchers and educators who, by combining their clinical expertise with a profound understanding of the basic sciences, promoted periodontics to new levels. In the second half of the century, the rise of the Scandinavian school of periodontal research played a key role in the development of new concepts in the basic understanding of, as well as clinical approach to, the solution of periodontal problems.

The increasing realization that periodontal disease was a leading cause of tooth loss and the understanding that more than mechanical and technical approaches were needed to solve this problem, led to investigations in the basic sciences. Researchers directed their attention to histology, pathology, microbiology, biochemistry, immunology, genetics, and many other areas, and followed, when pertinent, with efforts to transfer the basic science findings to clinical approaches and techniques. All these research activities in periodontics have been at the forefront of dental science in the twentieth century and have influenced other areas of dentistry. The chapters that follow present briefly the efforts by twentieth-century periodontal researchers.

## References

1. Carranza F. Revolucionarios de la Ciencia. Buenos Aires: Vergara, 1998.
2. Field MJ (ed). Dental Education at the Crossroads. Washington, DC: National Academy Press, 1995.
3. Hoffmann-Axthelm W. History of Dentistry. Chicago: Quintessence, 1981.
4. Kolata G. Flu: The Story of the Great Influenza Pandemic of 1918 and the Search for the Virus That Caused It. New York: Simon & Schuster, 1999.
5. Obituary, William Hoffman Gardiner Logan. J Am Dent Assoc 1943;30:968.
6. Orland FJ. William John Gies: His Contributions to the Advancement of Dentistry. The William J. Gies Foundation for the Advancement of Dentistry, 1992.
7. Pickard HM. Conservative Dentistry in the Past Century. Br Dent J 1980;149:5.
8. Ryan F. Virus X. Boston: Little, Brown, 1997.
9. Starr P. The Social Transformation of American Medicine. New York: Basic Books, 1984.

# 18

# Periodontal Histopathology 1900–1950

The technical and scientific advances in pathology and microbiology of the nineteenth century and early twentieth centuries were soon reflected in studies on periodontology. During the first half of the century studies in periodontal pathology were descriptive analyses of histological sections of human or, less frequently, animal specimens. Human material was obtained at autopsy and permitted a clear analysis and description of the normal periodontal tissues and their changes in pathological conditions. By mid-twentieth century excellent descriptions of tissue changes were available, and investigators turned their attention to identifying changes at the cellular level, using the recently developed electron microscope, and the effects of various experimental conditions on the periodontium of animals.

The first publication on periodontal histopathology appeared in 1902. N. N. Znamensky, professor of stomatology at the University of Moscow, shows clear understanding of the nature of periodontitis, and the interaction of local and systemic factors in its etiology. He offers the first description of the histopathology of periodontal disease, demonstrating the close association between calculus, the inflammatory response, and the migration of the junctional epithelium to produce a periodontal pocket.[77]

Znamensky relates one case obtained at autopsy of a 39 year old woman who had died of a hemorrhage after parturition. He traces the inflammatory infiltrate in the gingiva (Fig 44), its extension to the bone and the lacunar resorption of the bone with multinucleated osteoclasts, proceeding from the periosteal side of the alveolar crest and from the Haversian canals, leading to destruction of the socket (Fig 45). He summarizes his findings as follows[77]:

> The whole picture of the anatomo-pathological alterations exhibited in their gradual course, show very distinctly that the development of alveolar pyorrhea proceeds from the periphery to the centre, i.e., primarily inflammatory phenomena originate in the gum and then successively pass into the very bone and periosteum of the socket. This process is not an atrophical one, but a chronic inflammation; the secretion of pus (at the same time with the loosening of the tooth and a denuding of the root in consequence of the disappearance of the socket at a certain stage) I consider to be one of the cardinal symptoms of the ailment. …
>
> The above described microscopical pictures show that we have here to do with a rarefying inflammation-osteitis rarefaciens.

He goes on to differentiate between alveolar pyorrhea and atrophy of the socket, explaining how the latter occurs in the absence of inflammation, with a normal gum and no tartar and no pus discharge. Next Znamensky turns his attention to etiology, recognizing that there are two schools of thought[77]:

> [S]ome authors thought it a local expression of a constant and continual irritation of the gums, produced by mechanical, chemical, and other forms of irritation. Others took it for a manifestation of some common constitutional ailment.

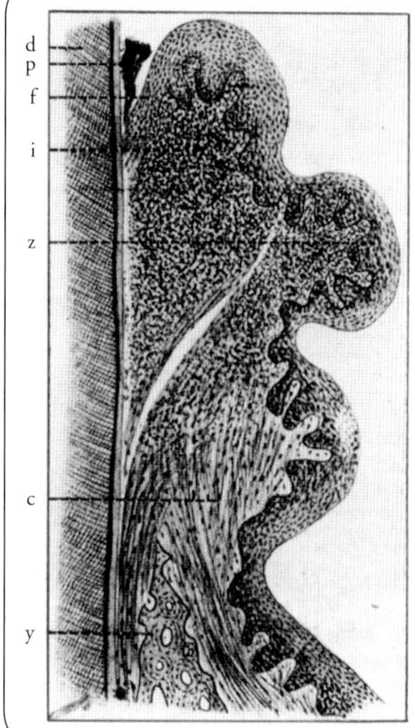


**Fig 44** Figure from Znamensky's article.[77] His legend follows: "d, dentine of the tooth; p, tartar; f, papillary layer of bone; z, epithelial covering; i, infiltration of the gum with white blood corpuscles; c, healthy part of the gum; y, healthy bone. Magnified 80 times."

**Fig 45** Another figure from Znamensky's article[77] showing osteoclasts in Howship's lacunae.

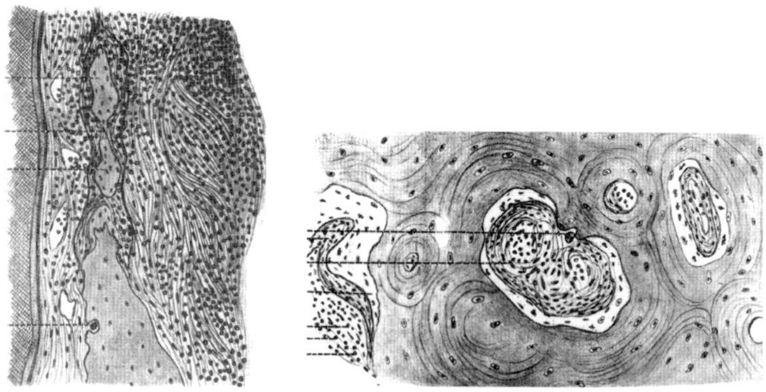

He believed that

> for the development of an alveolar pyorrhea in common constitutional ailments, on one side there is a prepared soil in the form of an osteoporous atrophy of the socket, and on the other a series of acting local conditions, the first place of which is given to tartar. But it must be noted, that not every constitutional disorder or exhausting disease is to be necessarily associated with atrophy of the sockets.

Znamensky realized that there are "some constitutional disorders which sometimes particularly quickly cause an atrophy of sockets, among such may be included rickets, tabes dorsalis and diabetes."

Early in the century (1901) the Viennese dentist Moritz Karolyi (1865–1945), a student of Joseph Arkövy, described grinding and clenching the jaws and blamed it for the destruction of bone associated with periodontal disease; he recommended occlusal correction to prevent it and the use of bite plates at night.[45]

In 1911, A. Hopewell-Smith of England, published two papers[36,38,39] describing the microscopic findings made in three human specimens. In the first paper[38] Hopewell-Smith details epithelial changes, mentioning the "hydropic degeneration," and proliferation of the basal cell layer; in the gingival connective tissue he describes the presence of "great masses of inflammatory cells—consisting of crowds of polymorphonuclear neutrophiles, eosinophiles, lymphocytes, and lymphoid cells, with numerous mast cells and Unna's plasma cells."

Hopewell-Smith describes massive bacterial invasion of the gingival tissues. Then he outlines changes in the periodontal membrane, pointing, in the cervical area, to hyperemia, cellular infiltration, hyperplasia of the fibrous elements, and an increase in width. In more apical areas he finds slight cellular proliferation, and "no great amount of round-cell infiltration or leukocytic invasion." He also notes the presence of "gland-like bodies."

In the cementum, Hopewell-Smith reports thickening and Howship's "foveolae" (lacunae) occupied by large "myeloplaxes" (osteoclasts). In the bone he discerns bone loss by three processes: osteoclastic resorption, halisteresis, and "by means of perforating canals," the first two being more common.

Hopewell-Smith concluded that

> pyorrhea alveolaris does not begin as a gingivitis ... and it is essentially dependent upon an osseous lesion, *an atrophy of the bone,* which in the thinnest parts causes the cervical margins of the teeth to become denuded through the halisteresis and osteoclastic resorption. ... The pus associated with it, is derived from débris of food, pyogenic bacteria and other extraneous elements. ... The presence of serumal calculus is not sufficient in itself to induce the condition, and may not be associated with it at all as a predisposing or exciting cause.[38]

In the second paper[39] Hopewell-Smith looks at another human specimen to conclude that

> Atrophy of the bony socket and shrinkage is followed by a widening of the gingival margin and broadening and deepening of the pockets, with hyperplasia of the periodontal membrane. If a pathogenic infection occurs, there is a lodgement of pathogenic bacteria in these already suitable pockets, and pyorrhea results, and it may or may not be accompanied by gingivitis and the production of tartar.

Eugene S. Talbot (1847–1924) was a prominent dentist and physician in Chicago. In 1913 he published *Interstitial Gingivitis and Pyorrhea Alveolaris,* based on investigations of the previous twenty-five years.[72] The book includes detailed microscopic descriptions of the periodontal tissues of one 60-year-old individual, and numerous dogs. Talbot rejects the name *pyorrhea alveolaris* because it "implies that there must always be a flow of pus, and hence that the disease must always result from infection with pus microbes."

He prefers the term *interstitial gingivitis.* The word *interstitial,* according to Talbot, who quotes various lexicographers, refers to "a condition disseminated through the substance of an organ or part, and to an inflammation affecting the connective tissue of an organ." Talbot contends that inflammation may be of bacterial origin but can also be caused by various "irritants or poisons circulating in the blood at any locality between the gum margin and the apical end of the root of the tooth."

Talbot defines interstitial gingivitis as a "local inflammatory condition of the gums, or alveolar process, or both, tending to accelerate the normal tendency to disappearance at certain periods of stress, or involution, of which involution the changes produced by old age are a type." He recognizes the important role of bacteria, although "there is no specific germ which is capable of producing the disease itself, and furthermore, that the pyorrhea stage is merely a complication due to pyogenic germ infection of the already diseased gums." Talbot argues for the existance of local predisposing factors and toxic agents.

Greene Vardiman Black (1836–1915), prominent researcher and educator, and dean of Northwestern University School of Dentistry in Chicago, published in 1915 a 489-page book covering in detail the diagnosis and treatment of periodontal and pulpal diseases.[11] After presenting the clinical and microscopic features of the periodontal tissues, Black describes gingivitis and pericementitis due to deposits of salivary calculus, its treatment by removal of the deposits, the removal of serumal calculus, and then chronic suppurative pericementitis (previously called *phagedenic pericementitis* by Black), which leads to the formation of "pus pockets." Clinical, radiographic, and histologic photographs (some in color) and diagrams illustrate the book. Black notes that gingivitis always precedes pocket formation, that only a very limited number of cases recognize a systemic causation, and that microorganisms, especially *Endameba buccalis,* are always associated with the lesions, although its etiologic role was yet undetermined.

G. V. Black's son, Arthur D. Black, (1870–1937), was a clinical dentist and scholar and also became dean of Northwestern University School of Dentistry and originated the *Index to Dental Periodical Literature.* In a 1920 paper he summarizes the pathological events leading to periodontal disease as follows:

> [G]ingival irritation allows a microbial invasion. Systemic conditions may reduce tissue resistance to bacterial invasion so that this may occur without apparent local irritation. The infection which penetrates the tissue is taken up by perivascular lymphatics and travels into the peridental membrane along the blood vessel walls. ... The cemental attachment of the periodontal fibers gradually disappears, leaving the cementum denuded. The rest of the fiber and the bone are absorbed and destroyed.[10]

He further argues that salivary calculus is unrelated to pocket formation, but that serumal calculus does cause pockets.

## The Vienna School

In the central European countries medical sciences evolved vigorously in the late nineteenth and early twentieth centuries. In Austria, dentistry was a specialty of medicine while in Germany it was an independent profession, as in the United States.[40]

A major part of the extraordinary progress in the understanding of the biological basis of dentistry and several of its subspecialties (periodontics, endodontics, and orthodontics), between 1920 and 1960, is attributable to a group of European scientists working at the University of Vienna. They were forced to emigrate to America as a result of Nazi persecution of Jews.

The leader of this group, Bernhard Gottlieb (Fig 46), was born in Poland in 1886 and received his MD from the University of Vienna in 1912. During World War I, Gottlieb was a distinguished officer in the Austro-Hungarian Army and, after the war, returned to Vienna where he organized his laboratory and opened a private practice with his student Balint Orban.[46,53,54]

Numerous investigations on the histopathology of periodontal disease started to appear in the German literature and many were translated into English in American journals.[22,26–30,60–62,74] These papers describe the mechanism of the union between the epithelium and the tooth (epithelial attachment), the microscopic tissue changes in periodontal pockets, effects of traumatic occlusion, and so on. The studies form the basis of periodontal biology as it is understood today. A book published by Gottlieb and Orban in 1938[33] synthesized their findings and concepts of periodontal histology and pathology. Their book also includes complete list of the Vienna group's publications until 1935.

Gottlieb's concept of the formation of the epithelial attachment[25] was as follows[28]:

> Before the eruption of the tooth, the outer layer of the enamel epithelium is attached to the enamel surface and the two are grown together. There is no space between the epithelium and the enamel surface. Before the enamel is visible, the epithelium of the mouth and the outer layer of the enamel epithelium grow together, and, through an opening at the point of union, the enamel comes into the mouth. Next, the epithelium detaches itself from the enamel surface as the tooth erupts. When the tooth reaches a position that is in occlusion with the opposing teeth, we speak of eruption as completed. We previously believed that the bottom of the pocket was now at the cemento-enamel junction. But not so: The detachment of the epithelium from the enamel surface has never, at this period, reached that point. Only about two thirds of the crown has really come through the gum. The last third is still one with the epithelium, and the saliva, for instance, or food or microorganisms cannot reach this part of the enamel surface. This part is really not yet erupted. In the years following, the detachment goes on. Between the ages of 20 and 30, the bottom of the pocket passes the cemento-enamel junction.

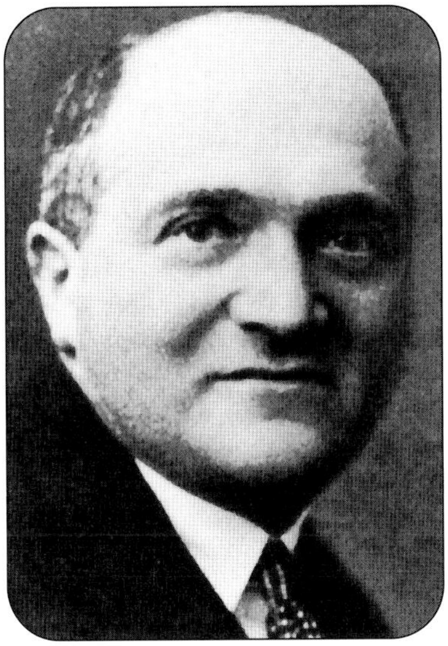

**Fig 46** Bernhard Gottlieb.

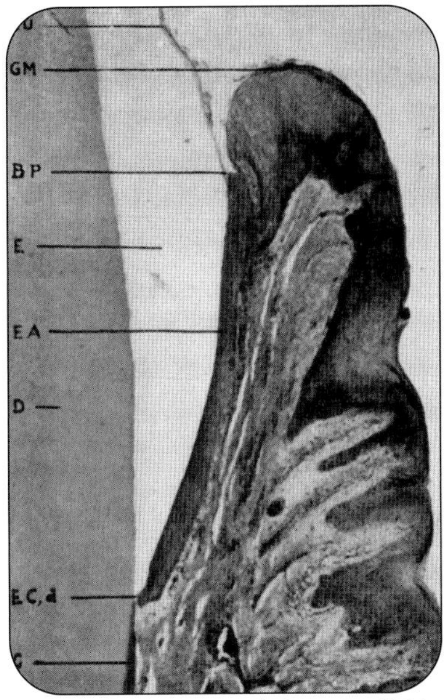


**Fig 47** Photomicrograph from Gottlieb's paper,[28] illustrating his description of the gingival attachment.

> I say passes, not reaches. It can never be seen either in man or in animals (we have studied thousands of teeth microscopically) that the bottom of the pocket is at any time around the whole tooth at the cemento-enamel junction. On the one side of the tooth, the bottom passes this point earlier, on another later. But it does not remain at this point any longer than at another point of the tooth surface. Before the bottom of the pocket reaches the cemento-enamel junction, a proliferation of the epithelium along the cementum begins so that the epithelium is always attached to the tooth surface, enamel or cementum.

Figure 47, from Gottlieb's article, illustrates his description. Gottlieb calls the epithelium that is attached to the tooth (enamel or cementum) the *epithelial attachment.* His concept was challenged in 1952 by Jens Waerhaug and finally clarified by the electron microscopic studies of Hubert Schroeder and Max Listgarten in 1971. After Schroeder and Listgarten's investigations, the meaning of the term *epithelial attachment* changed. It now refers not to the epithelium itself but to the mechanism of union, and the epithelium itself is now called the *junctional epithelium.*

Gottlieb envisioned the bottom of the gingival sulcus/periodontal pocket located at the coronal end of the epithelial attachment, where this tissue separates from the cuticle (*cuticula dentis*) that covers the enamel, and that is seen in histological sections by a short, thin line extending for a short distance over the empty space of the decalcified enamel.

Some of his contemporaries disagreed with this idea. German histologist Hermann Becks (1897–1962), who was professor at the University of California, San Francisco, contended that when the oral epithelium fused with the enamel epithelium, the degeneration of the enamel epithelium progresses apically, while the oral epithelium proliferates downward to cover the defect. This would mean that the normal pocket forms between the oral epithelium, which now forms the pocket epithelium and the more or less degenerate enamel epithelium.[7] Another researcher,

Oskar Weski (also discussed later in this chapter), suggested that the bottom of the sulcus was an intraepithelial split. William Skillen, of Northwestern University, carried out extensive research in support of Gottlieb's ideas.[67–70]

Gottlieb assigned a key role in pocket formation to the cementum. He believed that downgrowth of the epithelial attachment was a physiologic phenomenon, which occurred as part of the continuous eruption of the tooth, and that the continuous deposition of cementum acts as a barrier that slows down the rate of epithelial migration.

Gottlieb classified periodontal disease into four groups: *(1) Schmutzpyorrhea* (filth pyorrhea), characterized by calculus, infection, suppuration, and bone loss; *(2) paradental pyorrhea* (deep, irregular pockets); *(3) diffuse atrophy*, characterized by tooth mobility, extrusion, migration of teeth, with lack of inflammation (later called *periodontosis*, now called *aggressive periodontitis*); *(4) traumatic occlusion* identified by bone loss and tooth mobility.[36]

In 1938 Hitler invaded Austria, and Gottlieb was forced to leave the country. He sent his family to London while he went to Tel-Aviv, where he tried to create a research institute. The political situation, however, prevented him from reaching this goal, forcing him to change his plans and go to England. Unable to obtain a university position in the United Kingdom, Gottlieb emigrated to the United States, where he obtained an appointment at the University of Michigan. Gottlieb later became professor of pathology and dental research at Baylor College of Dentistry in Dallas, Texas. He was in difficult financial straits when he died in Dallas in 1950.[46,53,54]

Balint J. Orban (Fig 48) was born in Temesvar, Hungary, on March 24, 1899. Orban obtained his medical degree from the University of Budapest in 1922 and moved to Vienna where he became Gottlieb's student and coworker. In 1927 he was invited by Loyola University to head the Dental Research Institute of the Chicago College of Dental Surgery. He accepted the invitation and spent two years in Chicago before returning to Vienna in 1929. In 1930 he received a second medical degree from the University of Vienna.

Although Orban was born Jewish, he had converted to Catholicism many years previously. Correctly suspecting he would also be persecuted, he returned to the United States in 1938. His second immigration was highly successful. He was professor of oral pathology and director of research at Loyola from 1940 to 1947. Next he was research fellow at the University of Illinois until 1952, when he returned to Loyola as professor and chairman of periodontology, a position he retained until his death. Orban created a dental research foundation in Colorado Springs and died of a heart attack in 1960.[46,57,58]

Orban authored many research papers and several books that gave a solid biologic foundation to periodontics and other specialties. His greatest contribution to the world of science was the creation of a school, with numerous disciples that led the progress of world dentistry for many decades.

Orban continued and refined Gottlieb's theories of the epithelial attachment, continuous eruption, and pocket formation[61,62]; gave the first detailed microscopic description of the effect of trauma from occlusion on the human periodontium[60]; and provided the biologic basis for numerous clinical procedures. Several editions of his books on dental histology and embryology and on periodontics were published, and his disciples continued publishing them for several decades after his death.

Rudolph Kronfeld (Fig 49) was born in Vienna on December 10, 1901. As a child, he was fascinated by botany; at 10 years old he could identify all plants and flowers around Vienna. Regularly engaged in outdoor activities, Kronfeld was an excellent skier, mountain climber, and yachtsman and he won trophies in each sport.

Kronfeld obtained his medical degree from the University of Vienna in 1926. He conducted research under Gottlieb, before replacing Balint Orban as director of the Dental Research Institute of the Chicago College of Dental Surgery at Loyola University, in 1929. In 1933 he obtained the DDS degree from the University of Chicago. Moreover he published extensively

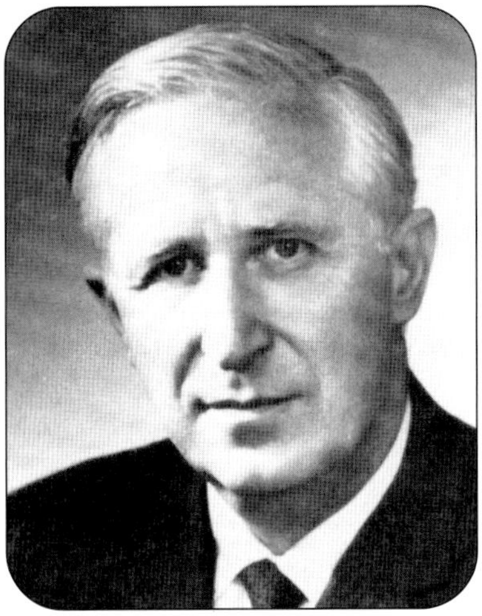

Fig 48 Balint J. Orban.

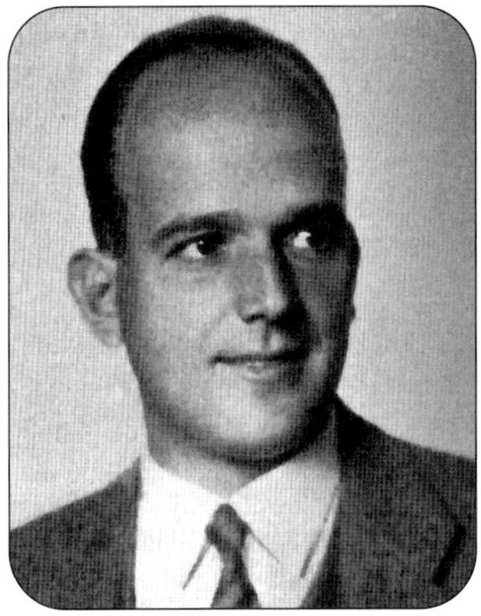

Fig 49 Rudolph Kronfeld.

in German and American journals and authored a classic text on periodontal histopathology.[49] Kronfeld was not only a gifted educator and a brilliant researcher, but also a leader in providing a biologic foundation for the diagnosis and treatment of oral diseases.

Rudolph Kronfeld's life ended tragically. In the winter of 1938, he contracted a serious chronic neurologic disease (possibly Lou Gehrig disease). Illness was unbearable for the active sportsman, and he could not endure the prospect of life as an invalid. On February 13, 1939, he was found dead in his laboratory. He had committed suicide. He was 37 years old.[55,56]

Two other members of the Vienna school merit attention (Fig 50). Harry Sicher (1889–1974) was an Austrian doctor, student of the renowned anatomist Julius Tandler. In Vienna he practiced oral surgery, before moving to the United States in 1939. Sicher was professor of anatomy and histology at Loyola University School of Dentistry. He published numerous research papers and a text, *Oral Anatomy*, which became the standard reference book in the field. In addition, Sicher co-authored *Bone and Bones* with Joseph Weinmann (see below). An outstanding teacher and investigator, Sicher was also an accomplished musician (he played the violin and directed chamber music groups) and had an impressive collection of butterflies.[59]

Joseph Peter Weinmann (1896–1960) was born in Bohemia, joined Gottlieb's laboratory after graduating with his MD in 1923, and emigrated to the United States in 1938. He was a faculty member at Columbia and Loyola universities and in 1946 joined the University of Illinois, becoming head of oral pathology in 1949. He was a prolific researcher, particularly in the area of bone biology and pathology. His book *Bone and Bones*, in collaboration with Sicher, provides an outstanding description of the anatomy, biology, physiology, and pathology of bone tissue. The text proved influential over the world and was translated into several languages.

Weinmann made two fundamental contributions to periodontal pathology. In 1941 he published a paper demonstrating that gingival inflammation follows the tissue around blood vessels in its progress to the supporting tissues.[74] In 1942 Orban and Weinmann introduced the term *periodontosis* (now called *aggressive periodontitis*) and described the three stages that, according to their theory, occur as the disease progresses (degeneration of cervical periodontal ligament fibers, epithelial migration, and pocket formation).[63]

The pathogenesis of aggressive periodontitis offers a useful example of the evolution of knowledge in the decades between 1920 and 1950. In 1923 Gottlieb reported on a patient who

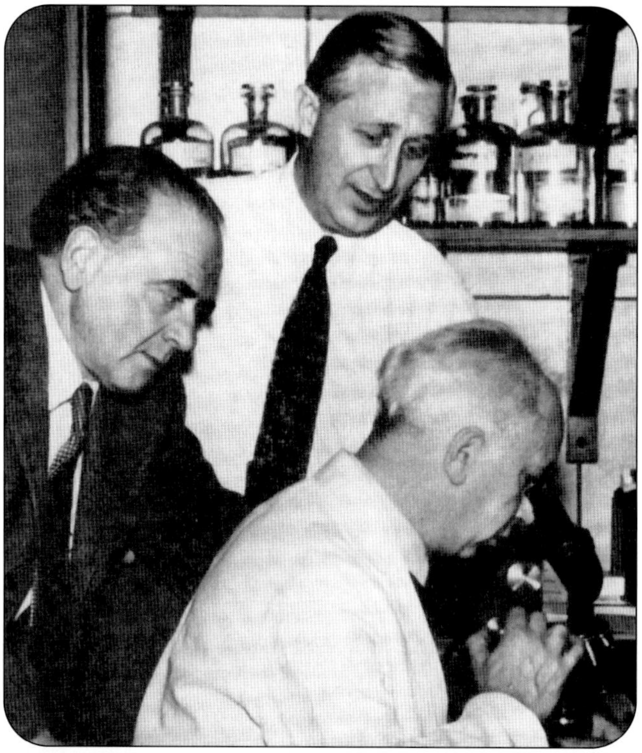

**Fig 50** Harry Sicher, Balint Orban, and Joseph Weinmann *(left to right)*. (Photo by Daniel Grant.)

had died of influenza and presented what he called "diffuse atrophy of the alveolar bone," which Gottlieb described as a loss of collagen fibers of the periodontal ligament, replaced by loose connective tissue and causing extensive bone loss; the gingiva was apparently uninvolved.[26] In 1928, Gottlieb hypothesized that this disease was caused by an inhibition of cementum formation and called it *deep cementopathia.*[31]

Ten years later E. Wannenmacher (1897–1974) described the disease as inflammatory in character and having an incisor–first molar distribution; he called it *parodontitis marginalis progressiva.* In 1940 Kurt H. Thoma and Henry M. Goldman, of Harvard University, suggested the initial abnormality occurs in alveolar bone, resulting in vascular resorption and halisteresis rather that osteoclastic resorption.[73] Finally, in 1942 Orban and Weinmann presented their theory (see above). It was not until the 1970s that the bacterial etiology of the disease was described by Michael G. Newman and Sigmund Socransky.[51]

The first measurements made on histological slides were those of Rudolph Kronfeld in 1931 and Edgar Coolidge in 1937. Kronfeld measured the width of the periodontal ligament in functioning and nonfunctioning teeth[48] while Coolidge measured the same parameter in fifteen human jaws in relation to age.[20]

Oskar Weski (1879–1952) (Fig 51) was born in Eastern Prussia, received his medical degree from the University of Eastern Prussia and then studied dentistry, deepening his studies in histology and specializing in radiology at the Charité Hospital in Berlin. Weski never held a university appointment,[37] but he conducted research that resulted in seventy publications, mainly in the area of radiology and periodontics,[76] correlating clinical, microscopic, and radiologic observations. He differed from Gottlieb locating the bottom of the sulcus/pocket, and he denied that eruption continued after the tooth reaches the plane of occlusion.

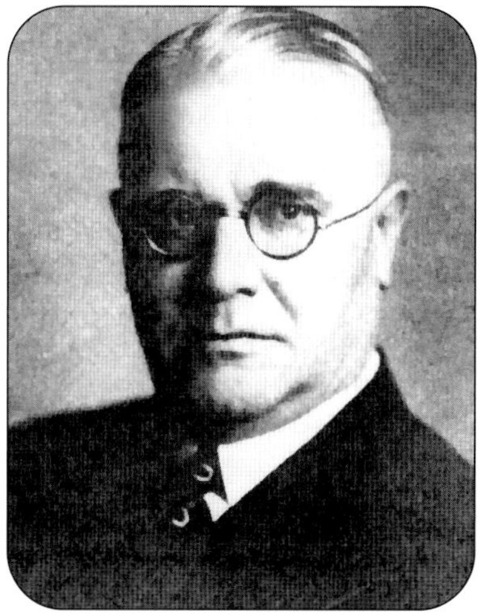

**Fig 51** Oskar Weski.

Weski conceived of a periodontal organ, which he called the *paradentium* (now *periodontium*), composed of gingiva, alveolar bone, periodontal ligament, and cementum. This novel concept was based on the common embryological origin of cementum, periodontal ligament and bone, and their common involvement in pathological processes. As a derivative of the term *paradentium*, the name *pyorrhea alveolaris* was gradually abandoned and replaced by *paradentosis* and *paradentitis*, terms that were used in many countries.

For Weski, the basic pathologic change in periodontal disease was a "dystrophic atrophy of the bone"; he did not accept gingival inflammation or infection as the initial change leading to periodontal destruction. Weski distinguished between horizontal and vertical bone losses (he called them *atrophies*), characterizing suprabony and infrabony pockets and also the existence of cases with or without pocket formation. On this distinction he based the classification of periodontal diseases, in total atrophy (early or juvenile and late or senile) and partial atrophy (horizontal or vertical, each with or without pockets). This classification was used in Europe and South America for decades, although authors like Wannenmacher, Haüpl, Kantorowicz, and others opposed it.

In Germany, Weski founded the institution for research in periodontology, called ARPA, after the initials of its name in German in 1923, and later the International ARPA, together with other scientists (see Chapter 26).

Weski lectured extensively in Europe and South America. While speaking in Argentina in 1949, he suffered a cerebrovascular accident that severely limited his activities. He died in Berlin in 1952.

Harold Keith Box (1890–1956), born in Canada, was associated with the University of Toronto as professor of dental pathology and periodontology (1920–1927) and as research professor of periodontology (1927–1956).[51] Box published extensively on periodontal histopathology,[13–18] describing in humans the normal periodontal tissues and their changes in disease. In an early paper[12] Box points out that early inflammatory reaction follows the initial invasion of bacteria, leading to loss of some of the epithelial lining and gingival ulceration. The resultant inflammatory response results in exudation of desquamated epithelial cells and leukocytes.

> Due to the action of ferments, either by the polymorphonuclear leucocytes or by bacteria, tissue solution takes place, resulting in the stripping of gingival tissue from the cementum and the formation of a small pocket. Penetration of this pocket into the deeper tissues, following further bacterial invasion, results in the complete loss of attachment of the cemental gingiva to the cementum, and in the establishment of ulceration and pocket formation in the pericementum.

Box suggests, too, that pocket deepening may be related to specific bacterial agents.

Two German investigators, Karl Haüpl (1893–1960) and F. J. Lang, argue, in a 1927 study, that all periodontal diseases are inflammatory in nature, albeit sometimes not clinically apparent, and call them *paradentitis marginale*.[35] Haüpl and Lang also mention the invasion of the periodontal ligament by inflammatory cells under the influence of trauma from occlusion.[34,35]

In 1928 British investigators W. W. James and A. Counsell[36,42] challenged Hopewell-Smith's concept of the osseous origin of the disease, placing the initial lesion in the gingiva. Their description of the marginal periodontal lesion, based on their histologic sections, is remarkably accurate, reporting an abundance of plasma cells in the lesions, but "the periodontal membrane remains singularly free from the presence of inflammatory cells."[42]

Early in the century, Alfred Kantorowicz (1880–1962), director of the Dental Institute of the University of Bonn, Germany, was first to clearly separate the inflammatory from the dystrophic changes, classifying periodontal diseases into *paradentitis* and *paradentosis*.[43,44]

E. Wilfred Fish, of St. Mary's Hospital in London, published a book in 1948, in which he describes "parodontal disease" as an inflammatory disease that he summarizes as follows:

> Commencing as persistent traumatic ulceration of the gum margin the epithelium becomes detached from the enamel—chronic marginal gingivitis. The parodontal fibres are progressively destroyed by diffusion of soluble proteolytic and toxic substances from these ulcers—pyorrhœa simplex. Bacteria become implanted traumatically in the parodontal membrane causing parodontal abscesses which on opening into the sulcus produce the deep pockets of pyorrhœa profunda.[21]

Fish describes bone changes as resorption and sclerosis, and says that bone is never infected.

Several other European investigators made important contributions to the histology and pathology of the periodontal tissues. Among them are German scientists H. Adrion, J. Lehner and H. Plenck, W. Meyer, R. Meyer, H. Euler, O. Lund, and F. Neuwirth; English investigators J. R. Toller, P. Pincus, and R. D. Emslie; and Italian researcher A. Beretta.

In Argentina, Rodolfo Erausquin (1883–1945), dentist, physician, and professor of pathology at the University of Buenos Aires Dental School, and Fermin Carranza Sr. (1900–1988), periodontist and later professor of periodontics at the same university, conducted important investigations in the pathology of periodontal disease, correlating the clinical (in vivo and postmortem), the microscopic, and the radiographic findings,[2–5,19] and presenting a statistical analysis of their results, using histometric techniques.[3–5] They classified the periodontium into the periodontium of protection (gingiva) and the periodontium of attachment (bone, periodontal ligament, and cementum). Unfortunately the untimely death of Erausquin, on January 2, 1945, prevented the continuation of the studies and eventual synthesis of the findings.

Alfonso Leng (1884–1974) was a Chilean dentist, professor of periodontics, and founding dean of the University of Chile Faculty of Dentistry. During the 1930s and 1940s, Leng pioneered investigations into the biochemical aspects of the periodontal tissues in health and disease. In addition, Leng was an accomplished musical composer; his music has been presented by such noted conductors as Erich Kleiber, Malcolm Sargent, and Fritz Busch. Leng earned several prestigious artistic awards in his country.

## References


1. Aisenberg MS, Aisenberg AD. A new concept of pocket formation. Oral Surg Oral Med Oral Pathol 1948;1:1047.
2. Ballbé R, Carranza FA Sr, Erausquin R. Los paradencios del caso número siete. Rev Odontol (Buenos Aires) 1941;29:600.
3. Ballbé R, Carranza FA Sr, Erausquin R. Los paradencios del caso número ocho. Rev Odontol (Buenos Aires) 1942;30:606.
4. Ballbé R, Carranza FA Sr, Erausquin R. Los paradencios del caso número nueve. Rev Odontol (Buenos Aires) 1943;31:313,398,451.
5. Ballbé R, Carranza FA Sr, Erausquin R. Los paradencios del caso número once. Rev Odontol (Buenos Aires) 1944;32:383.
6. Bass CC, Johns FM. Pyorrhea dentalis and alveolaris. JAMA 1915;64:553.
7. Becks H. Normal and pathologic pocket formation. J Am Dent Assoc 1929;16:2167.
8. Becks H. What determines the early stages of paradentosis (alveolar pyorrhea)? J Am Dent Assoc 1931;18:922.
9. Beckwith TD, Simonton FV, Williams A. A histologic study of the gum in pyorrhea. J Am Dent Assoc 1925;12:129.
10. Black AD. The pathology and treatment of diseases of the peridental membrane. Dent Cosmos 1920;62:820.
11. Black GV. Special Dental Pathology. Chicago: Medico-Dental, 1915.
12. Box HK. The evolution of the periodontal pus-pocket. Canadian Dental Research Foundation, Bulletin #1, May 1921.
13. Box HK. Studies in Periodontal Pathology. Canadian Dental Research Foundation, Bulletin #7, May 1924.
14. Box HK. Treatment of the Periodontal Pocket. Toronto: University of Toronto Press, 1928.
15. Box HK. Microscopic Studies of the Periodontal Pocket. Toronto: University of Toronto Press, 1928.
16. Box HK. Traumatic occlusion and traumatogenic occlusion. Oral Health 1930;20:642.
17. Box HK. Necrotic Gingivitis. Toronto: University of Toronto Press, 1930.
18. Box HK. The significance of recent findings in periodontal pathology. J Dent Res 1948;14:543.
19. Carranza FA Sr, Erausquin R. Primeros hallazgos paradentosicos. Rev Odontol (Buenos Aires) 1939;27:486.
20. Coolidge ED. The thickness of the human periodontal membrane. J Am Dent Assoc 1937;24:1260.
21. Fish EW. Surgical Pathology of the Mouth. London: Isaac Pitman & Sons, 1948.
22. Fleischmann L, Gottlieb B. A contribution to the histology and pathogenesis of pyorrhea alveolaris. Dent Cosmos 1921;63:215,375.
23. Glickman I. Clinical Periodontology. Philadelphia: Saunders, 1953.
24. Goldman HM. The relationship of the epithelial attachment to the adjacent fibers of the periodontal membrane. J Dent Res 1944;23:117.
25. Gottlieb B. Der Epithelansatz am Zahne. Dtsch Monattschr Zahnheilk 1921;39:142.
26. Gottlieb B. Die diffuse Atrophy der Alveolarknochens. Z Stomatol 1923;21:195.
27. Gottlieb B. Schmützpyorrhea, Paradentalpyorrhea und Alveolaratrophie. Vienna: Urban & Schwarzenberg, 1925.
28. Gottlieb B. What is a normal pocket? J Am Dent Assoc 1926;13:1747.
29. Gottlieb B. Traumatic occlusion. J Am Dent Assoc 1927;14:1276.
30. Gottlieb B. Tissue changes in pyorrhea. J Am Dent Assoc 1927;14:2178.
31. Gottlieb B. The formation of the pocket: diffuse atrophy of the alveolar bone. J Am Dent Assoc 1928;15:462.
32. Gottlieb B. Continuous deposition of cementum. J Am Dent Assoc 1943;30:842.
33. Gottlieb B, Orban BJ. Biology and Pathology of the Tooth and Its Supporting Mechanism. Diamond M (trans). New York: Macmillan, 1938.
34. Hanford WH, Patten CO, Westbay C, Simonton FV. A contribution to our knowledge of pyorrhea from the standpoint of histo-pathology. Dent Cosmos 1923;65:12.
35. Haüpl K, Lang FJ. Marginale Paradentitis. Berlin: Meusser, 1927.
36. Held A-J. Periodontology. From Its Origins Up to 1980: A Survey. Basel: Birkhäuser, 1989.
37. Held A-J. Oskar Weski (1879–1952). Bull Hist Dent 1991;39:77.
38. Hopewell-Smith A. Pyorrhea alveolaris—Its patho-histology. I. Preliminary note. Dent Cosmos 1911;53:397.
39. Hopewell-Smith A. Pyorrhea alveolaris—Its interpretation. II. Concluding note. Dent Cosmos 1911;53:981.
40. Huff DW. A comparison of American and German dentistry, 1850–1900. Bull Hist Dent 1985;33:47.

41. James WW, Counsell A. A histological investigation into so-called pyorrhea alveolaris. Br Dent J 1927;48:1237.
42. James WW, Counsell A. The primary lesion in so-called pyorrhœa alveolaris. Br Dent J 1928;49:1129.
43. Kantorowicz A. Fundamentos anatomopatológicos de la odontología conservadora. In: Bruhn C, Kantorowicz A, Partsch C (eds). La Escuela Odontologica Alemana, vol 2. Barcelona: Editorial Labor, 1937.
44. Kantorowicz A. Das Wesen und die Behandlung der Paradentitis. Zahnärzt Rdsch 1925;26:393.
45. Karolyi M. Beobachtungen über Pyorrhoea alveolaris. Öst-ung Vjschr Zahnheilk 1901;17:279.
46. Kremenak NW, Squier CA. Pioneers in oral biology: The migrations of Gottlieb, Kronfeld, Orban, Weinmann and Sicher from Vienna to America. Crit Rev Oral Biol Med 1997;8:108.
47. Kronfeld R. The epithelial attachment and the so-called Nasmyth's membrane. J Am Dent Assoc 1930;17:1889.
48. Kronfeld R. Histologic study of the influence of function on the human periodontal membrane. J Am Dent Assoc 1931;18:1242.
49. Kronfeld R. Histopathology of the Teeth and their Surrounding Structures. Philadelphia: Lea & Febiger, 1933.
50. Kronfeld R. Condition of alveolar bone underlying periodontal pockets. J Periodontol 1935;6:22.
51. Newman MG, Socransky SS. Predominant cultivable microbiota in periodontosis. J Periodontal Res 1977;56:545.
52. Obituary, Harold Keith Box. J Periodontol 1956;46:225.
53. Obituary, Bernhard Gottlieb. J Am Dent Assoc 1950;40:607.
54. Obituary, Bernhard Gottlieb. J Periodontol 1950;21.
55. Obituary, Rudolph Kronfeld. J Am Dent Assoc 1940;30:648.
56. Obituary, Rudolph Kronfeld. J Periodontol 1940;11:99.
57. Obituary, Balint J. Orban. J Periodontol 1960;50:86.
58. Obituary, Balint J. Orban. J West Soc Periodontol Abstr 1960;8:45.
59. Obituary, Harry Sicher. Anat Record 1975;183:145.
60. Orban BJ. Tissue changes in traumatic occlusion. J Am Dent Assoc 1928;15:2090.
61. Orban BJ, Köhler J. Die physiologische zahnfleischtasche, epithelansatz und epitheltiefenwucherung. Z Stomatol 1924;22:353.
62. Orban BJ, Mueller E. The gingival crevice. J Am Dent Assoc 1929;16:1206.
63. Orban BJ, Weinmann JP. Diffuse atrophy of alveolar bone. J Periodontol 1942;13:31.
64. Sicher H, Tandler J. Anatomie für Zahnärzte. Vienna: J. Springer,1928.
65. Simonton FV. Pyorrhea: definition and classification. Dent Cosmos 1926;68:158.
66. Skillen WG. The morphology of the gingiva of the rat molar. J Am Dent Assoc 1930;17:645.
67. Skillen WG. Normal characteristics of the gingiva and their relation to pathology. J Am Dent Assoc 1930;17:1088.
68. Skillen WG. Normal anatomic and physiologic gingiva and its relation to pathologic processes. J Am Dent Assoc 1931;18:600.
69. Skillen WG. A contribution to the anatomy and pathology of the human gingiva. J Dent Res 1931;11:727.
70. Skillen WG, Mueller E. Epithelium and the physiologic pocket. J Am Dent Assoc 1927;14:1149.
71. Stewart FE. Recent discoveries concerning the etiology and treatment of pyorrhea alveolaris. Dent Cosmos 1915;57:605.
72. Talbot ES. Interstitial Gingivitis and Pyorrhea Alveolaris. Toledo, OH: Ransom & Randolph, 1913.
73. Thoma KH, Goldman HM. Wandering and elongation of the teeth and pocket formation in paradontosis. J Am Dent Assoc 1940;27:335.
74. Weinmann JP. Progress of gingival inflammation into the supporting structures of the teeth. J Periodontol 1941;12:71.
75. Weinmann JP, Sicher H. Bone and Bones: Fundamentals of Bone Biology. St. Louis: Mosby, 1947.
76. Weski O. Röntgenologische-anatomische Studien aus dem Gebiete der Kieferpathologie. Vjschr Zahnheilk 1921;37:1 and 1922;38:1.
77. Znamensky NN. Alveolar pyorrhea—Its pathological anatomy and its radical treatment. J Br Dent Assoc 1902;23:585.

# 19

# Etiology of Periodontal Disease 1900–1950

The different conceptions of the etiology of periodontal disease, namely the "localist" and the "constitutional" or "generalist" schools of thought developed in previous centuries, continued into the twentieth century. The first decades of the century saw confusion regarding the etiology of periodontitis and the periodontal manifestations of systemic diseases. This was further complicated by the theory of focal infection, which described systemic diseases originating in a periodontal or oral infection (see Chapter 23).

From Fauchard, in the early eighteenth century, to the beginning of the twentieth century, many systemic diseases were considered the cause of periodontal disease. This concept was particularly popular in Europe where Emile Magitot, of France, and J. Arkövy, of Hungary, were its major proponents (see Chapter 13). The most common disease considered was scurvy, since this nutritional deficiency obviously has periodontal manifestations, that are now known to be triggered by a gingivitis of bacterial origin. Other systemic diseases that were repeatedly mentioned in all considerations of periodontitis etiology were other nutritional and metabolic diseases and arthritis.[37]

In a review article published in 1920, Arthur Merritt[30] (Fig 52) mentions that

> those who hold to the *"constitutional theory"* have furnished almost no support for their belief; nothing of an exact nature is known regarding the influence of disease, heredity, diet, etc., upon the causation of periodontoclasia. ... The *"parasitic theory"* ... has had its strongest supporters abroad [but] there has never been any evidence to show that there is a specific infective organism.

Merritt further opines that there are great quantitative differences but no qualitative differences between the bacterial flora in health and disease. He then states:

> The advocates of the *"local-disease theory"* have furnished what seems to be convincing proof of the reasonableness of their claims as applied to most cases, in achieving a considerable measure of success in its treatment.

Merritt subdivides the factors involved in the latter theory into primary and secondary causes. Primary causes act directly on the tissues and are irritative in nature (uncleanliness, food impaction, overhanging margins of restorations, ill-fitting crowns), or they act through a "traumatic occlusion." Secondary causes are abnormal systemic conditions, chemical irritations, and so on.

In 1950, Samuel Charles Miller wrote:

> It is doubtful that any one influence could, by itself, produce periodontal disease. A combination of factors which both lower the tissue resistance and acts upon this weakened tissue is necessary to establish disturbances of the periodontium. It is for this reason that the constant search by investigators for a single factor as the cause of periodontal disease has been to no avail. Treatments directed at factors which are thought to be causing the disease, but which actually only contribute to it, have been responsible for the many failures in handling this condition.[31]

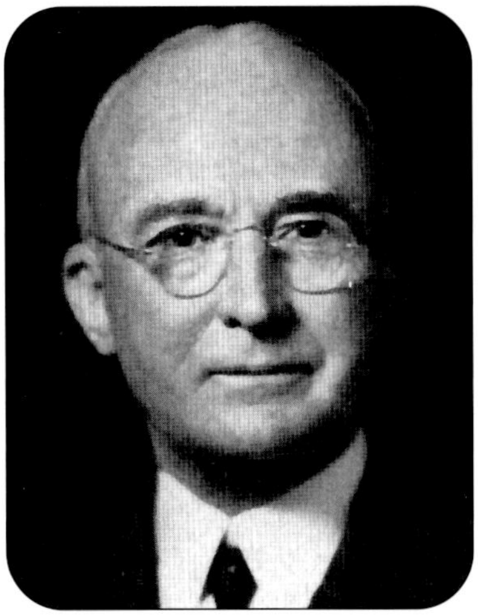

**Fig 52** Arthur Hastings Merritt.

## Calculus and Other Local Irritants

As previous chapters show, calculus had been recognized as an etiologic factor of gingival and periodontal disease for many centuries. The mechanisms of its formation were thought to be physical, bacterial, and systemic (dietary or emotional).

During this era, most researchers gave little if any consideration to the mechanism or mechanisms by which calculus and so-called local irritants became deleterious to the tissues. Of course, the concept of bacterial plaque or a biofilm forming on a tooth surface was decades in the future, and microbiological studies were very incipient, interest being focused more on tissue changes than their causes. In general calculus was considered a consequence, not a cause of pocket formation. Gottlieb and Orban, in 1938, wrote:

> The commonly prevailing opinion that calculus is a direct cause for the deepening of the gingival crevice, is incorrect. ... One must, on the contrary, begin with the concept that the depth of the crevice is practically zero, that therefore the primary factor is the deepening of the crevice in which debris is retained.[9]

Most authors describe extensively "irritational factors" caused by abnormal tooth anatomy, food impaction, prosthetic, restorative or orthodontic inadequacies, chemical irritants, and mouth breathing.

## Periodontal Microbiology

Search for a specific bacteria responsible for periodontal disease went on in the first part of the twentieth century. Several investigators (Barrett,[1] Bass and Johns,[2] and others[14,19,32,38,40]) blamed a protozoan organism, the *Endameba buccalis* (today called *Entamoeba gingivalis*) as the etiologic agent of periodontal disease. Most of these investigators were physicians, and their publications appeared in medical journals. The concept of the entameba playing a key role led to the use of ipecac, and its chief component emetin, as a therapeutic agent for periodontal disease because of its amebicidal effect.[2,3,35]

The role of the ameba as an etiologic agent was, however, strongly disputed by other scientists.[13] Percy Howe, of the Forsyth Dental Infirmary in Boston,[18] and J. Mendel, in France,[26] presented evidence on the harmless nature of entameba and against the use of emetin in periodontal treatment. The treatment, however, remained in vogue for a few years before it was abandoned.

Spirochetes and fusiform bacilli were also considered in the search for an etiologic agent of periodontal disease.[5] In 1912 Noguchi[33,34] described a spirochete isolated from periodontal lesions, while Kritchevsky and Seguin, in 1924, recovered spirochetes from every case of destructive periodontal disease they studied.[22] However, the Salvarsan they attempted as intravenous treatment resulted in limited success unless calculus was removed by scaling, so they assumed that the spirochetes were secondary invaders.[6,22]

Keilty[19] in 1922 and Glynn[7] in 1923 described fusiform bacilli in the oral cavity. And in 1946 H. S. Klein[21] reported the presence of spirochetes in normal mouths and their increase in disease, particularly in destructive conditions. In 1936, Tunnicliff[43] reported that fusiform bacilli and spirilla became pathogenic when tissue vitality was reduced. Other microorganisms that were considered a possible culprit were the streptococci. Hartzell and Henrici[14] described the presence of *Streptococcus viridans* in all periodontal infections.

Interest in microbiology resulted in the search for a vaccine to prevent the disease. K. Goadby of London, in a book published in 1903, focused attention on the possible bacterial etiology of periodontal disease but opined that a low immune response against the oral flora initiated the lesions. He advanced the idea that therefore vaccines might be effective.[4,8] In 1904 H. C. Boenning suggested the use of antistreptococcus vaccines and sera.[23] From cultures obtained from pyorrhea pockets, vaccines were made and injected directly, or animals were injected until a high antibody blood content was supposedly built up and the animal serums injected into human pyorrhea cases. Later the opsonic index was used as a means of determining which of the many microorganisms found in pyorrhea pockets were the pathogenic ones.[23]

Two types of vaccines were considered: the autogenous vaccine and the stock vaccine. Vaccines were recommended only if local therapy had not been successful. In 1913, Thomas B. Hartzell concisely summarized this position:

> Vaccines are needed only when recurrence occurs in a clean mouth, or when the patient's resistance is extremely low, and then only when such tonics as peptomangan fortified by strychnine and iron (Blaud's pills) or phosphorus have failed, or when joint infection will not yield after the initial focus in the mouth has been eliminated, at which juncture an autogenous vaccine is indicated.[17]

The use of autogenous vaccines seems to have been preferred. George Harris, of Detroit,[11] explained that infection in pyorrhea is always mixed and that autogenous vaccines utilize the "beneficial effects" derived from all bacteria. Some practitioners, however, used a combination of autogenous and stock vaccines,[25] while others who did not have access to laboratories preparing autogenous vaccines for their patients had to rely on stock vaccines.[24]

Between 1916 and 1918 Merritt published several papers[27–29] discouraging the use of vaccines, which were gradually abandoned. However, as late as 1946, their use was recommended in the European literature.[44]

The interest in microbiological research declined slowly after the 1920s, and almost disappeared by the mid 1930s. The nonspecific hypothesis, espoused half a century earlier by W. D. Miller, was supported by Hemmens and Harrison in 1942.[17] Theodore Rosebury, initially at Columbia University and then at Washington University School of Dentistry, led one of the few groups that investigated periodontal microbiology in this period. They believed that bacteria aggravated a preexistent inflammation initiated by local irritating factors such as calculus or occlusal trauma.[36]

Analyses of the etiology of periodontal disease returned to consideration of constitutional factors and trauma from occlusion, bacteria being thought of as secondary invaders. Not until the late 1950s and 1960s, influenced by Jens Waerhaug and the Scandinavian school, would interest in bacteriology be reborn.

*Necrotizing ulcerative gingivitis.* Identification of bacteria associated with necrotizing ulcerative gingivitis had been determined in the last decade of the previous century. The exact role of these bacteria and other factors was not clear. In 1939 British scientist J. D. King performed an experiment that not only helped clarify this problem, but showed his personal devotion to research.[20] His experiment was as follows, as summarized by Ronald Emslie[4]:

> In 1939 he traumatized his interdental gingiva between the lower right canine and first premolar, and forced down between these teeth a pledget of cotton-wool; impregnated with ulcerative debris from a severe case of acute ulcerative gingivitis. 24 hours later, smears from various parts of the gums showed very large numbers of fusiform bacilli and spirochetes, but these disappeared on the third day and at no time did any clinical lesions develop. Exactly a year later, in December 1940, the experiment was repeated, dental hygiene having been purposely neglected during the intervening period. This time failure to transmit the disease again seemed likely, although some fusospirochætal organisms had been found in his mouth prior to inoculation. However, a month later, following two severe colds, increasing gingival bleeding was noted, culminating five months later during a further cold in a "severe flaring subacute ulcerative gingivostomatitis" around several teeth in both jaws.

## Trauma from Occlusion

First described by the Viennese dentist Morris Karolyi in 1901, trauma from occlusion was an important topic of study and analysis by practitioners and investigators. Paul R. Stillman, of New York City, and John Oppie McCall, of Buffalo, New York, created the term *traumatic occlusion*, which they defined as an abnormal occlusal stress capable of producing or having produced injury to the periodontium. They clarified the possibility of tissue to become reinforced and adapt to the forces or to be damaged and break down. Stillman and McCall also described a number of gingival changes supposedly caused by traumatic occlusion (Stillman clefts, McCall festoons, and several others) that later were found not to be of traumatic origin.[41,42] During the period, numerous other investigators analyzed the tissue changes induced in humans and animals by trauma from occlusion (see Chapters 18 and 20).

## References

1. Barrett MF. Preliminary report. Dent Cosmos 1914;56:948.
2. Bass CC, Johns FM. Pyorrhea dentalis and alveolaris. JAMA 1915;64:553.
3. Beall EN. The present status of emetin in the treatment of pyorrhea. Dent Cosmos 1916;58:406.
4. Emslie RD. A century of British periodontology. Br Dent J 1980;149:3.
5. Fisher JH. Pyorrhea alveolaris: The role of certain microorganisms found in the lesions. Am J Pathol 1927;3:169.
6. Glickman I. Clinical Periodontology. Philadelphia: Saunders, 1953.
7. Glynn EE. The organisms found in the periodontal infections and their relation to the "toxemia." Br Dent J 1923;44:601,698.
8. Goadby K. The Mycology of the Mouth. London: Longman, Green, 1903.
9. Gottlieb B, Orban B. Biology and Pathology of the Tooth and Its Supporting Mechanism. New York: Macmillan, 1938.
10. Greve C. Alveolarpyorrhoe, Riggs' disease. Dtsch Zahnärztl Wschr 1911;14:653. Cited in: Held A-J. Periodontology. From Its Origins Up to 1980: A Survey. Basel: Birkhäuser, 1989.

11. Harris GB. The treatment of pyorrhea by bacterial vaccines, and the results of animal experimentation. Dent Cosmos 1913;55:391.
12. Hartzell TB. The operative and postoperative treatment of pyorrhea. Dent Cosmos 1913;55:1101.
13. Hartzell TB. The use of emetine in the treatment of periodontal disease. J Allied Dent Soc 1915;2:143.
14. Hartzell TB, Henrici AT. A study of streptococci from pyorrhea alveolaris and from apical abscesses. JAMA 1914;64:2023.
15. Hecker F. Experimental studies with Endamœba Gros. J Infect Dis 1916;19:729.
16. Held A-J. Periodontology. From Its Origins Up to 1980: A Survey. Basel: Birkhäuser, 1989.
17. Hemmens ES, Harrison RW. Studies on the anaerobic bacterial flora of suppurative periodontitis. J Infect Dis 1942;70:131.
18. Howe PR. The Endamœba and pyorrhea alveolaris. Dent Cosmos 1916;58:369.
19. Keilty RA. Focal infections: A bacteriological study of the gums in 200 cases. J Med Res 1922;43:377.
20. King JD. Nutritional and other factors in "trench mouth" with special reference to the nicotinic acid component of the vitamin B2. Br Dent J 1943;74:113,141.
21. Klein HS. Spirochetes in normal mouths, gingivitis and suppurative periodontitis. Acta Odontol Scand 1946;7:92.
22. Kritchevsky B, Seguin P. The unity of spirochetes of the mouth. Dent Cosmos 1924;66:511.
23. Leonard HJ. Diagnosis and treatment of periodontoclasia. J Periodontol 1940;11:67.
24. McGehee WHO. Stock vaccines in the treatment of pyorrhea alveolaris. Dent Cosmos 1913;55:997.
25. Medalia LS. Chronic alveolar osteomyelitis (pyorrhea alveolaris): Its treatment by vaccines. Dent Cosmos 1913;55:708.
26. Mendel J. Quelques recherches sur l'etiologie et la pathogenie de la pyorrhée alvéolaire. Odontologie 1919; 39:235,283.
27. Merritt AH. Irrationality of bacterial vaccines in the treatment of pyorrhea alveolaris. Dent Cosmos 1916;58:62.
28. Merritt AH. Vaccines in pyorrhea. J Allied Dent Soc 1916;11:639.
29. Merritt AH. The pathology, etiology and treatment of pyorrhea alveolaris. Dent Cosmos 1918;60:574.
30. Merritt AH. Progressive Dentistry and Stomatology. 2. Periodontology, with special reference to Periodontoclasia. J Dent Res 1920,3.77.
31. Miller SC. Textbook of Periodontia, ed 3. Philadelphia: Blakiston, 1950.
32. Mitchell OWH, Culpepper WL, Ayer WD. *Endamœba buccalis* in the mouths of institutionalized children. J Med Res 1916;35:51.
33. Noguchi H. Cultural studies of mouth spirochete (*Treponema microdentium* and *macrodentium*). J Exp Med 1912;15:81.
34. Noguchi H. *Treponema mucosum* (new species), a mucin producing spirochete from pyorrhea alveolaris grown in pure culture. J Exp Med 1912;16:194.
35. Prinz H. A contribution to the history of emetin. Dent Cosmos 1915;57:313.
36. Rosebury T. The nature and significance of infection in periodontal disease. Am J Orthod Oral Surg 1947;33:658.
37. Roy M. La Pyorrhée Alvéolaire. Paris: J.-B Baillière et Fils, 1935.
38. Sandford AH, New GB. The relation of amœbiasis to pyorrhea alveolaris. Surg Gynecol Obstet 1916;22:27.
39. Socransky SS, Haffajee AD. Evidence of bacterial etiology: A historical perspective. Periodontol 2000 1994;5:7.
40. Smith AJ, Barrett MT. The parasite of oral endamœbiasis. Science 1915;42:354.
41. Stillman PR. Occlusion. J Am Dent Assoc 1930;17:81.
42. Stillman PR, McCall JO. A Textbook of Clinical Periodontia. New York: Macmillan, 1922.
43. Tunnicliff R. The life cycle of *Bacillus fusiformis*. J Infect Dis 1923;33:147.
44. Vincent R. La Pyorrhée dans le cadre de la Médecin Générale. Paris: Masson et Cie, 1946.

# 20

# Clinical Periodontology 1900–1950: Diagnosis

## Clinical Examination

Periodontal diagnosis in the nineteenth century was limited to obvious clinical findings. Controversy over the local or systemic origin of periodontal disease confused the distinction between periodontal disorders and systemic diseases with periodontal manifestations. Suppuration was considered a key finding. In the latter part of the nineteenth century, John Riggs (see Chapter 15) and William Younger, in 1901, detailed clinical gingival changes, tooth mobility, and tooth migration in advanced disease.[30]

*Gingiva.* The assessment of gingival changes in color, size, contour, position, and shape have long been part of clinical oral examination. In 1915, G. V. Black delineated the redness and slight swelling of the gingiva, areas of food impaction, suppuration and pain, and calculus deposits.[2] The advent and subsequent improvement of electrical lighting in dental offices in the twentieth century, and particularly after the 1920s, helped in detecting gingival changes and analyzing their importance.[6]

*Pocket probing.* The third edition of G. V. Black's *Special Dental Pathology*, published in 1924 after his death, mentions "the use of very thin flat explorers to determine the depth of pockets" (cited by Gold[6]). These instruments were not calibrated and they were used for decades.

The periodontal probe and its use was first described by F. V. Simonton, of the University of California, San Francisco, in 1925.[24] Simonton refers to the periodontal probe as a "periodontometer" and credits W. H. Hanford and C. O. Patten for its invention (Fig 53). There were right-sided and left-sided calibrated probes. Simonton gives the exact measurements of the probe and detailed instructions on its use. Simonton defines detachment ("loss of periodontal membrane that takes place, as measured gingivoapically, along the root surface"), pocket ("space that intervenes between the denuded root surface and the circumjacent investing tissues"), and recession ("apical retrogression of the free margin of the gum from an assured normal"). Then he explains how to measure each of these parameters and how to record the measurements in a chart. He also explains how to indicate in the chart the presence of caries, missing teeth, condition of investing tissues, root and apical conditions, atrophy, abrasion, and erosion, and previous dental procedures such as restorations, crowns, bridges, and so on. In a subsequent paper[25] Simonton analyzes the possible sources of error in pocket measurement and the reliability of the method. Simonton insists that the only way to determine the existence and extent of pyorrhea is the measurement of the depth of pockets, either instrumentally, roentgenographically, or both. Acceptance of routine periodontal probing in diagnosis was slow. Periodontal books published in the 1930s make brief mention of probes and probing, and the charts they propose have no space for pocket depth recordings.[4,16,18]

*Occlusion.* Analysis of the occlusion in the first half of the century was carried out mostly by prosthodontists, restorative dentists, and orthodontists. These analyses were, overall, detailed

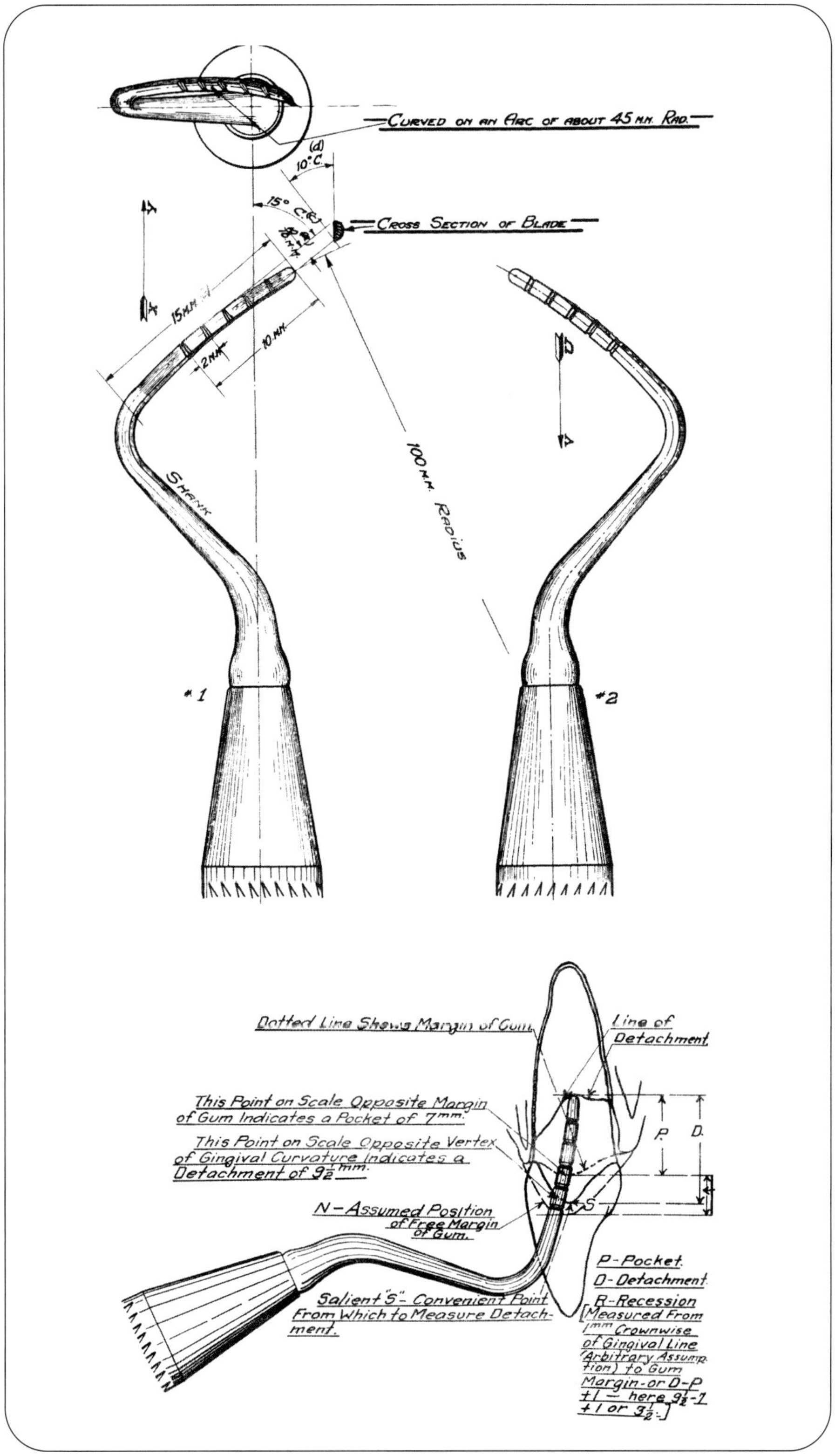


**Fig 53** Periodontal probe (periodontometer) developed by Hanford and Patten.

anatomical descriptions of human teeth and comparative anatomy of carnivorous ruminants and rodents. In 1930, Canadian periodontist Harold K. Box attributed primary and secondary occlusal trauma to increased forced or reduced periodontium, respectively.[3]

A number of gingival changes—traumatic crescents, gingival congestion and recession, McCall's festoons, Stillman's clefts, loss of stippling, and others—were ascribed to trauma from occlusion.[3,27] None of these changes is accepted today as being of traumatic origin. The technique for correction of occlusal disharmonies proposed by Clyde H. Schuyler in 1935 and 1947 was the most popular method.[22,23] Sidney Sorrin, of New York University, in 1935 called attention of the etiologic role of various habits in periodontal disease.[26]

Isador Hirschfeld (see Chapter 21), of Columbia University, published in 1930 a classic paper on food impaction, describing vertical and horizontal impaction, and analyzing and classifying its causes, effects, and treatment.[9] His 1939 book, *The Toothbrush, Its Use and Abuse*, details oral hygiene methods and their effects on all types of gingival and oral diseases.[10] Six decades after its publication this book continues to be a valuable source for those interested in prevention of oral diseases.

## Radiographic Examination

Dentistry became the first medical specialty, outside of the military, to adopt the use of radiography.[13] Dental radiographs were used from the beginning to identify the dead, and increasingly bone radiographs also proved useful to determine the cause of death.[13]

The first use of radiographs for periodontal diagnosis was reported by William Herbert Rollins in December 1896.[20] Rollins had a medical degree from Harvard University and practiced dentistry in Boston. He and his brother-in-law, Francis H. Williams, a medical doctor with a degree in chemistry from the Massachusetts Institute of Technology (MIT), had been experimenting with an X-ray machine at MIT. Williams used the machine to differentiate radiographically, and with contrasting substances, such lung diseases as pneumonia, emphysema, and tuberculosis.[13]

Rollins developed an intraoral cassette and an X-ray tube for use in dental offices (see Chapter 14). He later developed radiation burns on his hand and advocated the use of protective shields.[1] Rollins performed experiments on guinea pigs to study the effects of radiation and determined that X-ray tubes should be shielded with lead and placed as far as possible from the patient, and that the least amount of necessary radiation should be used. He also devised a badge of film to indicate when the wearer had been dangerously exposed to X rays.[13] Rollins never patented his inventions and his papers were not widely read by those who could have profited from his advice.

At the beginning of the new century (1903) X rays started to be used also as a therapeutic agent in periodontics and for other problems such as thermal sensitivity and facial neuralgia.[7,17,21] Although some investigators reported success, the practice was discontinued due to incidents of radiation dermatitis.

The first X-ray unit for dental use was the Record, made in Europe in 1905 (Fig 54). It was manufactured by Reinger-Gebbert and Schall of Germany, predecessors of the Siemens Company. Although the X-ray tube was shielded, the high voltage wires were exposed.[1,5] In the United States, the first commercially manufactured X-ray machine appeared in 1913, made by the American X-ray Equipment Company of Mount Vernon, New York.[1,5] The first commercial dental radiographic film packet was marketed by Eastman Kodak in 1913, and the same company introduced high-speed dental radiographic film in 1941.[5]

In 1913, MIT physicist William David Coolidge invented the high-vacuum, hot-cathode, tungsten-target X-ray tube, which signified a great step forward. The Coolidge tube was marketed by General Electric.[13]

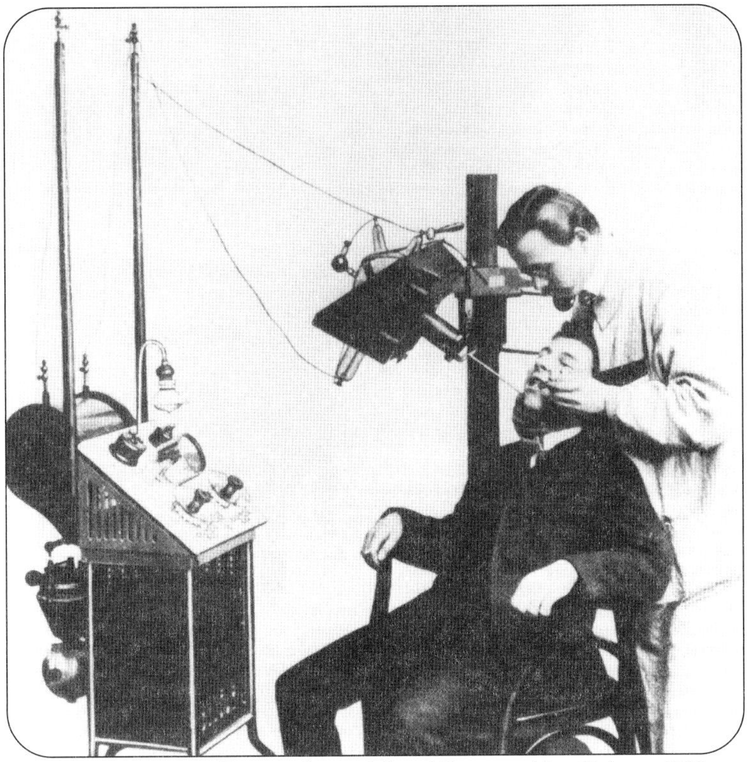

**Fig 54** First commercially manufactured dental X-ray machine (Reinger-Gebbert and Schall, Germany, 1905).

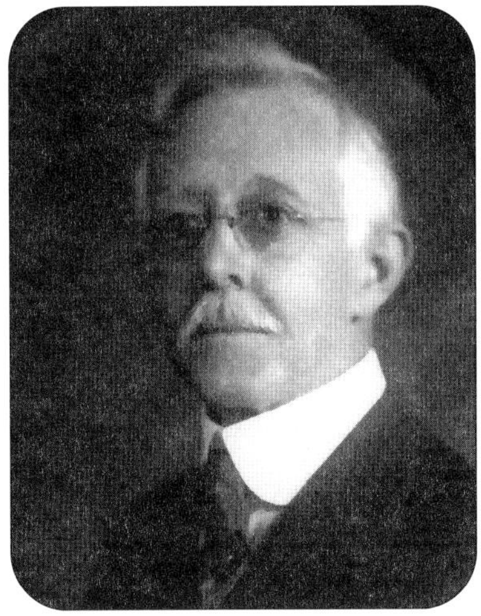

**Fig 55** C. Edmund Kells.

Since the 1910s the use of radiographs has been recommended as an adjunct to periodontal diagnosis. Arthur Merritt in 1916 described the radiographic features of bone loss in pyorrhea.[15] The following year Kurt H. Thoma published *Oral Roentgenology*,[28] in which he recommends the Roentgen method for the diagnosis and prognosis of the disease, but cautions that it does not improve understanding of its etiology or duration.

C. Edmund Kells (Fig 55) pioneered the use of radiographs in dentistry (see Kells' biography in Chapter 14). He soon realized, however, that radiographs alone were of little value in periodontal diagnosis and said bluntly in 1920 that the periodontist who cannot diagnose without the aid of radiographs should undoubtedly better engage in another specialty.[11] Howard Riley Raper and others disagreed with Kells. In 1920, F. McCormack argued that radiographs were useful to show widened periodontal ligaments, alteration or obliteration of the periodontal lamella, granuloma, cyst, pyorrhea alveolaris, necrosis, osteosclerosis, and osteitis serrata.[19]

In 1924 Raper invented the bitewing radiograph. Again Kells was skeptical. He wrote:

> [I]f an operator cannot find cavities in the crowns of teeth, without the use of X-ray, what he needs is a competent dental assistant to make the examination for him and not a roentgen-ray machine.[12]

German scientist Oskar Weski (see Chapter 18) published, in 1921, an atlas documenting patterns of bone loss (horizontal and vertical) and correlating them to the clinical findings.[29]

Then, in a paper published in 1926,[12] Kells presented an interesting review of the evolution of X rays—physical traits as well as clinical, dental application—over the first quarter of the century.

## References


1. A review of dental radiography. J Am Dent Assoc 1984;108:552.
2. Black GV. Special Dental Pathology. Chicago: Medico-Dental, 1915.
3. Box HK. Traumatic occlusion and traumatogenic occlusion. Oral Health 1930;20:642.
4. Coolidge ED. Clinical Pathology and Treatment of the Dental Pulp and Periodontal Tissues. Philadelphia: Lea & Febiger, 1939.
5. Glenner RA. The Dental Office: Pictorial History. Missoula, MT: Pictorial Histories, 1984.
6. Gold SI. Diagnostic techniques in periodontology: A historical review. Periodontol 2000 1995;7:9.
7. Guy W. X rays in the treatment of pyorrhea alveolaris. Dent Cosmos 1903;45:498.
8. Hirschfeld I. Diagrammatic recording of periodontal disease. J Am Dent Assoc 1931;18:1927.
9. Hirschfeld I. Food impaction. J Am Dent Assoc 1930;17:1504.
10. Hirschfeld I. The Toothbrush: Its Use and Abuse. New York: Dental Items of Interest, 1939.
11. Kells CE. The X rays in dental practice. J Am Dent Assoc 1920;7:241.
12. Kells CE. Thirty years' experience in the field of radiography. J Am Dent Assoc 1926;13:693.
13. Kevles BH. Naked to the Bone. Medical Imaging in the Twentieth Century. New Brunswick, NJ: Rutgers University Press, 1997.
14. McCormack F. A plea for a standardized technique for oral radiography with an illustrated classification of findings and their verified interpretation. J Dent Res 1920;2:467.
15. Merritt AH. The Roentgen ray in dental practice. Dent Cosmos 1916;58:948.
16. Merritt AH. Periodontal Diseases: Diagnosis and Treatment. New York: Macmillan, 1935.
17. Parker CH. The treatment of interstitial gingivitis (pyorrhea) by the X ray and high frequency currents. Dent Cosmos 1903;45:947.
18. Pucci FM. El paradencio, su patologia y tratamiento. Montevideo: Ed Médica Garcia Morales, 1939.
19. Raper HR. Notes on the early history of Radiodontia. Oral Surg Oral Med Oral Pathol 1953;6:70.
20. Rollins W. Radiography in pyorrhea alveolaris. Int Dent J 1897;18:140.
21. Saterlee FL Jr. The X ray in dentistry. Dent Cosmos 1906;48:260.
22. Schuyler CH. Fundamental principles in the correction of occlusal disharmony, natural and artificial. J Am Dent Assoc 1935;22:1193.
23. Schuyler CH. Correction of occlusal disharmony of the natural dentition. N Y J Dent 1947;13:445.
24. Simonton FV. Examination of the mouth—with special reference to pyorrhea. J Am Dent Assoc 1925;12:287.
25. Simonton FV. Technic involved in measuring destructive changes of investing tissues of teeth. J Am Dent Assoc 1925;12:448.
26. Sorrin S. Habit, an etiologic factor of periodontal disease. Dent Dig 1935;41:290.
27. Stillman PR, McCall JO. Textbook of Clinical Periodontia, ed 2. New York: Macmillan, 1937.
28. Thoma KH. Oral Roentgenology. Boston: Ritter, 1917.
29. Weski O. Roentgenologische-anatomische studienen auf dem Gebiete der Kieferpathologie. Vjschr Zahnheilk 1921;37:1.
30. Younger WM. Pyorrhea alveolaris. Dent Cosmos 1901;43:394.

# 21

# Clinical Periodontology 1900–1950: Nonsurgical Therapy

## Instrumentation

The development of local anesthesia and the discovery of X rays at the turn of the twentieth century brought new ideas and possibilities for periodontal surgical procedures and resulted in great progress in this therapeutic procedure. However, many practitioners continued to use only the so-called conservative method, rejecting the surgical approach.

The importance of removal of all accretions from the tooth surface had been recognized and practiced for centuries (see Chapters 3, 6, and 11). Pierre Fauchard in the eighteenth century developed a technique for this purpose, and in the nineteenth century several investigators recommended that each practitioner should construct his own instruments since those "sold in shops are ill suited for the purpose."

James Snell, of London, (cited by Glenner[14]), in an 1832 study entitled *A Practical Guide to Operations on the Teeth*, writes:

> The instruments sold in the shops as scaling instruments are without doubt the most awkward things for the purpose that can be conceived. ... [To do a good job of scaling] the operator must possess suitable instruments, a light hand, a good eye and a certain mechanical tact in the use of instruments that can be acquired only by practice.[14]

Snell recommends a set of six scalers, mostly spear-shaped and of different sizes, and explains that the technique for their use requires placing the tip of the instrument under the calculus and dislodging it with a flipping motion.

Chapin Harris, cofounder of the Baltimore College of Dental Surgery in 1839, describes the scaling technique in *The Dental Art*, published the same year.[14] Harris opines that most instruments sold are ill-suited for their purposes, and the dentist should have a variety of scalers and develop the skill necessary to remove calculus, a task which is more difficult than most persons imagine. (Harris's biography can be found in Chapter 15.)

Paul Goddard, of Pennsylvania, developed in 1844 a set of eleven instruments, and in 1859 Jonathan Taft, of Ohio, later to be the first dean of the University of Michigan School of Dentistry, writes that calculus removal is an "operation that does not involve a great amount of skill, but, with suitable instruments, is easily performed."[14] Taft describes calculus removal by scraping or by application of an acid, and says he prefers the former (cited by Glenner[14]).

Glenner[14] also mentions the methods of James Dexter in 1876 and A. W. Harlan in 1887. Harlan describes instruments to be used with a pull motion and with a push motion, and he concludes that

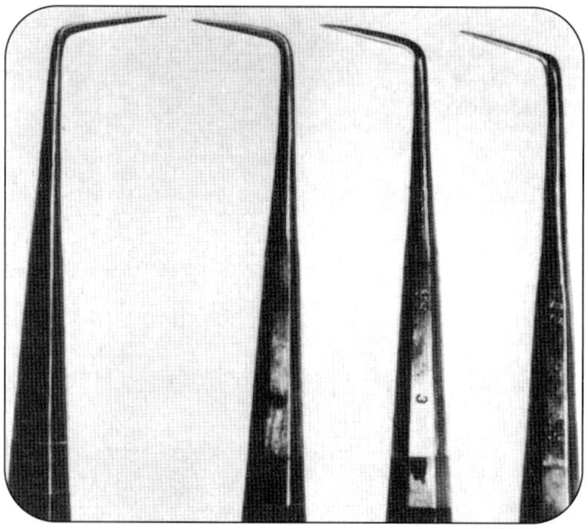

**Fig 56** Riggs' set of scalers.

> While it is undoubtedly true that tartar may be removed from the teeth with large chisels and scalers, or even with excavators if sufficient time is given to the performance of the operation, still it is always at the expense of great laceration of the gums, the production of much pain, and the mental determination of the patient to not submit to such a dreadful ordeal in the future.[14]

John W. Riggs later in the century designed a series of six instruments, refined the technique, and promoted its use. (See Chapter 15 for a biography of Riggs.) Riggs' original set of six instruments was the first to have various instrument designs for the different tooth surfaces to be treated (Fig 56). The instruments were essentially sickles, but were still large and clumsy and not suitable for fine scaling,[16,27] and there was little regard for the damage that the instrument could cause to the tooth surface or the gingiva. Riggs' instruments were later modified and improved by several clinicians.

Already in the nineteenth century the difference between scaling and root planing was understood, including the rationale of removing bacteria that may have penetrated the cementum via the collagen fiber remnants. Some researchers, however, opposed root planing to avoid injury to the cementum and soft tissues. William Crenshaw, of Atlanta, Georgia, writes against the use of chisels and hoes, favoring a set of seventeen instruments he designed. In addition, Crenshaw advocates the use of dull instruments to dislodge calculus without nicking the root surface.[9]

William J. Younger, who practiced in San Francisco, Chicago, and, for the last twenty years of his life, in Paris, devised a set of instruments that represented real improvement over those of his mentor, John Riggs. (See Chapter 15 for a biography of Younger.) Younger's set included curette-style instruments with more delicate blades and slender shanks, but the tools still lacked a contra-angle.[11,17]

This instrument set, later modified by Robert Good, was a big step forward; the so-called Younger-Good set was in general use until the 1950s (Fig 57) (see Chapter 15). These instruments came in a variety of shapes that allowed access to all parts of the mouth.[27] Their weakness continued to be the lack of a contra-angle, which meant that the working tip was not in line with the handle, making it difficult to manage successfully, except with expert hands.[27]

The hoe scalers were developed by Henry Tompkins, although experiments into this instrument design had been performed by A. W. Harlan and Frank Abbott. Tompkins' design introduced several different types of hoes, but they also lacked a contra-angle.[27] At about the same time, David D. Smith developed the files—some with a slight, inadequate contra-angle.[27] R. G. Hutchinson also designed a set of delicate curettes and files; however, they were not contra-angled and therefore difficult to use.[27]

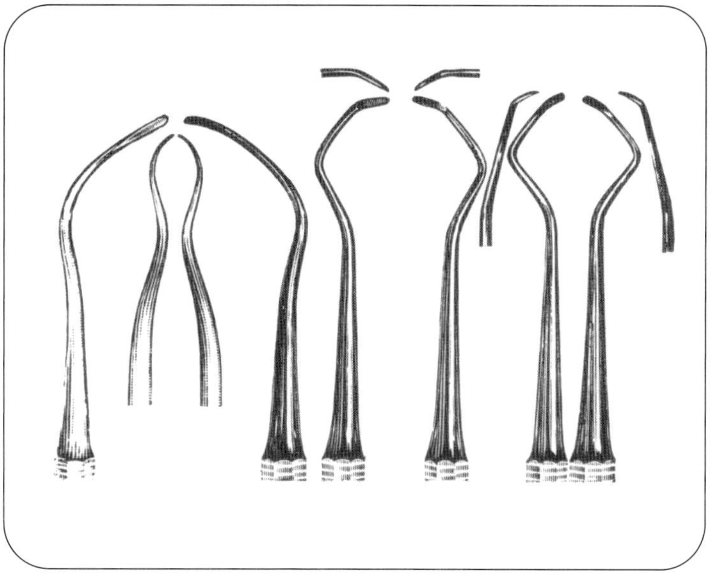

**Fig 57** Younger-Good scalers.

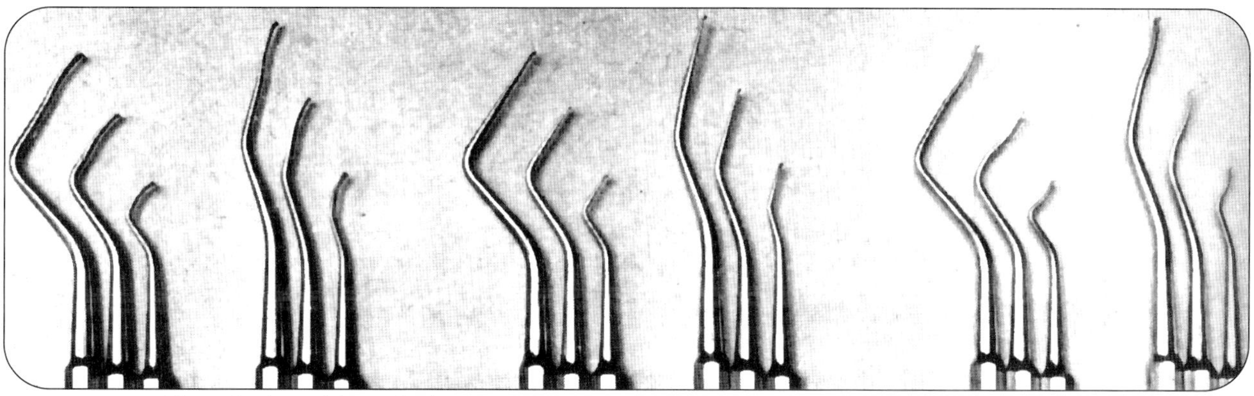

**Fig 58** Carr's partial set of scalers.

C. M. Carr made major improvements in instrument design, with suggestions from Thomas Hartzell and Austin James.[27] McCall[27] credits Carr with the following:

> exact contra-angle, even in instruments of the greatest curvature for reaching posterior teeth; two-point contact, on the root surface, of instrument blade and shank; rotation of the blade on the axis of the shank to permit convenient application to all surfaces around the circumference of the tooth; shank design in straight, concave and convex shapes for adaptation to root surfaces of different contours; refinement of the design of the hoe with most favorable angulation of blade to shank, and constancy of such angulation through the development of a true flat surface for the proximal surface or the face of the blade [(Fig 58)].

Another of Carr's important contributions was the improved technique for tempering scalers, making them extremely hard while maintaining a sharp cutting edge.[27] In addition, he devised a tool to maintain a uniform bevel of the cutting edge while sharpening the instrument.

The entire Carr set consisted of 150 instruments: 144 hoes and 6 sickle scalers. The set was popular among practitioners, in spite of the fact that the large number of instruments made instrument selection rather cumbersome.

Merritt lists in his 1935 book[28] four different sets of instruments: the Younger-Good-Hutchinson set; the McCall set, consisting of eight planes, three sickles, one chisel, and eighteen curettes, which was a simplified Carr set; the Towner "periodontomes"; and the Austin James planes. This last set brought about the concept of "two-point contact" for instrumentation. The Austin James planes consisted of 150 instruments that required special training for its purchase and use.

In the 1930s, Clayton H. Gracey of Michigan, designed the curettes used by most practitioners today. They are characterized by being area specific, with an "offset" blade that is curved in two planes. Current periodontology texts give detailed descriptions of these instruments, their many variants, and other instruments developed in recent years.[33]

Periodontics began in this period to attain the relevance of a true specialty, and numerous practitioners started to limit their practice to it. In the United States, the following were among the outstanding periodontists: Frank E. Beube, of Columbia University; Edgar D. Coolidge, of Ann Arbor, Michigan; Thomas B. Hartzell, of Minneapolis; Maynard K. Hine, of Indianapolis; Isador Hirschfeld, of Columbia University; Austin F. James, of Chicago; Harold J. Leonard, of Columbia University; Arthur Hastings Merritt, of New York City; John Oppie McCall, of Buffalo, New York; Samuel Charles Miller, of New York University; Sidney Sorrin, of New York City; Edward B. Spalding, of Detroit; Paul R. Stillman, of New York University; A. W. Ward, of San Francisco; James L. Zemsky, of New York City.

The champion of nonsurgical therapy in the United States during this period was Isador Hirschfeld (Fig 59). Born in 1882, he was founder and first chair of the Department of Periodontics at Columbia University, in 1928. Author of a classic, *The Toothbrush, Its Use and Abuse*,[19] Hirschfeld also published important papers, many of them pioneering topics such as food impaction and unreplaced missing teeth (see Chapter 20). Hirschfeld conducted a practice in Manhattan for more than fifty years, and a paper by his son, Leonard Hirschfeld, and Bernard Wasserman recorded the treatment results of mostly nonsurgical methods used on patients followed over a period of fifteen to fifty-three years.[20] Isador Hirschfeld died February 5, 1965.

In Europe Hans Sachs was a pioneer periodontist and strong advocate of conservative treatment.[14] Sachs was born in Breslau, then part of Germany, in 1881 and died in 1974. His father and grandfather were dentists. Sachs studied general medicine and physics before entering dentistry in Berlin and Breslau, and completed his dental studies in the United States, where he was a student of Robert Good, of Chicago. In 1908 Sachs returned to Germany and practiced in Berlin. In 1938, Sachs, a Jew, returned to the United States, where he obtained a dental degree and practiced in New York until 1962.

Sachs' treatment consisted of scaling and curettage using the Younger-Good instruments, which he modified. In addition, he used medicaments (50% lactic acid) originally described by Younger and prescribed meticulous oral hygiene.

Other prominent European periodontal researchers and clinicians of this period were Maurice Roy, René Vincent, Chactas Hulin, and Andrée Chaput, of France; E. Wilfred Fish, W. G. Cross, and A. B. Wade, of Great Britain; Arthur-Jean Held, René Jaccard, Louis J. Baume, Mario Spirgi, and Giorgio Cimasoni, of Switzerland; Otto Loos, Robert Neumann, and Oskar Weski, of Germany; Stefan Loos, of Austria; Silvio Palazzi, and Carlo Zerosi, of Italy; and many others.

In Latin America the leading periodontists were Pedro B. Ayllon, of Peru; Fermin Carranza, Sr, and Juan Bilbao, of Argentina; Alfonso Leng and Juan José Villavicencio, of Chile; and Jorge S. Mazzoni, of Uruguay.

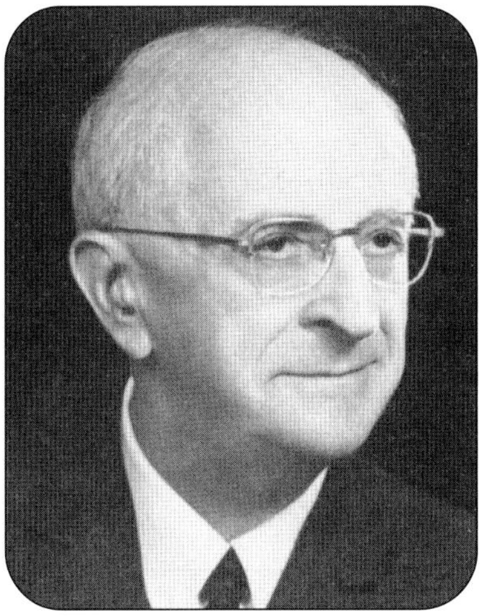

**Fig 59** Isador Hirschfeld.

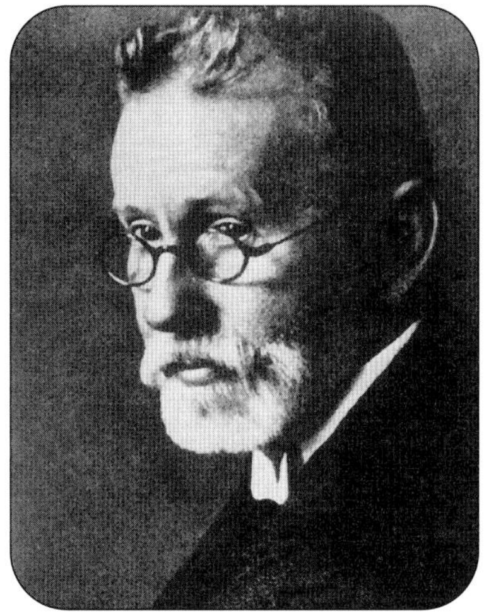

**Fig 60** Paul Ehrlich.

## Antimicrobial Agents

Scientists had searched for antimicrobial agents for the treatment of periodontal disease since the germ theory of disease became an accepted fact. It was Paul Ehrlich's pioneering work in chemotherapeutic drugs that revolutionized the treatment of infectious diseases.

Paul Ehrlich (1854–1915)[4,25] (Fig 60) was born in Prussian Silesia (today, Poland) and obtained his medical degree in 1878 at the University of Leipzig. His first interest was the use of anilines to stain tissue sections, particularly blood cells. He analyzed the cytoplasmic granules, which he classified according to their staining properties, as acidophiles, neutrophiles, and basophiles—a classification system still in use.

In the first decade of the twentieth century, Ehrlich, then director of the Institute for Experimental Therapy in Frankfurt, began extensive chemical and biological experiments, searching for therapeutic agents against infectious diseases. The idea that specific chemical substances could attach to specific cells (or microbes) stemmed from his original work with dyes.

Ehrlich tested literally hundreds of synthetic agents, concentrating on arsenical compounds, and in 1909 found that preparation No. 606 (Salvarsan), had excellent spirocheticidal properties. Later, in 1912, Ehrlich found an improved agent, No. 914 (Neosalvarsan). Ehrlich's work opened the field of antimicrobial pharmacological agents, which, decades later, with Alexander Fleming's discovery of penicillin (see Chapter 25), changed the practice of medicine and dentistry.

Scores of antibacterial agents have been advocated over the years for the treatment of gingivitis and periodontitis. Among them are spirocheticidal agents such as neoarsphenamin, novoarsenobenzol, bismuth salts, Fowler's solution (potassium arseniate), salvarsan, and neosalvarsan; bactericidal-bacteriostatic agents such as various iodine and mercury compounds, methylene blue, and sodium perborate; fungicidal agents such as mercury and arsenic preparations; and various dyes.[23,34] Many of these were used until not too long ago, and may still be used in some parts of the world, for treatment of acute necrotizing ulcerative gingivitis.

The treatment of necrotizing gingivitis was also performed with caustic drugs including potassium bicromate, chromium anhydride, mercuric chloride, silver nitrate, trichloracetic acid, chromic acid, iodo-glycerol solution, etc.[8]

*Vaccinotherapy.* Many dentists advocated the use of vaccines to supplement the local treatment of periodontal disease (see Chapter 19).

## New Attachment

Although Eustachius in the sixteenth century hinted at the problem of reattachment (see Chapter 8), William Younger appears to have been the first to mention, in 1893, the possibility of reattachment.[17] Younger was followed, in 1899, by Stewart. Younger recognized that reattachment was the ideal outcome of pocket therapy. He understood, too, that the persistence of the pocket epithelium was a potential barrier to obtaining reattachment. He used acid solvents for this purpose, recommending applications of lactic acid (50%) after scaling.

Other clinicians, such as D. D. Smith in 1902, advocated devitalization of the teeth with advanced periodontal disease, assuming that the blood supply that normally goes to the pulp would be diverted to the periodontium and would favor tissue regeneration and reattachment.[24]

In a book published in 1913, Friedrich Hecker clarifies the need for removal of the pocket epithelium.

> The tartar having been removed from the root, the next step is to rid the lining of the pocket of the epithelium, because no union can occur between the gum and the peridental membrane unless a raw bleeding surface is present. This is generally accomplished with an acid solution or by a normal solution of potassium hydroxyde (40 grams in 1,000 c.c. of distilled water). The author has secured the best results by the use of antiformin.[16]

In 1926 through 1928 John Oppie McCall, of New York, advocated the use of sodium sulphide for the removal of the epithelial lining of the pocket.[24,26] This technique was later evaluated by Samuel Charles Miller and Sidney Sorrin,[29] of New York University, and by Frank E. Beube,[5] of Columbia University, with conflicting results.

## Other Nonsurgical Methods

In the first half of the twentieth century, several methods were advocated as adjuncts to scaling and curettage or as separate methods of treatment. The Italian Piergili, in 1911, and W. F. Dunlop, in 1914, recommended the use of packing procedures to expand the pocket lumen, thus facilitating the removal of accretions. Piergili used a bismuth paste while Dunlop used paraffin. After a few days the paste was removed and scaling performed.[24]

The Dunlop method also included an oxygen spray and a special syringe for the application of the paraffin. The method was later adopted by Harold K. Box, Bernhard Gottlieb, and Balint Orban. Various drugs have also been suggested to induce shrinkage and cauterization of the gingival tissue. Among them are trichloracetic acid, silver nitrate, copper sulphate, potassium hydroxyde, phenol, zinc chloride, sulphuric acid/ether, silver nitrate, paraformaldehyde, and patent medicines such as the French product *Skapior.*[32,34]

Numerous methods were advocated in France and other European countries to obtain a so-called reactivation therapy, aimed at increasing blood circulation with special machines. Reactivation therapy included dietary modification, biostimulants obtained from extracts of placenta and other tissues, osteogenic stimulation with patent medicines (Alveoactiv, Herostéon. L. 3532, Vaduril, Eboson), and oral hygiene. Of course, oral hygiene was the only one that had any positive effect and is the only one that has persisted.[18] Ionic medication, employing a machine to send an electrolyte moving in a definite direction, was also proposed.[36,38]

## Plaque Control

Personal oral hygiene has been advocated since biblical times and its relation to periodontal health and disease was understood. Many of the previous chapters of this book refer to oral hygiene as a recommended method to treat and prevent periodontal diseases.

Early tooth cleaning devices included toothpicks (metallic and wood) and wooden chewsticks. Toothpicks were used by Greeks and Romans, and probably before them by Babylonians and Chinese.[10,19,22] In the thirteenth to seventeenth centuries toothpicks were made of precious metals and jewels, being ornamental in addition to utilitarian.[10,19,21] The Persian poet and mathematician Omar Khayyam (1025–1123), the Dutch philosopher Erasmus of Rotterdam (1466–1526), and William Shakespeare (1564–1616) mention toothpicks in their writings.[21]

The use of a chewstick, called *siwak*, was recommended by Muhammad and is still used by many Muslims, as well as other peoples in rural areas of Asia and Africa. It is effective and certainly more hygienic than the toothbrush since the chewstick is discarded after a single use.[1,21]

The first bristle toothbrushes date back to the fifteenth century, possibly earlier. They were introduced in China and reinvented in the West in the late eighteenth or early nineteenth century.

Since the beginning of the twentieth century, public awareness of the importance of oral hygiene, particularly to keep teeth clean and free of caries and stains and to maintain cleaner breath, has been the center of sweeping campaigns by dentifrice manufacturers. The concept of the "pink toothbrush" for prevention and detection of gingivitis was introduced by The Ipana Company. This campaign was decades ahead of dentists' advocacy of disease prevention.[12]

Toothbrushing methods used in the first decades of the twentieth century were the vertical technique, the horizontal technique, and the rolling technique. The last consisted of placing the brush horizontally against the gingivae and moving it vertically toward the crown. This method was most commonly used in the United States.[19]

Alfred Fones, in 1934, described the circular technique, known as the Fones method, which moves the brush in a circular or oblong manner, from the upper to the lower vestibule.[13] Fones was born in Bridgeport, Connecticut, in 1869, graduated from New York University in 1890, and founded the first clinic for the instruction of dental hygienists (see Chapter 26). He died in Bridgeport in 1938.[30]

Paul R. Stillman (1870–1945) received his dental education at the Baltimore College of Dental Surgery, graduating in 1899. He taught at Columbia University and later became clinical professor of periodontics at New York University. Stillman published extensively on periodontal diseases and their treatment. In 1932 he outlined the so-called Stillman method, which places the brush with its bristles obliquely into the gingival sulcus/pocket, with sufficient pressure to bend the bristles slightly, perceptibly blanching the tissues. The brush is then lifted and the procedure repeated. This was supposed to activate the circulation of blood.[19,37] The method was later modified when some practitioners added a vibratory motion.

William J. Charters (1872–1951), of Ankeny, Iowa, was an 1898 graduate of the Chicago College of Dental Surgery, Loyola. In 1935 he proposed a method that was widely used for several decades. It consisted of placing the brush obliquely toward the crown, with the sides of the bristles against the gingiva, and giving it a slightly rotary or vibratory motion. The effect was to be a stimulating massage to the gingiva.[6] At that time gingival massage was thought to be of primary importance to periodontal health and disease prevention, and the concept of plaque and its importance was not yet widely known. The introduction of chlorhexidine by Harald Löe and coworkers in their experimental gingivitis studies, revealed that gingival massage was not needed—that removal of plaque was the real purpose of oral hygiene. This revived the technique described years before by Charles C. Bass.

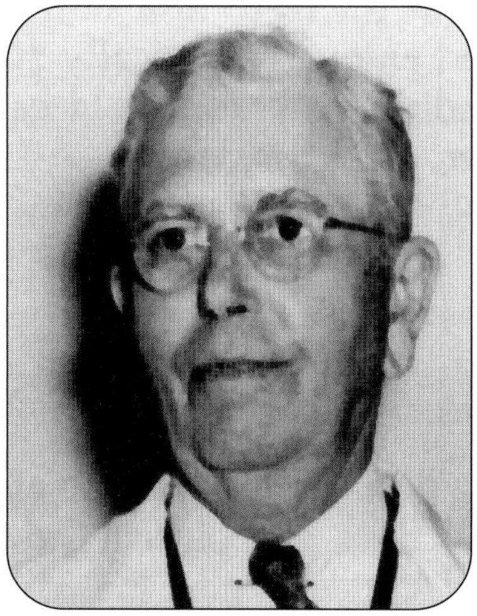

**Fig 61** Charles C. Bass, 1951.

Charles C. Bass (Fig 61), born in Lumberton, Mississippi, in 1875, was a physician and medical educator, and a graduate and later dean of Tulane University Medical School, in New Orleans. Bass worked in microbiology of malaria and hookworm diseases and investigated periodontal microbiology. In the 1910s Bass was a proponent of the ameba as the etiologic agent of periodontal disease.

Upon his retirement in 1940, Bass turned his attention again to oral microbiology and oral hygiene. He devised a method of brushing for which he developed the first synthetic-bristle brush, called the "Right Kind," which he sold at wholesale or at cost to dentists who had learned to demonstrate its proper use. The Bass method uses a soft brush placed at a 45-degree angle into the gingival sulcus, activated with short back-and-forth strokes. Bass was also a strong advocate of the use of dental floss to remove plaque from interproximal tooth surfaces.[2]

Bass was an open opponent of fluoridation in any form for the prevention of caries. He had a hostile and opinionated attitude toward the dental profession and its leaders in education and public health, believing that oral cleanliness was the only true preventive measure. Most of his articles were published in the medical literature. Among Bass' followers was Sumter S. Arnim, of the University of Texas, Houston, who expanded Bass' work by studying the dental microcosms with phase contrast cinemicrographs.[7] Bass died in 1975, at 100 years of age.[3]

Powered toothbrushes were invented in 1939. Numerous types have been marketed since then, with technological advances that have made them a valuable part of the oral hygiene armamentarium.

As noted in Chapter 15, dental floss was invented in the early 1800s by the New Orleans dentist Levy Spear Parmly, who recommended use of "waxed silk thread" in addition to thorough brushing.

Yeretsky mentions that S. T. Beal wrote in 1847:

> Those persons who brush or rub away daily all accumulations of saliva or food from between the teeth by passing back and forth, a piece of floss silk, ribbon, tape, towel or the like, and pay particular attention to cleanliness of those organs, never have them thus affected, except in those parts that cannot be reached.[39]

In 1939, Isador Hirschfeld described the importance of flossing and the technique for its use, including the use of floss holders, but flossing did not come into practice until gingival massage was proven to be unimportant in maintaining gingival health. Flossing then acquired primary importance.

## References


1. Asgis AJ. History of the toothbrush. Dent Dig 1929;35:307.
2. Bass CC. The necessary personal oral hygiene for prevention of caries and periodontoclasia. New Orleans Med Surg J 1948;101:52.
3. Bass CC. Collected Papers Relative to Dental Health 1941-1968. Chicago: John Butler, 1984.
4. Bäumler E. Paul Ehrlich — Scientist for Life. New York: Holmes & Meier, 1984.
5. Beube FE. Experimental study of the use of sodium sulphide solution in the treatment of periodontal pockets. J Periodontol 1939;10:49.
6. Charters WJ. Eliminating mouth infections with the toothbrush and other stimulating instruments. Dent Dig 1932;38:130.
7. Christen AG. Charles C. Bass, M.D. (1875–1975): That Cantankerous Genius of Preventive Dentistry. Bull Hist Dent 1990;38:8.
8. Coolidge ED. Clinical Pathology and Treatment of the Dental Pulp and Periodontal Tissues. Philadelphia: Lea & Febiger, 1939.
9. Crenshaw W. Pyorrhetic instrumentation. Dent Cosmos 1913;55:1015.
10. Davies GN. Social customs and habits and their effect on oral disease. Dent Cosmos 1963;42(suppl):209.
11. Fales MH. History of periodontology and the role of the dental hygienist. In: Perry DA, Beemsterboer PL, Taggart EJ (eds). Periodontology for the Dental Hygienist. Philadelphia: Saunders, 1996.
12. Fischman SL. The history of oral hygiene products: How far have we come in 6000 years? Periodontol 2000 1997;15:7.
13. Fones AC. Mouth Hygiene, ed 4. Philadelphia: Lea & Febiger, 1934.
14. Glenner RA. The scaler. Bull Hist Dent 1990;38:31.
15. Gold SI. Hans Sachs: Pioneer periodontologist and dental historian. Bull Hist Dent 1986;34:28.
16. Hecker F. Pyorrhea alveolaris. St. Louis: Mosby, 1913.
17. Held A-J. Periodontology. From Its Origins Up to 1980: A Survey. Basel: Birkhäuser, 1989.
18. Held A-J, Chaput A. Les Parodontolyses. Paris: Julien Prélat, 1959.
19. Hirschfeld I. The Toothbrush: Its Use and Abuse. New York: Dental Items of Interest, 1939.
20. Hirschfeld L, Wasserman B. A long-term survey of tooth loss in 600 treated periodontal patients. J Periodontol 1978;49:225.
21. Kanner L. Folklore of the teeth. VII. The folklore and cultural history of the toothpick and toothbrush. Dent Cosmos 1926;68:691.
22. Kimery MJ, Stallard RE. The evolutionary development and contemporary utilization of various oral hygiene procedures. J West Soc Periodontol Abstr 1968;16:90.
23. Kolmer JA. The chemotherapy of gingivitis. Dent Cosmos 1926;68:354.
24. Leonard HJ. Diagnosis and treatment of periodontoclasia. J Periodontol 1940;11:67.
25. Marquardt M. Paul Ehrlich. London: W. Heineman Medical Books, 1949.
26. McCall JO. The measure of success in periodontic practice. J Am Dent Assoc 1928;15:279.
27. McCall JO. The evolution of the scaler and its influence in the development of Periodontia. J Periodontol 1939;10:69.
28. Merritt, AH. Periodontal Diseases. Diagnosis and Treatment. New York: Macmillan, 1935.
29. Miller SC, Sorrin S. The action and use of sodium sulphide solution as epithelial solvent. Dent Cosmos 1927;69:1113.
30. Obituary, Alfred C. Fones. J Am Dent Assoc 1938;25:798.
31. Obituary, Paul R. Stillman. J Am Dent Assoc 1946;32:278.
32. Orban B. Gingivectomy by chemosurgery. J Am Dent Assoc 1943;30:198.
33. Pattison AM, Pattison GL, Takei HH. The periodontal instrumentarium. In: Newman MG, Takei HH, Carranza FA (eds). Carranza's Clinical Periodontology, ed 9. Philadelphia: Saunders, 2002.
34. Pucci FM. El Paradencio. Su Patologia y Tratamiento. Montevideo: Médica García Morales, 1939.
35. Sanoudos M, Christen AG. Levy Spear Parmly: The apostle of dental hygiene. J Hist Dent 1999;47:3.
36. Smith TS. Inflammatory diseases of the gingival margin and periodontal membrane (pyorrhea alveolaris): Dealing with the clinical signs, local treatment and treatment by ionic medication and vaccines. Dent Cosmos 1916;63:1239.
37. Stillman PR. A philosophy of the treatment of periodontal disease. Dent Dig 1932;38:314.
38. Sturridge E. Periodontal Disease and Its Treatment by Ionic Medication. Philadelphia: Lea & Febiger, 1919.
39. Yeretsky W. A historical review of oral prophylaxis. J Periodontol 1940;11:81.

# 22

# Clinical Periodontology 1900–1950: Periodontal Surgery

In the first half of the twentieth century, as in centuries past, techniques for the treatment of periodontal diseases were proposed on the basis of clinical experience and the ingenuity of the proponent to develop new technical approaches and design new instruments. This, of course, gave great importance to personal opinions, experience, and the prestige and position of the person proposing the method. While from the perspective of a century later this may seem unscientific and unsound, one should not underestimate the fact that this undoubtedly resulted in great progress with a clear benefit to the patients. This approach to the development of treatment methods was the same throughout all the medical sciences. Determination of the advantages and disadvantages of the different techniques based on the study of series of cases of similar characteristics, treated with different (standardized) techniques and analyzed using clinical measurements or other objective criteria, was not used until the last decades of the century.

## Surgical Techniques

Periodontal surgical techniques used in the nineteenth century (see Chapter 11) were essentially gingivectomies with a straight line incision followed by an aggressive curettage to remove the crestal bone, and thorough scaling of the root surface. Riggs had called these techniques barbaric, although apparently he practiced them.

Such operations were usually performed while the patient was under general anesthesia with chloroform. The surgical wound was not protected postoperatively since periodontal dressings were not developed until the 1920s. Neither were effective analgesics available to reduce postoperative pain, until the beginning of the twentieth century. German chemist Felix Hoffman (1868–1946) in the 1890s developed acetylsalicylic acid, which proved to have analgesic and anti-inflammatory properties and in 1899 received the name *aspirin.* In 1900 it was marketed worldwide by the German pharmaceutical company Bayer.[33]

The advantages provided by local anesthesia and knowledge of the underlying bone topography, as obtained with the advent of radiographs, led to the use of flap surgery. Carl Partsch (1855–1932), professor of oral surgery at the University of Breslau, developed a technique in the last years of the nineteenth century, performed under cocaine local anesthesia, for the surgical treatment of periapical lesions and cysts. The procedure involved a curved incision with the convexity toward the crown of the teeth, known to this day as the *Partsch incision.* After separating the tissues and elevating a flap, a cyst could be removed and the flap returned to its original position. After 1907, Partsch recommended that the flap be sutured.[20]

Most of the progress in periodontal surgery in this period came from Germany and other central European countries, and is associated with three names: Robert Neumann, Leonard Widman, and A. Cieszinski. Robert Neumann[15] (Fig 62) was born in 1882, in the town of Patschkau, in what was then eastern Germany (now Poland). He studied medicine and dentistry

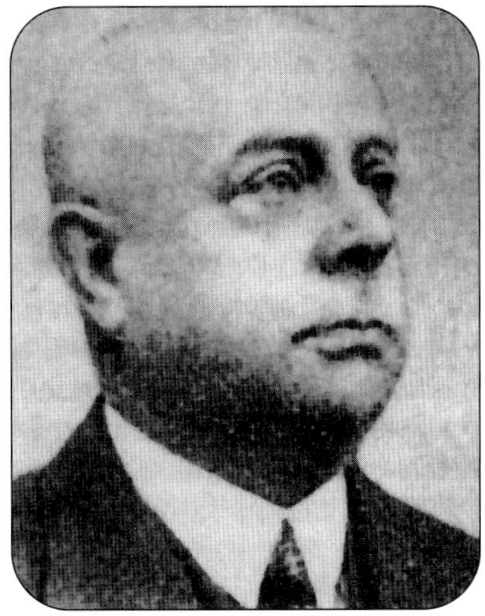

**Fig 62** Robert Neumann.

at the University of Berlin. After graduating, he assisted in the surgery department under Professor Willinger and worked also with Professor Partsch.

Neumann published several papers on various surgical subjects but early in his career became interested in periodontal disease, lecturing about the subject in the 1910s.

The surgical treatment Neumann proposed in 1912[15,28] and refined in subsequent publications was done in sextants and consisted of vertical incisions—not bisecting the interdental papilla—followed by crevicular incisions to the bone margin to separate a flap that was then elevated to gain clear view of the entire field of operation. While the flap was held open with retractors, all granulations and calculus were removed and the bone margin smoothed with chisels and burs to reshape it to its normal topography (Fig 63). (In later editions of his book, Neumann followed Weski, advocating transformation of all vertical bone losses into horizontal ones, meaning to eliminate all vertical losses.) The margin of the flap was then trimmed and scalloped with scissors to reach exactly the bone margin, and sutured using straight and curved needles and silk thread. Neumann's flap operation had wide diffusion in North and South America in the 1920s.[3,8]

Neumann also performed frenotomies to prevent the flaps from being separated from the tooth and advocated taking radiographs with gutta-percha points in the pocket, presurgical scaling, provisional splinting prior to surgery, and toothbrushing with horizontal strokes. Robert Neumann died in 1958.

Leonard Widman[14] (1871–1956) (Fig 64) was a Swedish dentist who published two papers on the surgical treatment of periodontal disease, one in 1917 and the other in 1923. Widman's technique was similar to Neumann's. Widman recommended surgery to obtain access to root deposits for their complete removal and for complete elimination of granulation tissue.

Widman's surgical technique[14] consisted of oblique vertical incisions outlining an area of about three to four teeth, followed by a festooned incision about 1 mm from the gingival margin; this makes him the first to advocate the internal bevel incision currently used. Widman then elevated the flap by sharp dissection, thinning the flap to separate it from the granulation tissue, "but not too much to avoid flap necrosis," as far as the edge of "sound bone." After the flap was retracted, all granulation tissue and calculus were removed, and "rough" bone projections rounded off with burs to obtain a normal anatomical topography. The flap was then returned to its place and sutured with interdental silk sutures.

A. Cieszinski was a Polish dentist. Little is known about his life and work except that he published two papers, one in 1914 and another in 1926.[10]

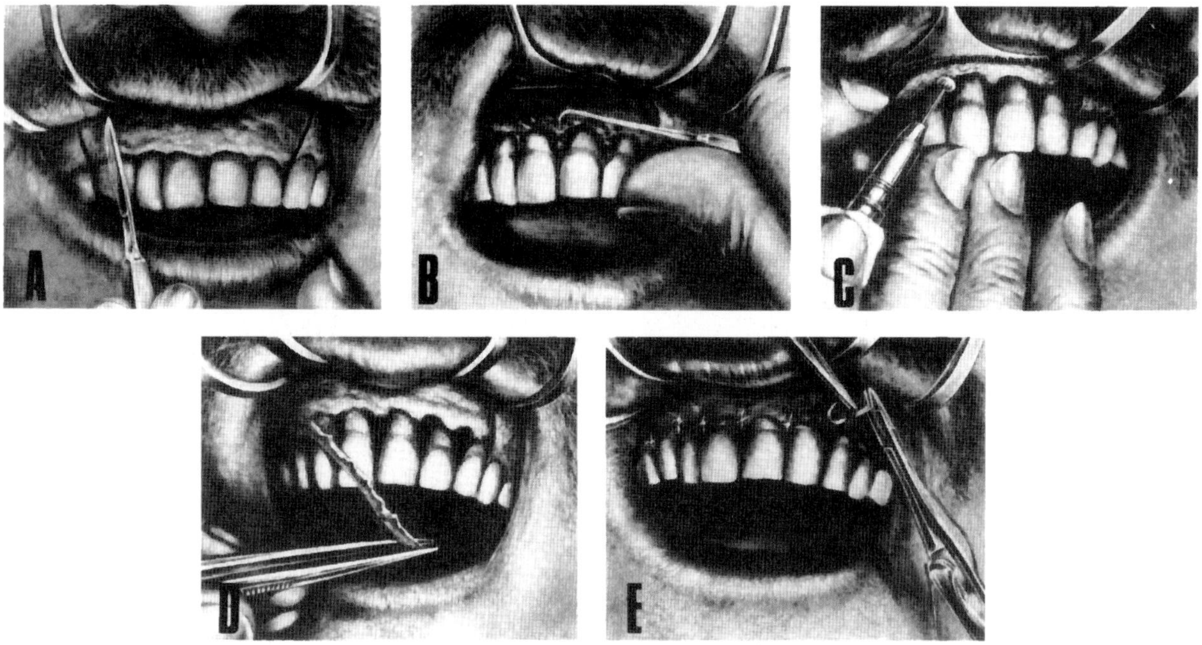


**Fig 63** Neumann's surgical technique.[15]

In the 1920s a bitter controversy arose between Neumann and Widman. Cieszinski and dentist Arthur Zentler later joined this fray over who was the first to describe the flap operation.[11,29] During World War I, communications between scientists were difficult if not impossible[12]; furthermore, all scientific developments are seldom the work of one person in isolation but the concurrent work of many individuals.[15] The exact assignment of priority is therefore difficult. Neumann and Widman probably could share the credit for the development of the flap operation.

In the United States several clinicians also advocated surgical techniques for the treatment of periodontal disease. G. V. Black, famous for his development of a systematized approach to cavity preparation for the treatment of dental caries, also turned his interest to periodontal therapy and proposed a surgical technique for the treatment of periodontal pockets. Black's technique was a gingival resection operation, using a straight incision following the bottom of the pockets at the bone margin. He recommended use of cautery or a knife. Black admitted that in some cases pockets may recur but usually will be shallower, allowing more effective cleaning by the patient. The treatment is contraindicated in maxillary incisors "on account of the unsightly appearance of the denuded root." Black also mentions that "there is little hope for those cases in which pockets of considerable depth have formed on proximal surfaces."[6]

In 1918, Arthur Zentler, a New York dentist affiliated with Columbia University, described a technique similar to Neumann's, as two parallel vertical incisions and scalloped incisions "following the original festoons of the gums," lifting a flap to allow root scaling and curettage to remove all granulation tissue from the pocket area and the underside of the flap, and trimming and smoothing, with chisel and mallet, all "infected bone."[42] He then cut away with scissors the margin of the flap and sutured the vertical and interdental incisions. Zentler claimed his treatment produced a successful and permanent cure in a short number of visits, and was not painful.[43]

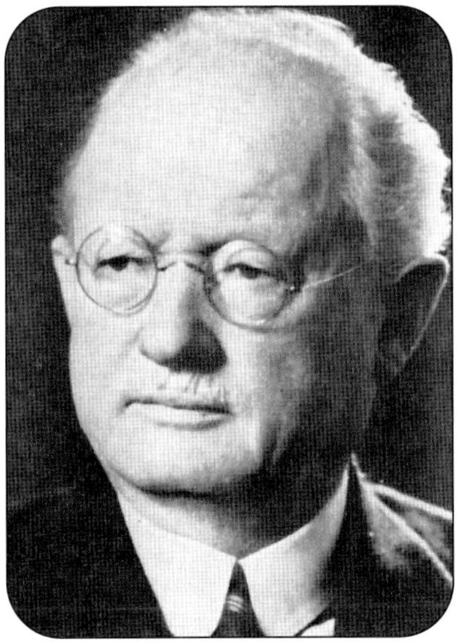

**Fig 64** Leonard Widman.

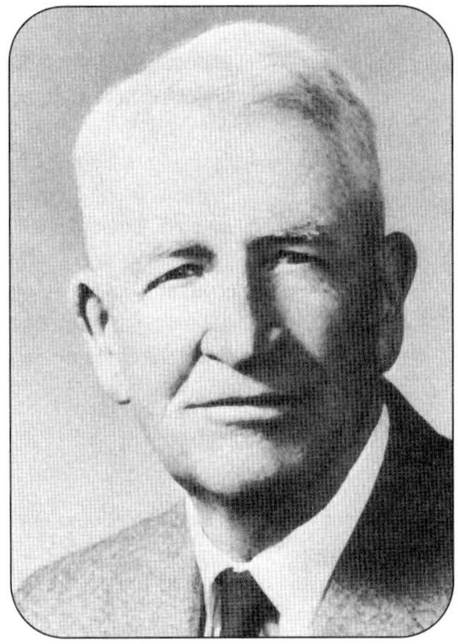

**Fig 65** A. W. Ward.

William Ziesel, of Philadelphia, presented in 1920[44] a gingivectomy technique using specially designed instruments. Then in 1923 Abraham Wesley Ward (1880–1973) (Fig 65), of San Francisco, developed a surgical dressing that he called *Wondr-Pak,* to be applied on surgical gingival wounds. This improved the post-operative care of the gingivectomy technique.[39,40] The dressing consisted largely of zinc oxide and eugenol, and, with modifications, is still used.

In 1926, James L. Zemsky (1884–1951), of New York City, presented a technique that he called *open view* operation, which was a flap technique with removal of "infected and sharp edges of bone."[41]

Olin Kirkland (1876–1969) (Fig 66), a prominent dentist in Montgomery, Alabama, presented in 1932, a technique that he called a *modified flap* operation.[23,24] It was used for isolated deep periodontal lesions. The procedure consisted of splitting mesiodistally the papilla of the involved space and retracting the gingiva using separators to keep the area open, followed by root scaling and removal with nippers of all granulation tissue on the soft tissue flap, and closure of the wound with one suture. A dressing consisting of one part sticky wax and three parts beeswax was applied over the area with a camel-hair brush. Kirkland also designed some widely used periodontal instruments, such as the Kirkland gingivectomy knives.

In 1934, A. B. Crane and Harry Kaplan, of Washington, DC, described a technique[12] that they indicated for pockets extending beyond the middle third of the root. The procedure consists of probing and marking the bottom of the pockets on the outer gingival surface, making a horizontal scalloped incision connecting the bleeding points, removing the excised tissue, curetting the exposed osseous surface using specially designed sawlike instruments to obtain a horizontal interdental bone margin, scaling the root surface, and finally applying surgical dressing.

Many periodontists continued to reject all kinds of surgical periodontal therapy and advocated only the "scaling and curettage" technique. The periodontal world divided into two camps: those recommending conservative treatment (scaling and curettage) and those using the radical approach (surgery). The latter group had two subgroups: the gingivectomy proponents and the flap surgery advocates. Several decades passed before indications for each procedure were determined and a more rational approach to therapy followed. The gingivectomy technique continued to be the more widely recommended and practiced technique. Toward the late 1930s and 1940s, the procedure was refined and the aggressive curettage of the osseous margin—an attempt to remove "diseased bone"—was ceased.[16,22,25,31,32]

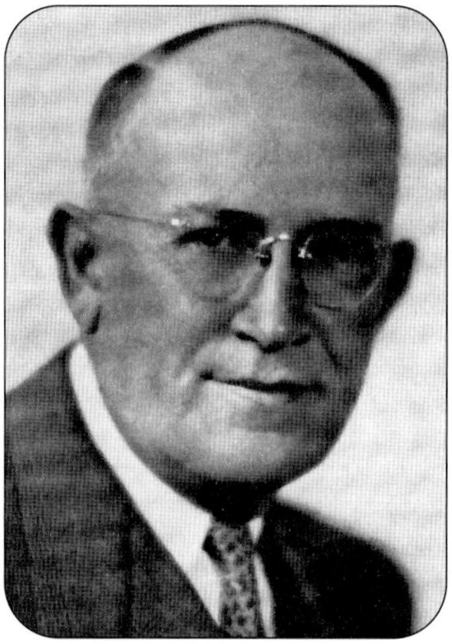

**Fig 66** Olin Kirkland.

In 1950 Henry M. Goldman (1911–1991), of Boston, described gingivoplasty,[17] a concept that would attain wide acceptance in the following decades and lead to periodontal plastic surgery. Goldman recommended reshaping the gingiva for the purpose of attaining a more desirable form and not for pocket eradication.

## Management of the Alveolar Bone

The concept prevalent in the nineteenth and early twentieth centuries, that the bone margin was infected or diseased, made necessary in all surgical techniques a step to remove the osseous margin. This was carried out with the gingivectomies proposed by Robicsez, Riggs, and Black, by means of aggressive curettage after removing the pocket wall.

With the introduction of the flap operation, which opened the operative area to full view, the bone margin could be removed with burs, or with chisels and mallets. The concept, however, continued to be removal of diseased bone, although Neumann and Widman also spoke of smoothing the "rough" osseous margin.

In 1935, Rudolph Kronfeld (1901–1939), of Chicago (formerly of Vienna, Austria), finally clarified the condition of the bone underlying periodontal pockets.[26] He described the osteoclastic resorption of the alveolar bone, occurring on the bone surface adjacent to the inflammatory process in the pocket but also on the deeper bone trabeculae, mentioning also that the bone is neither decalcified nor necrotic. This new concept eliminated the need to remove "diseased" bone, but clinicians continued to find recurrence of disease when irregular bone edges were left in place. The result was a new rationale for osseous resection: that bone contouring is necessary, particularly in the case of vertical and irregular bone losses, in order to avoid recurrence of the pocket. This idea was developed by two clinicians, independently of each other.

Fermin Carranza, Sr. (1900–1988) (Fig 67), of Buenos Aires, Argentina, developed the rationale for osseous resection in a paper published in 1941. Carranza described and illustrated the cases in which this treatment was recommended: vertical bone loss, interdental craters, and irregular bone margins (Fig 68). The fact that this approach would remove useful bone with a normal periodontal ligament attachment was recognized but deemed necessary for pocket removal.[9]

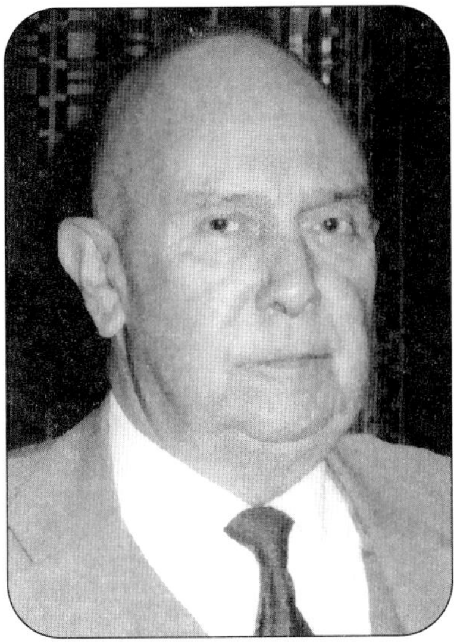

Fig 67 Fermin A. Carranza, Sr.

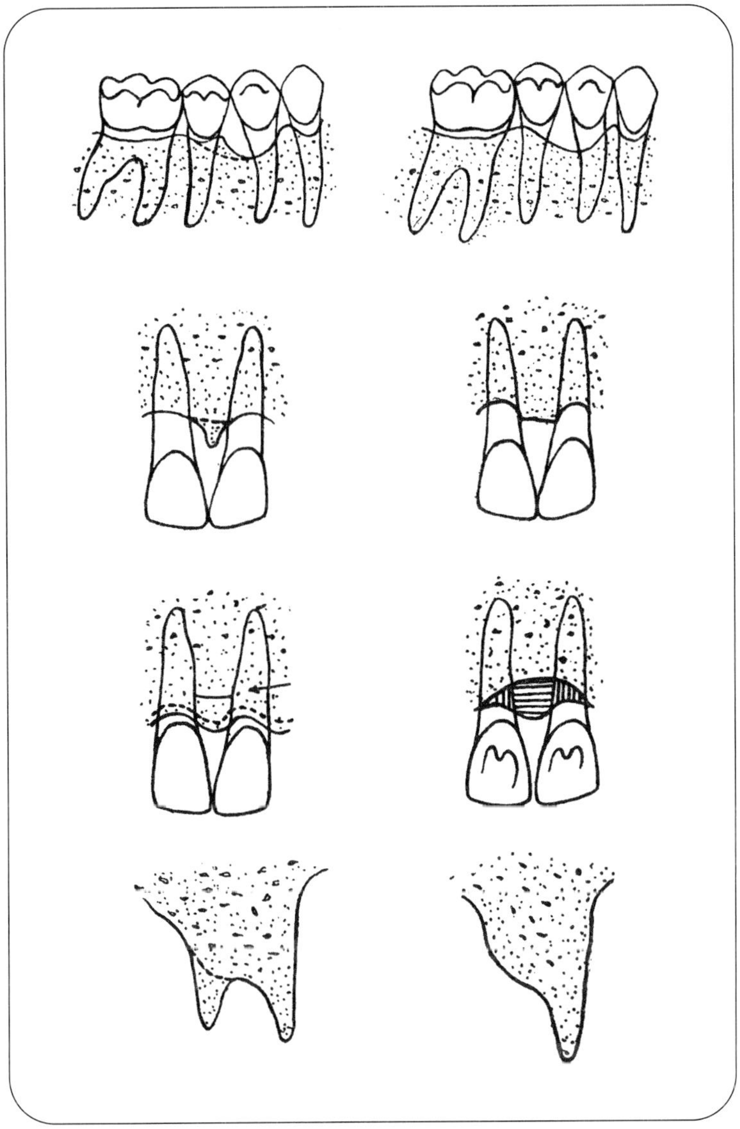

Fig 68 Indications for osseous removal as determined by Carranza.[9]

A few years later, in 1949, not knowing of Carranza's work (published in Spanish in a little-known journal), Saul Schluger[36] (1908–1990; see biography of Schluger in Chapter 25), of Columbia University, New York, and later of Seattle, Washington, described a similar technique, with the indication of bone contouring in isolated infrabony pockets on facial or lingual surfaces, interdental craters, and deep pockets on the mesial aspect of tilted second molars where the first molar has been lost and not replaced. Schluger's rationale for osseous resection in periodontal surgery added the fact that the gingiva follows the bone contour during healing and therefore the latter must be contoured to a physiologic shape in order to attain proper gingival morphology.

In 1923, a new approach to the treatment of osseous defects, seeking to rebuild rather than eliminate them by surgical recontouring, had begun to appear with the work of Zoltán Hegedüs, of Budapest, Hungary.[19] Hegedüs proposed to rebuild the lost alveolar bone by "utilizing the bone-building and regenerative property of the periosteum." He further explained:

> Relying on this fact, we have transplanted a periosteo-cortical band in the place of the destroyed alveolar processes. The transplanted periosteum, having grown together with the neighboring sound periosteum, there begins a new bone formation. ...
>
> In our first efforts we tried to take the transplant from the neighborhood: In the case of the upper teeth, from the corpus maxillæ; in the lower from the mandible. This procedure was attended by great technical difficulties on the one hand, and on the other, the tissue preparation had to extend deeply, in order to obtain a transplant of adequate size, which was also disadvantageous on account of the successive severe pains. We found it much simpler to take the transplant from the tibia, which is technically much easier, and in healing within a week, it was attended by less pain.

Hegedüs goes on to describe the importance of a correct diagnosis, differentiating between "pyorrhea and atrophia alveolaris praecox" since the latter "being a regressive disease is not amenable to surgical treatment." Next he elucidates the technique to obtain bone from the tibia, under "strictest sterilization, for in the case of infection there may occur osteomyelitis of the tibia." The periodontal surgery he advocates is a Neumann-type flap, careful removal of all "concretions adhering to the roots," scraping off the granulation tissues with a chisel, and removing the softened parts of bone until sound bone is reached. The surface of the sound bone is "freshened" and the transplanted bone is placed on it, fixed with one or two stitches of catgut, and the flap placed back in its position and sutured. Hegedüs reports on six cases, illustrated with radiographs taken preoperatively and four to ten weeks after.

In the following decade, Frank Beube, of Columbia University, investigated in dogs[5] and in humans[4] the use of devitalized heterogeneous bone powder for periodontal bone regeneration. Other early investigators of the problem of reattachment were William Skillen and G. A. Lundquist,[38] who experimented with it in 1937, reporting reattachment of epithelial and connective tissue fibers during pocket healing.

These were the first attempts to understand and promote regeneration and reconstruction of bone lost to periodontal disease. Only after several decades would they attain great clinical relevance and become an extremely important aspect of periodontal therapy.

## Esthetic Surgery

Techniques to solve esthetic problems also interested periodontists in the early years of the twentieth century. William Younger (1838–1920), a disciple and contemporary of John Riggs, presented a case before the American Dental Club of Paris on December 6, 1902. The minutes of the meeting read as follows[1]:

> Dr. Younger reported a case of extensive absorption of gum and alveolar tissue, from the upper left canine to the molar, due to former pyorrhea. He attempted to restore the gum by grafting a piece taken from behind the third molar of the same mouth; he scarified the surface to receive the graft by rubbing with cotton saturated with lactic acid, making a raw surface for granulations; upon this he fixed his gum graft and fastened it in place with a coating of celluloid solution, but the piece came off. The he tried another piece and stitched it into place, using fine cambric needles bent to proper curve after drawing the temper. That operation was a success. The graft contracted greatly, but he obtained an increase of tissue about equal to one-fourth of the bulk of the graft. He proposes to try transplanting gum from the mouth of a rabbit.

During the same session Younger related another experiment that can be considered the first attempt at guided tissue regeneration. The minutes continue[1]:

After cleansing the root of tartar, etc., and treating them with lactic acid, I dry the parts as perfectly as possible, then rubbing with alcohol, to dry the roots; I then place over the parts bits of Japanese paper saturated with liquid celluloid, so as to form a protecting wall over the roots and edge of the gum. After that is done I take a thread and wing it around and tie it, to prevent all possibility of the paper getting out of position. The covering hardens and forms a perfect shield to the granulations, which grow up and fill the spaces between the roots. I have several cases in which the gums are growing in nicely.

On June 8, 1906, A. W. Harlan, presented a paper in Washington, DC,[2,18] in which he describes the following technique for root coverage of isolated gingival recessions[2]:

I first cleanse the surface of the exposed root and carefully dissect the gum from the root to about one-quarter to three-eighths of an inch in depth, carefully wiping away the blood, keeping the mouth open until the hemorrhage ceases spontaneously or through the use of an adrenaline solution. I then make three incisions into and through the gum tissue. When the bleeding has almost ceased, I fill these cuts with dried zinc iodid, allowing the blood to liquefy it so that it may be carried around the gingival margin. This will create a profound irritation of the gum, which must be left undisturbed. The patient should use for a few days some mildly antiseptic wash—an antacid one—composed of such agents as sodium bicarbonate or milk of magnesia. After the lapse of three weeks the scar tissue which will grow in these incisions will be hard enough to permit of repeating the operation in a new locality. The exposed face of the root should be roughened to permit close adherence of the gum to this surface, as it is slowly pushed downward over the root.

It is no wonder that this strange technique did not gain any followers, but it is interesting to see that the esthetic problem created by tooth recession, "especially in the mouth of a lady, or of a man whose teeth are not hidden from view by a mustache," was already recognized and solutions sought. A more reasonable root coverage technique was engineered a few years later (1911) by the French researcher P. Rosenthal.[2,35] The procedure is somewhat similar to the semilunar coronally repositioned flap devised seven decades later by Dennis Tarnow, of New York. Nevertheless, root coverage techniques did not attract the interest of the profession until the latter part of the century.

## References


1. American Dental Club of Paris. Meetings of December 1902 and January and March 1903. Dent Cosmos 1904;46:39.
2. Baer PN, Benjamin SD. Gingival grafts: A historical note. J Periodontol 1981;52:206.
3. Berger A. The surgical treatment of periodontoclasia. J Am Dent Assoc 1927;14:1013.
4. Beube FE. A study on reattachment of the supporting structures of the teeth. J Periodontol 1947;18:55.
5. Beube FE, Silvers HF. Influences of devitalized heterogeneous bone powder on regeneration of alveolar and maxillary bone of dogs. J Dent Res 1934;14:15.
6. Black GV. Special Dental Pathology. Chicago: Medico-Dental, 1915.
7. Blanquie RH. Fundamentals and technic of surgical periodontal packing. J Oral Surg 1946;4:227.
8. Carranza FA Sr. La cirujia en el tratamiento de la piorrea alveolar. Trib Odontol 1928;12:17.
9. Carranza FA Sr. Cuando y porque sacrificar hueso en el tratamiento de la paradentosis. An Ateneo Inst Munic Odont Buenos Aires 1941;1:311.
10. Cieszinski A. Bemerkungen zur radical chirurgischeen Behandlung der sogennanten Pyorrhoealveolaris. Dtsch Monattschr Zahnheilk 1914;11:36.
11. Cieszinski A. Radikal chirurgische Behandlung der parodontale Erkrankungen nach Cieszinski-Widman-Nodine-Zentler-Neumann oder Operation Neumann's? Dtsch Monattschr Zahnheilk 1926;23:80.
12. Crane AB, Kaplan H. The Crane-Kaplan operation for the prompt elimination of pyorrhea alveolaris. Dent Cosmos 1931;73:643.

13. Denton GB. History of diseases and treatment of the investing tissues of the teeth. In: Black GV (ed). Operative Dentistry, vol 4. Chicago: Medico-Dental, 1936:51–67.
14. Everett FG, Waerhaug J, Widman A. Leonard Widman: Surgical treatment of pyorrhea alveolaris. J Periodontol 1971;42:571.
15. Gold SI. Robert Neumann: A pioneer in periodontal flap surgery. J Periodontol 1982;53:456.
16. Goldman HM. Gingivectomy: Indications, contraindications and method. Am J Orthod Oral Surg, Oral Surg Sect 1946;32:323.
17. Goldman HM. The development of physiologic gingival contours by gingivoplasty. Oral Surg Oral Med Oral Pathol 1950;3:879.
18. Harlan AW. Restoration of gum tissue on the labial aspect of teeth. Dent Cosmos 1906;48:927.
19. Hegedüs Z. The rebuilding of the alveolar processes by bone transplantation. Dent Cosmos 1923;65:736.
20. Held A-J. Les Paradentoses et Leur Traitement. Paris: Masson et Cie, 1939.
21. Hoffmann-Axthelm W. History of Dentistry. Chicago: Quintessence, 1981.
22. Johnson RE. Gingivectomy in the treatment of suppurative periodontoclasia. J Am Dent Assoc 1931;18:1455.
23. Kirkland O. The suppurative periodontal pus pocket: Its treatment by the modified flap operation. J Am Dent Assoc 1931;18:1462.
24. Kirkland O. Modified flap operation in surgical treatment of periodontoclasia. J Am Dent Assoc 1932;19:1918.
25. Kirkland O. Modern techniques in surgical periodontia. J Am Dent Assoc 1942;29:817.
26. Kronfeld R. The condition of alveolar bone underlying periodontal pockets. J Periodontol 1935;6:22.
27. Mann JB, Crane AB, Kaplan H. Pyorrhea alveolaris: Histopathology and results of radical surgical treatment. Dent Cosmos 1934;76:432.
28. Neumann R. Die Alveolarpyorrhea and ihre Behandlung. Berlin: Meusser, 1912.
29. Neumann R. Erwiderung zu Widmans aufahrungen über die Prioritätfrage betreffs der radikalchirurgischen Behandlung der sogennanten Alveolarpyorrhoe. Vjschr Zahnheilk 1923;39:170.
30. Nodine AM. Surgical treatment of pyorrhea. Dent Cosmos 1921;63:345.
31. Orban BJ. Gingivectomy or flap operation? J Am Dent Assoc 1939;26:1276.
32. Orban BJ. Indications, technique and post-operative management of gingivectomy in the treatment of the periodontal pocket. J Periodontol 1941;12:89.
33. Porter R. The Greatest Benefit to Mankind. New York: Norton, 1997.
34. Pucci FM. Paradencio—Patologia y Tratamiento. Montevideo: Médica Garcia Morales, 1939.
35. Rosenthal P. Recovering the exposed necks of teeth by autoplasty. Dent Cosmos 1912;54:377.
36. Schluger S. Osseous resection—A basic principle in periodontal surgery. Oral Surg Oral Med Oral Pathol 1949;2:316.
37. Simonton GW. The treatment of pyorrhea by surgical exposure of the tissues involved. J Am Dent Assoc 1925;12:329.
38. Skillen WG, Lundquist GA. An experimental study of peridental membrane reattachment in healthy and pathological tissues. J Am Dent Assoc 1937;24:175.
39. Ward AW. Inharmonius cusp relation as a factor in periodontoclasia. J Am Dent Assoc 1923;10:471.
40. Ward AW. Postoperative care in the surgical treatment of pyorrhea. J Am Dent Assoc 1929;16:635.
41. Zemsky J. Surgical treatment of periodontal disease with the author's open view operation for advanced cases of dental periclasia. Dent Cosmos 1926;68:465.
42. Zentler A. Suppurative gingivitis with alveolar involvement. JAMA 1918;71:1530.
43. Zentler A. The surgical treatment of suppurative gingivitis, so-called pyorrhea. J Dent Res 1920;2:xvii.
44. Ziesel W. Pyorrhea extermination: Gingivo-ectomy. Dent Cosmos 1921;63:352.

# 23

# Focal Infection

The concept of focal infection—the spread of infections to remote tissues or organs—has been known since antiquity. Seventh-century BC Assyrian clay tablets found in Nineveh, capital of ancient Assyria on the river Tigris, mention that the king's child had a fever caused by tooth eruption.[10,15] Three centuries later, Hippocrates (460–370 BC) notes a case of rheumatism cured after extraction of an infected tooth.[33] The Babylonian Talmud (third century AD), also refers to diseases caused by oral infections, as did Italian scholar Girolamo Cardano (1501–1576) and German researcher Walter Hermann Ryff (d. 1562), in the sixteenth century.[15,25] In the nineteenth century Benjamin Rush (1745–1813), noted physician and signer of the American Declaration of Independence, recognized the relation of oral infection to general health. Rush relates several cases in point, among them an incident of rheumatism that did not respond to current medications and disappeared without recurrence after the extraction of an aching tooth.[33] Leonard Koecker (1785–1850), in 1828, recognized the role of oral sepsis in rheumatic and other diseases.[19]

Later in the century (1891), W. D. Miller (1853 1907) mentioned oral infections as the cause of many diseases:

> During the last few years the conviction has grown continually stronger, among physicians as well as dentists, that the human mouth, as a gathering-place and incubator of diverse pathogenic germs, performs a significant role in the production of varied disorders of the body, and that if many diseases whose origin is enveloped in mystery could be traced to their source, they would be found to have originated in the oral cavity.[23]

Miller describes in this long paper many diseases that could originate in oral bacteria. Among them are septicemia, pyemia, meningitis, encephalitis, abscess of the brain, disturbances of the alimentary tract, lung diseases, tuberculosis, and syphilis.

Miller presented this paper at the International Congress of Hygiene in London, at a session presided by Lord Lister. British physician Sir William Hunter was part of the audience.[25] Hunter was interested in this problem since he had studied the mouth as a possible source of infection in pernicious anemia; his interest was increased by Miller's presentation.[25]

Hunter's paper, published in 1900,[16] and a decade later his lecture at McGill University in Montreal, published in *Lancet*,[17] caused considerable confusion and increased interest in the topic. Hunter (1861–1937), a lecturer in pathology at the Charing Cross Hospital in London, indicted dentistry as the cause of what he called *oral sepsis* which in turn caused rheumatic and other chronic diseases.

> In my clinical experience septic infection is without exception the most prevalent infection operating in medicine, and a most prevalent cause and complication of many medical diseases. Its ill-effects are widespread and extend to all systems in the body. The relations between these effects and the sepsis that causes them are constantly overlooked, because the existence of the sepsis is itself overlooked. For the chief seat of that sepsis is the mouth; and the sepsis itself, when noted, is erroneously regarded as the result of the various conditions of ill-health with which it is associated—not, as it really is, an important cause or complication.

> The causal connexion between the two sets of processes—the sepsis and its ill-effects—can be demonstrated by the simple expedient of removing the sepsis, and noting the striking effect which the removal has upon the existence, character, and intensity of its ill-effects.

Hunter locates "the chief seat of that sepsis" in "septic lesions of streptococcal and staphylococcal infection found in the mouth" and suggests two potential origins: "follicular tonsillitis ... [and] a foul, septic, suppurating condition of the gums, with deposition of calcareous 'crusts and scabs' (so-called tartar), covering and hiding septic wounds and ulcers—loaded, as microscopic examination shows, with staphylococci and streptococci."

He notes, too, that follicular tonsillitis is rare while gum infections are "exceedingly common."

> My clinical experience satisfies me that if oral sepsis (and naso-pharyngeal) could be successfully excluded, the other channels by which "medical sepsis" gains entrance into the body might almost be ignored. Sepsis as an important and prevalent cause of disease would almost cease to exist, instead of being, as in my judgement is at the present time, a more important and prevalent cause of disease.
>
> Even if the teeth were not subject to a very marked septic infective process—that which we term caries and carionecrosis ... the septic infection in the gums and in the periosteum of the sockets, constitute very important septic wounds and are a great source of sepsis to the body. As a matter of experience, this is often the case. The teeth remain intact or at least free from obvious caries or cario-necrosis; but the gums and periosteum of the sockets are the seat of numerous septic wounds. These effects are shown by septic suppuration, by deposits of tartar, sometimes in great masses on the teeth, on the gum margin and beneath the gum margins, by the formation of pockets (septic ulceration of periodonteum [sic]—periostitis, absorption of bone, loosening of the teeth, suppuration—sometimes, however, by very slight suppuration.

Hunter goes on to say that this is most common in poor patients who have had "no care" of their mouths. But he also indicts dentistry:

> No one has probably had more reason than I have had to admire the sheer ingenuity and mechanical skill constantly displayed by the dental surgeon. And no one has had more reason to appreciate the ghastly tragedies of oral sepsis which his misplaced ingenuity so often carries in its train. Gold fillings, gold caps, gold bridges, gold crowns, fixed dentures, built in, on, and around diseased teeth, form a veritable mausoleum of gold over a mass of sepsis to which there is no parallel in the whole realm of medicine and dentistry.

Recognizing the infective nature of dental restorations, Hunter recommends the following protocol:

> to swab the edges of the gums and teeth with cotton-wool and 1 in 60 carbolic in order to clean off pus and to enable me to see the character and extent of the underlying wounds. The wounds are thereby dressed at the same time that they are being examined, and all the superficial sepsis is got rid of. This antiseptic dressing of the gums should be carried out daily, so long as open wounds are present.[17]

In addition, Hunter describes cases of septic gastritis, colitis, anemia, tuberculosis, chronic nephritis, and various fevers.

It is clear that to William Hunter the major infectious oral focus was the periodontium and not periapical disease. His principal indictment of "American dentistry" was not aimed at faulty endodontic treatments or the lack thereof, but at restorative procedures performed on untreated periodontally diseased teeth. Publication of Hunter's 1911 paper[17] in the prestigious *Lancet* unleashed a strong reaction, mostly because of the use of the phrase "American dentistry" to refer to ill-conceived and ill-prepared restorative procedures. Edward Cameron Kirk, professor of clinical dentistry at the University of Pennsylvania and for many years editor of *Dental Cosmos*, wrote in 1911 that the dentistry that Hunter indicted "must have been done by an advertising quack," and "a so-called American dentist, who had never seen America and of whom cult London is full."[10] In general, however, Hunter's message was well-received and generated a great deal of basic and applied research and reconsideration of clinical techniques. G. V. Black[5] saw it as an "opportunity before the dental profession to take an important part in the preservation of the general health … almost without parallel in medical advancement."

Frank Billings, of the Rush Medical College and Presbyterian Hospital in Chicago,[1–4] and Edward C. Rosenow, of the Memorial Institute for Infectious Diseases in Chicago,[29–31] published several clinical and microbiologic papers to clarify the role of focal infection in systemic disease. Charles H. Mayo, of the Mayo Clinic in Rochester, Minnesota, was also interested in the problem and published several papers.[20,21]

The bacteriologic investigations, perhaps influenced by the increasing use of radiographs in clinical dentistry,[26] gradually centered more on periapical disease rather than on periodontal disease.[7,11–13,32] The advocated solution was to extract all teeth with periodontal or periapical infections, to prevent systemic diseases. This led to wholesale extractions of all infected teeth (and removal of tonsils), unnecessarily mutilating many patients. Countless millions of teeth were extracted under the erroneous assumption that they put the life of the patient in danger.

After a quarter century of tremendous influence in the practice of medicine and dentistry, the focal infection theory fell into disrepute, partly due to the excesses committed in its name.[9] In 1938, R. Cecil, who had been a proponent of the theory of focal infection, published a study of 200 patients with rheumatoid arthritis who had not improved appreciably after having the tonsils removed and teeth extracted.[7] A review published by Williams and Burkett found no good scientific evidence to support the focal infection theory.[34] An editorial published in the *Journal of the American Medical Association* in 1952 explains it on the basis of the following[9]:

1. Many patients with diseases presumably caused by foci of infection have not been relieved by removal of the foci.
2. Patients with same diseases may not have detectable foci of infection.
3. Foci of infection can occur in healthy persons with no ill effects.

Moreover, improvements in dental restorative procedures, endodontic and periodontal treatments, and the advent of the antibiotic era in the late 1940s solved many oral infections while preserving the teeth.[9,23,25,26]

The problem with focal infection caused by dental procedures was not that it was not true. The trouble was that it led to the unwarranted and unnecessary extraction of teeth when the elimination of the oral infection, whenever possible, by adequate periodontal and endodontic therapy, and the prevention of "oral sepsis" by improved restorative procedures would have been a better, nondestructive solution.

The focal infection theory remains viable, although the mere presence of infection in periapical, periodontal, tonsillar, or other regions is not in itself sufficient to cause disease in remote areas. The well-known transitory bacteremia that occurs after manipulating infected tissues such as a periodontal pocket, demonstrates that the body defenses can handle these brief aggressions. When the body defenses are low, increasing the risk of disease, antibiotic premedication is used.

In the last decade of the century, strong epidemiologic evidence began to suggest that oral infections influence many systemic conditions and diseases, by mechanisms not yet fully clarified. These include an increased risk for cardiovascular diseases such as coronary heart disease, cerebrovascular accidents, infective endocarditis; respiratory diseases; the birth of low-weight, preterm babies; and poor control of diabetes mellitus.[28] These new research findings, constituting an area now called *periodontal medicine*, are a new insight into the old problem envisioned in the Assyrian clay tablets.

## References


1. Billings F. Chronic focal infections and their etiologic relations to arthritis and nephritis. Arch Intern Med 1912;9:484.
2. Billings F. Chronic focal infection as a causative factor in chronic arthritis. JAMA 1913;61:819.
3. Billings F. Focal infection. JAMA 1914;63:899.
4. Billings F. Mouth infection as a source of systemic disease. JAMA 1914;63:2024.
5. Black GV. Special Dental Pathology. Chicago: Medico-Dental, 1915.
6. Carr JG. Relationship between dental and cardiovascular disease. J Am Dent Assoc 1937;24:1979.
7. Cecil RL, Angevine DM. Clinical and experimental observations on focal infection, with an analysis of 200 cases of rheumatoid arthritis. Ann Intern Med 1938;12:577.
8. Cook TJ. Focal infection of the teeth and elective localization in the experimental production of ulcerative colitis. J Am Dent Assoc 1931;18:2290.
9. Editorial. JAMA 1952;150:490.
10. Francke OC. William Hunter's "oral sepsis" and American odontology. Bull Hist Dent 1973;21:73.
11. Galloway CE. Focal infection. Am J Surg 1931;14:643.
12. Gilmer TL, Moody AM. A study of the bacteriology of alveolar abscess and infected root canals. JAMA 1914;63:2023.
13. Grieves CJ. Dental periapical infections as the cause of systemic disease. Dent Cosmos 1913;55:52.
14. Hartzell TB. Review of the literature regarding infected teeth. J Am Dent Assoc 1926;23:441.
15. Hoffman-Axthelm W. History of Dentistry. Chicago: Quintessence, 1981.
16. Hunter W. Oral sepsis as a cause of disease. Br Med J 1900;1:215.
17. Hunter W. An address on the role of sepsis and antisepsis in Medicine. Lancet 1911;1:79.
18. Jastrow N. The medicine of the Babylonians and Assyrians. Proc Soc Med London 1914;7:109.
19. Koecker L. An essay on the devastation of the gums and the alveolar processes. Philadelphia J Med Phys Sci 1821;2:282.
20. Mayo CH. Mouth infection as a source of systemic disease. JAMA 1914;63:2025.
21. Mayo CH. Focal infection. J Am Dent Assoc 1925;22:970.
22. Meisser JG. Further studies on elective localization of bacteria from infected teeth. J Am Dent Assoc 1925; 22:554.
23. Miller WD. The human mouth as a focus of infection. Dent Cosmos 1891;33:689,789,913.
24. Miloslavich EL. A critical review of dental focal infection from the point of view of human pathology. J Am Dent Assoc 1926;23:472.
25. O'Reilly PG, Claffey NM. A history of oral sepsis as a cause of disease. Periodontol 2000 2000;23:13.
26. Pollia JA. Newer concepts of focal infection. J Dent Res 1931;11:83.
27. Price WA. Fundamentals suggested by recent researches for diagnosis, prognosis, and treatment of dental focal infections. J Am Dent Assoc 1925;22:641.
28. Proceedings of the Sunstar-Chapel Hill Symposium 1997 on Periodontal Diseases and Human Health: New Directions in Periodontal Medicine. Ann Periodontol 1998;3:1–387.
29. Rosenow EC. Experimental infectious endocarditis. J Infect Dis 1912;11:210.
30. Rosenow EC. Mouth infection as a source of systemic disease. JAMA 1914;63:2026.
31. Rosenow EC. Oral sepsis in its relationship to focal infection and elective localization. J Am Dent Assoc 1927;24:1417.
32. Sand RA. Periodontal sepsis in relationship to systemic disease. J Periodontol 1940;11:18.
33. Thoma KH. Oral Pathology. St. Louis: Mosby, 1941.
34. Williams NB, Burkett LW. Focal infection—A review. Philadelphia Med J 1951;46:1509.

# 24

# After World War II: The Researchers

The majority of microscopic studies performed on periodontal tissues in the first half of the twentieth century centered around descriptive analysis of lesions examined under light microscopy using conventional staining techniques. This provided a sound biologic understanding of the microscopic features of normal tissues and their changes in disease.

By the end of World War II, this approach had provided the necessary information, and a new generation of researchers took over: the experimental pathologists. The new approach consisted of animal experimentation to analyze the periodontal tissue response to a large variety of insults, local and systemic, as well as the healing of wounds of various types. It required a different, carefully planned research protocol, with adequate controls and more exact methods of observation. Histometric measurements, the use of histochemistry and electron microscopy, and other new methods gradually entered the realm of techniques used to clarify the questions that were asked. Most of these studies were performed between 1945 and 1970, and this period is addressed on the basis of the major contributors to research, in the United States and Europe.

In the following period, from around 1970 to the end of the century, studies on etiology and pathogenesis, based on the work of some of the previous investigators, brought bacteriology and immunology to the forefront of periodontal research. This period is addressed more succinctly because the historic distance from these findings is shorter and its impact on the future of periodontics cannot be adequately judged.

## United States

Five names define this period: Irving Glickman, Henry M. Goldman, Sigurd P. Ramfjord, and Helmut A. Zander were academicians who trained in pathology and oral medicine and practiced clinical periodontics in addition to their research and teaching activities. Balint J. Orban belonged to an older generation and his major contributions were in the area of descriptive pathology (Orban's biography and accomplishments are presented in Chapter 18), but he can also be considered, in the latter part of his career, an experimental pathologist. Many of Orban's students and collaborators had estimable careers in research, teaching, and practice; among them Surindar Bhaskar; Anthony Gargiulo; Daniel Grant; Harold Grupe, Sr; John and Claude Nabers; Harry Staffileno; S. Sigmund Stahl; Harold Ray; and Frank Wentz.

Following World War II, Glickman, Goldman, Ramfjord, Zander, and Orban, along with their students and coworkers, created the major thrust in basic and clinical research based on sound principles. All these scientists have published literally hundreds of papers, and it would be impossible to review them here. Only their most salient publications will be discussed in the context of the era. Readers are referred to current scientific reviews for detailed analysis of their contributions.

Irving Glickman (Fig 69) was born in Brooklyn, New York, January 17, 1914. He attended Brooklyn College and obtained his dental degree from Tufts College Dental School (now Tufts University School of Dental Medicine), where he later became professor and chairman of periodontology and research professor of oral pathology, as well as director of one of the

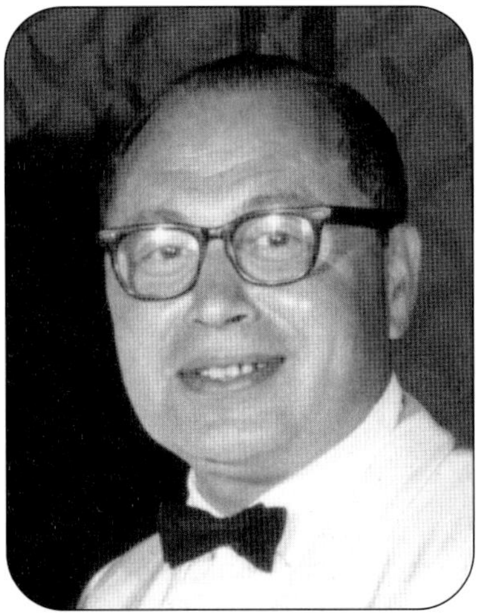

**Fig 69** Irving Glickman.

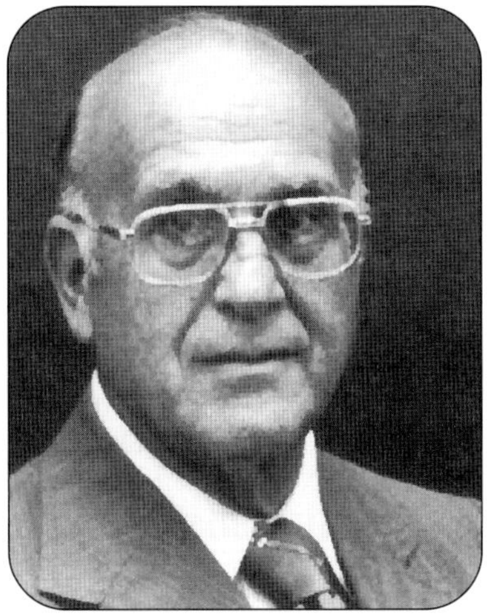

**Fig 70** Henry M. Goldman.

first postdoctoral periodontal programs in the United States. Glickman had a profound knowledge of the basic sciences relevant to periodontics, extensive clinical and research experience, and a stimulating influence on his students and audiences.[27]

Glickman's numerous contributions dealt with the effect of various systemic diseases on the periodontal structures of laboratory animals (nutritional deficiencies and endocrine dysfunctions), analyzing particularly the interaction of systemic and local factors, and clinical studies (phenytoin, Paget disease, biometric studies of surgical techniques, etc).[3] His studies on the effect of trauma from occlusion, including his intraoral occlusal telemetry, were and still are controversial, but provide lucid analyses of an important topic.[5,6] He also studied periodontal histochemistry, and plaque and calculus formation.

In the area of periodontal therapy, Glickman defended the gingivectomy as the surgical technique of choice, opposing osseous contouring and the flap operation. At the time esthetics was not a primary consideration and in the witty words of Irving Glickman the choice for the patient was to have the teeth "longer or no longer." The increased attention to esthetics in the 1970s and 1980s, as well as the development of regenerative techniques based on flap surgery, relegated the gingivectomy to a minor role in therapy.

Glickman was the author of a widely used book on periodontology and a leader at the American Academy of Periodontology. He also called for a reorientation of the role of periodontology in the dental curriculum as a way to improve the general practitioner's understanding of periodontal problems.[4] Glickman received numerous awards and honors. He was a brilliant speaker, a vigorous and even vehement debater, with a sharp wit and a quick mind. Debates in early years between Glickman, Goldman, Zander, Orban, Schluger, and others enlivened many a meeting of the American Academy of Periodontology, as well as other institutions.

Among Irving Glickman's students and collaborators are Samuel Turesky, Jerome Smulow, Benjamin Patur, O. Walter Donnenfeld, Max Perlitsch, Mario Martignoni, Arthur Gold, and many others, including the authors of this book. Glickman died in Boston of a massive heart attack at 58 years old, on October 2, 1972.

Henry Goldman (Fig 70) was born in Boston on September 12, 1911. He attended Brown University and received his dental degree from Harvard University in 1935. He continued at Harvard as a research fellow in oral pathology with renowned oral surgeon and pathologist Kurt H. Thoma. Goldman published his first book on periodontology in 1942, at 31 years of age.

During World War II he served at the Armed Forces Institute of Pathology, where he solidified his knowledge of oral pathology.[2]

Back in Boston he was chief of dentistry at Beth Israel Hospital, where he started a postdoctoral program in conjunction with the University of Pennsylvania. In 1960 Goldman became the first dean of the Boston University School of Graduate Dentistry. This school was later named the Henry Goldman School of Dentistry, in honor of its founding dean. Goldman continued to publish; credits include several books, with various co-authors (D. Walter Cohen, Saul Schluger, Lewis Fox, Robert Genco) and innumerable scientific articles.[7,8] Moreover, he earned many awards. He was an outstanding teacher and educator whose leadership and dedication created a school of clinical periodontics that, in great measure, shaped clinical thinking and promoted progress in this field in the remainder of the century. Goldman died in Boston on July 23, 1991. Among his students and collaborators, the following gained renown: D. Walter Cohen, Morris Ruben, Gerald Kramer, Arthur B. Novaes, Simao Kon, and Myron Nevins.

Sigurd P. Ramfjord (Fig 71) was born in Kolvereid, Norway, on June 6, 1911, and obtained his dental degree from the University of Oslo in 1934. After twelve years of general dentistry practice, with particular interest in reconstructive dentistry, he became a graduate student in periodontics at the University of Michigan, and then went on to earn a PhD in general and oral pathology. After graduation, Ramfjord returned to Norway with the aim of teaching periodontics in his native country. However, there were no university openings at the time, and Ramfjord returned to Michigan, where he joined the faculty. Eventually he was made chair of periodontics, a position he retained until his retirement.[11]

Ramfjord pioneered the use of controlled clinical research trials, comparing on different quadrants of the same mouths the results obtained with different therapeutic modalities.[28,29] At the time this was a novel approach to clinical research, but it developed a following and resulted in important findings. Results of Ramfjord's clinical research, known as the *Michigan longitudinal studies*, supported flap surgery with the purpose of exposing the root surfaces for a thorough scaling and planing, contouring bone only for a better adaptation of the flap. He called this technique a *modified Widman flap*. He also supported the concept of a "long epithelial attachment," or "epithelial adaptation" as an acceptable solution when followed by adequate maintenance.[1] These ideas were often in conflict with current opinion, but they strongly influenced the practice of periodontics.

Ramfjord and his group also conducted a number of experimental studies, exploring the healing of periodontal tissues after different treatment procedures, the effect of systemic diseases on the periodontium, and the effect of trauma from occlusion. They used electromyographic methods to study muscle action in relation to occlusal and temporomandibular joint function and dysfunction. Ramfjord developed an epidemiological index (using six selected teeth as representative of the whole dentition) that was used in many studies.[28] He also published one book on occlusion and another on periodontics, both with co-author Major Ash, that went through several editions and were widely used.

Ramfjord was above all a respected, albeit demanding, teacher profoundly devoted to his students, and a relentless investigator. Before his death in Ann Arbor, Michigan, on July 4, 1997, he received numerous awards, including four honorary doctorates. Many of his students and collaborators have attained noteworthy positions. Among them are Major Ash, Raul G. Caffesse, E. Barrie Kenney, Kenneth Kornman, Niklaus Lang, Walter Loesche, and Bruce Pihlstrom.

Helmut A. Zander (Fig 72) was born in Bautzen, Germany, on October 25, 1912, and received a DMD degree from the University of Würzburg. In 1935 he emigrated to the United States, and received another dental degree from Northwestern University in 1938, and a master's degree in 1940. His initial research interests were in children's dentistry, and he was professor and chairman of oral diagnosis and then of pediatric dentistry at Tufts University, from

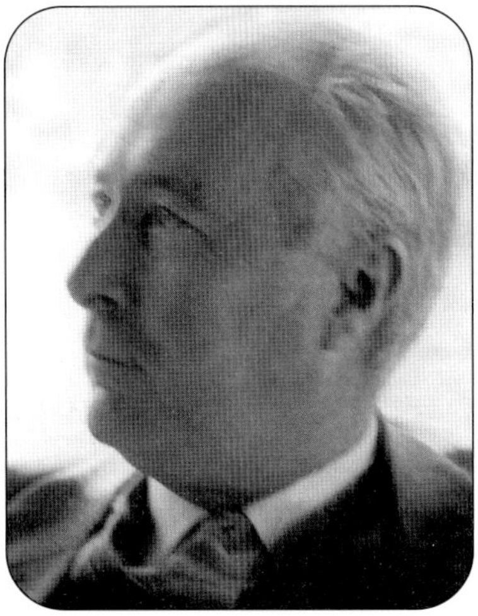

**Fig 71** Sigurd P. Ramfjord.

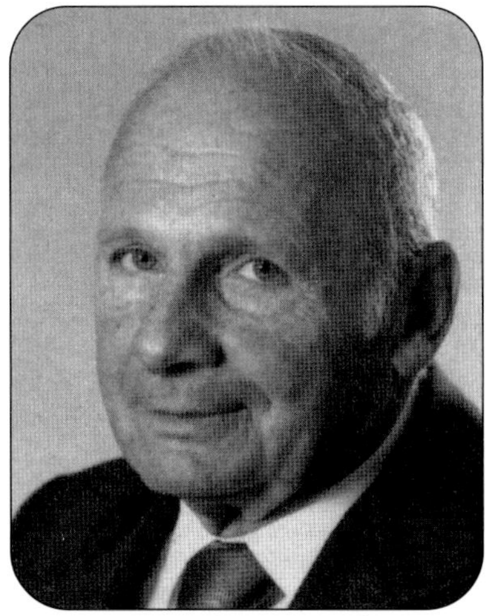

**Fig 72** Helmut A. Zander.

1942 to 1951, when he became professor and chairman of periodontics at the University of Minnesota. In 1957 he moved to Eastman Dental Center, in Rochester, New York, as founding chairman of the center's Department of Periodontology.[20]

Zander's research in periodontology focused on the role of calculus and its attachment to root surfaces, use of antibiotics, cellular turnover, functional contacts during mastication, the role of occlusion in periodontal disease, as well as other areas of interest.[38,39] Zander's work earned him numerous honors and awards, as well as honorary doctoral degrees from several universities. Students and collaborators of Helmut Zander were, among many others, Alan Polson, Jack Caton, James Kennedy, Richard Ranney, James Butler, and David Vandersall. Zander died in Naples, Florida, on November 30, 1991.

## Europe

The major researcher in Europe during this period was Jens Waerhaug, who changed the biologic foundation of periodontology, starting a new era in the clinical approach to therapy. Waerhaug is the major exponent of the Scandinavian school. Another European investigator was Swiss scientist Hans Muhlemann, who at about the same time started another important line of research.

Jens Waerhaug (Fig 73) was born near Oslo, Norway, on May 3, 1907. He received the dental degree from the University of Oslo in 1933 and his doctoral degree twenty years later. His long professional career was centered always at the University of Oslo, with long visits to the University of Stockholm, University of Minnesota, and the National Institute of Dental Research, National Institutes of Health.[10]

Waerhaug's 1952 doctoral thesis, entitled *The Gingival Pocket*,[37] presented a revolutionary new concept that challenged the existing views on periodontal biology derived from the investigations made in the 1920s and 1930s by Gottlieb, Orban, and others.

Waerhaug studied human and animal periodontal tissues; made detailed measurements of the depth of penetration of "ad hoc" probes into the sulci/pockets, determining also the forces used; analyzed the tissues with a stereomicroscope; and studied the location of the "secondary cuticle." He contended that the epithelium is not "organically connected" to the tooth, but that there is only a weak union by adhesion. Additionally he pointed out that the bottom of the sul-

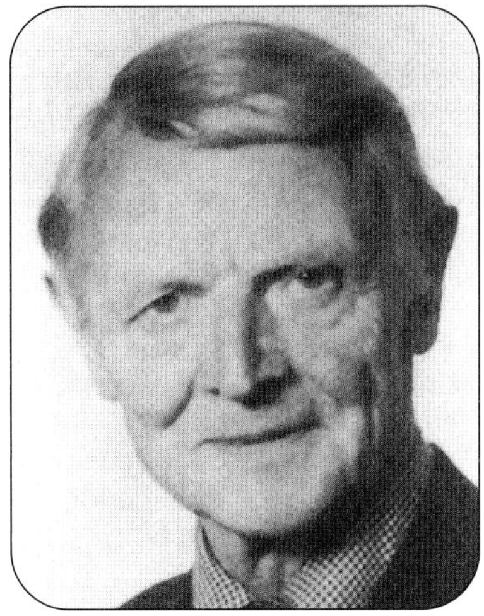

**Fig 73** Jens Waerhaug.

cus/pocket is located at the apical part of the so-called epithelial attachment and not at its coronal end, as the Vienna school believed. Waerhaug suggested that the term *epithelial attachment* be replaced by *epithelial cuff*.

According to Waerhaug, the adhesive connection between epithelium and tooth surface is normally sterile. A pathological pocket develops when calculus and bacteria form below the gingival margin. The complete removal of subgingival calculus eliminates all bacterial irritants and a sterile physiological pocket results.

Orban and coworkers in 1956 repeated Waerhaug's experiments and found that the strength of the union between epithelium and tooth surface is stronger than the union between epithelial cells. They also discovered that it is mechanically impossible to detach the gingiva from the tooth without tearing the epithelium.[24] This controversy was at the time unsolvable because of the inadequate technology at their disposal.[31] Twenty years later, when more advanced methods became available, Hubert Schroeder and Max Listgarten were able to clarify the problem.[32] Using electron microscopic sections of carefully prepared specimens, they described the union of the epithelium to the tooth by hemidesmosomes and a basal lamina. They proposed the term *junctional epithelium*, now in use, to refer to this epithelium and *epithelial attachment* to the mechanism of union.

Another important point that Waerhaug challenged was the concept of passive eruption, also proposed by the Vienna school. According to Gottlieb, the dentogingival junction normally migrates apically, accompanied by gingival recession. This theory was finally disproven by Harald Löe.[16]

Waerhaug's research findings recognized that plaque control was essential for successful periodontal treatment, thus creating a renewed interest in the role of bacteria in periodontal etiology and resulting in the rebirth of periodontal bacteriology. Epidemiologic studies by Waerhaug and coworkers, and by Löe (see below) proved that controlling plaque formation prevents periodontal destruction.

Jens Waerhaug continued to contribute to periodontal literature on topics such as avitaminosis C, epidemiology, trauma from occlusion, and so on. In all his publications, oral presentations, and discussions, his approach to the problem at hand, the reasoning behind his findings, and his interpretation of their meaning consistently offered new and refreshing views that clarified many clinical problems.

The Scandinavian school resulted from Jens Waerhaug's challenging research and ideas. Many important researchers belong to this group: Harald Löe, Jan Lindhe, Jorgen Slots, Jan Egelberg,

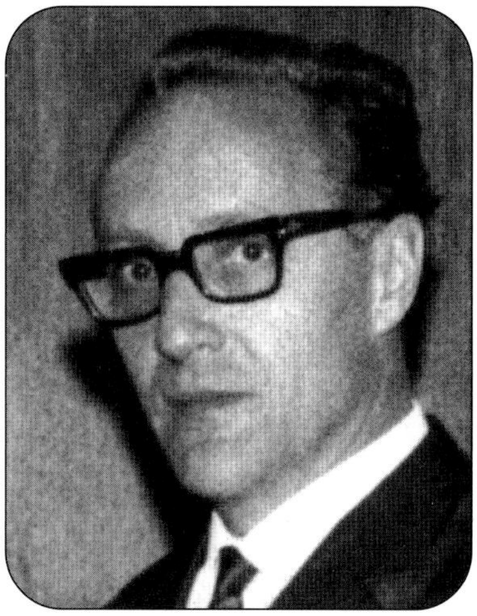

**Fig 74** Hans Mühlemann.

Jan Johansen, Sture Nyman, and Reynaldo Saglie, to name a few. Waerhaug retired from the University of Oslo in 1975, but continued his research until the day he died, September 26, 1980.

Hans R. Mühlemann (Fig 74) was born in Switzerland in 1917. His formal education included medical and dental degrees and specialization in orthodontics, oral surgery, periodontics, and radiology, and clinical research training in the United States. In 1953 he was appointed chairman of the Department of Periodontics, Cariology and Preventive Dentistry at the University of Zurich.[9]

Mühlemann's research and leadership attracted numerous scholars and investigators and transformed his department into a respected international center. Mühlemann developed a method to measure tooth mobility, created the sulcus bleeding index still in use today, and introduced dentifrice formulations for prevention of caries and calculus, among many accomplishments[21–23] that resulted from his innovative and profound knowledge of many fields. Among Mühlemann's students and collaborators were Thomas Hassell, Klaus Rateitschak, and Jean-Pierre Bernimoulin. Mühlemann died in Zurich in 1997.

## The Next Generation

In the 1960s and 1970s a new generation of periodontal scientists emerged. During this period microbiology and immunology gradually became the basis for an understanding of the causes and mechanisms of gingival inflammation and bone loss. Many postdoctoral periodontal students sought PhDs in both bacteriology or immunology, and research in these areas soared to new levels. In the 1980s and 1990s, molecular biology and genetics also became key research areas.

Lacking historical perspective it is difficult to decide whom to mention from a long list of respected scientists whose contributions have shaped present-day periodontics. Although there are many, only eight scientists born between the mid 1920s and late 1930s have been chosen as major contributors. They are S. Sigmund Stahl, Harald Löe, Roy C. Page, Hubert Schroeder, Sigmund S. Socransky, Max A. Listgarten, Jan Lindhe, and Robert Genco.

S. Sigmund Stahl was born in Berlin, Germany, on June 16, 1925, and emigrated to the United States in 1938. He obtained his dental degree from the University of Minnesota in 1947 and his graduate degree at the University of Illinois under Balint Orban, Joseph Weinmann, and Isaac Schour. He then went to New York University under Samuel Charles Miller and in 1971 became chairman of the Department of Periodontology until his retirement in 1991. After his retirement, Stahl moved to Florida, where he renewed his interest in studies of Judaism, founding a school for adult Jewish education in Palm Beach, Florida. In 1995 he became professor of periodontics and associate dean at Nova South Eastern University, in Fort Lauderdale, Florida.

Stahl extensively researched experimental periodontal pathology, studying gingival healing,[36] exfoliative cytology, and the effects of systemic diseases on periodontal tissues,[35] and, in later years, performing histologic evaluation of bone regenerative materials.

Harald Löe was born in Norway, on July 19, 1926. He obtained his dental degree from the University of Oslo and, in graduate school, trained under Jens Waerhaug in Oslo, and under Joseph Weinmann at the University of Illinois. He was professor of periodontics at the University of Århus in Denmark, and then moved to the United States, where he was, successively, director of the Dental Research Institute of the University of Michigan, dean of the School of Dentistry of the University of Connecticut, and director of the National Institute of Dental Research, National Institutes of Health at Bethesda, Maryland. Löe was also the founding editor of the *Journal of Periodontal Research*, which became an important avenue of expression for the vast amount of research that was beginning to appear on both sides of the Atlantic Ocean.

Harald Löe made many fundamental research contributions. Among them are the experimental gingivitis papers, which prove incontrovertibly the role of bacteria in the etiology of gingivitis.[18] These studies resulted in the use of chlorhexidine for treatment and prevention of gingival inflammation. Löe's studies on the natural history of periodontal disease[17] proved the existence of rapid, moderate, and no loss of attachment as a result of plaque accumulation. His many other contributions deal with diabetes, epidemiology, and healing, as well as other issues.

Roy C. Page was born in Campobello, South Carolina, in 1932 and obtained his dental degree from the University of Maryland in 1957. He then moved west and enrolled at the University of Washington, in Seattle, Washington, where he completed his periodontal training in 1963, and obtained a PhD in experimental pathology in 1967.

Roy Page has been a pioneer in studies of immunology and molecular biology as applied to periodontal problems. His 1982 *Periodontitis in Man and Other Animals*,[26] co-authored with Hubert Schroeder, is a milestone in periodontics. Page and Schroeder challenge the era's prevailing concept of a universal distribution of human periodontal disease. They established that the destructive manifestations of the disease are rare. In addition, they presented a comparative study of periodontitis in a broad range of animals, supporting the view that the polymorphonuclear leukocyte is the principal defensive cell of the periodontium, describing as the basic pathologic change in pocket formation the conversion of the junctional epithelium to pocket epithelium and its ulceration, and the clinical implications of these findings, recognizing different types of disease.

Page is director of the Center for Research in Oral Biology at the University of Washington. He succeeded Harald Löe as editor of the *Journal of Periodontal Research*, and was co-author of the Schluger textbook on periodontics. His numerous publications and presentations at symposiums and scientific congresses have been at the forefront of scientific knowledge, guiding periodontists, educators, and students in their search for understanding periodontal disease and its clinical treatment.

Hubert E. Schroeder was born in Königsberg, Germany, on February 17, 1931, graduated in 1956 from Goethe University School of Dentistry, in Frankfurt/Main, Germany, and completed his graduate training at the universities of Zürich, New York, Aarhus, and Harvard. In 1972 he was appointed professor and chairman of the Department of Oral Structural Biology, Dental Institute, University of Zürich.

Along with Listgarten, Schroeder made the definitive histological descriptions of the mode of attachment of the epithelium to the tooth.[32] Likewise, with Page, Schroeder outlined the experimental and clinical knowledge on all basic science aspects of periodontitis in man and animals.[26] His other books include *Differentiation of Human Oral Stratified Epithelia* (1981), which presents extensive original material on the structure and function of oral epithelium, combining morphological and quantitative stereological methods. In addition, his *Oral Strukturbiologie* (1976) and *Pathobiologie oraler Strukturen* (1983), published only in German, provide detailed descriptions of oral histology and embryology, and oral pathology, respectively.

Schroeder's book *The Periodontium*, published in 1986, presents a complete description of the normal periodontal tissues. He relies on all available methodologies, descriptive and quantitative, from histology to electron microscopy to monoclonal antibodies, from humans to animals, to clarify and integrate present knowledge on the subject in an unprecedented way.[31]

Sigmund S. Socransky was born in Toronto, Canada, on December 2, 1934. Socransky obtained his dental degree from the University of Toronto in 1957, and he completed his training in periodontics and microbiology at Harvard University in 1961. He is head of periodontology and microbiology at the Forsyth Dental Center, in Boston. In the last decades of the twentieth century, Socransky was the leading American periodontal microbiologist.

From the 1940s to the 1960s, investigators such as Theodor Rosebury (1904–1985), at Columbia University; John B. Macdonald (b. 1918), at Forsyth Dental Infirmary and Harvard, then at Columbia University; and others made important contributions to the study of periodontal bacteriology. They argued that periodontal disease is due to mixed infections. In the 1960s Paul H. Keyes (b. 1917) and Harold V. Jordan (b. 1924), at the National Institute of Dental Research, in Bethesda, Maryland, demonstrated the transmissibility of hamster periodontal disease. Walter Loesche (b. 1935), of the University of Michigan, described the nonspecific and the specific plaque hypotheses. Finally, bacterial specificity in the etiology of periodontal diseases was recognized after Michael Newman (b. 1947), of UCLA, along with his mentor, Sigmund Socransky, and Jorgen Slots independently identified a bacterium now called *Actinobacillus actinomycetemcomitans* as the predominant species in periodontal pockets of individuals with localized aggressive periodontitis. Later, Ann R. C. Tanner and others in Socransky's group extended this concept to chronic periodontitis.[25,33] The findings from Sigmund Socransky's group at Forsyth have provided the keys to sustained progress in periodontal bacteriology in the last few decades.

Max A. Listgarten was born in Paris, France, on April 14, 1935 and emigrated to Canada in 1962, obtaining his DDS from the University of Toronto in 1959, and a certificate in pediatric dentistry in 1960. In 1963 he completed his training in periodontology at Harvard University and was appointed professor of periodontology at the University of Pennsylvania in 1968, where he was chairman of the Department of Periodontology and director of research.

Listgarten is essentially an electron microscopist who is particularly interested in the periodontal tissues and bacterial plaque.[13,32] His book with Schroeder, *Fine Structure of the Developing Epithelial Attachment of Human Teeth*[32] provides the definitive description of the mechanism of union of the epithelium to the tooth, settling the dispute between the Vienna school (Gottlieb, Orban) and the Scandinavian school (Waerhaug). Among his contributions, Listgarten described (in 1965) the tissue penetration by spirochetes in necrotizing gingivitis,[12] clearly analyzed the real information provided by pocket probing,[14] and carried out numerous studies on the electron microscopy of bacterial plaque.

Jan Lindhe was born in Helsingborg, Sweden, on June 29, 1935 and obtained his dental degree from the Royal School of Dentistry, in Malmö, Sweden, in 1959. His postdoctoral training in roentgenology, oral surgery, and periodontology was at the University of Lund, between 1957 and 1965.

Lindhe's professional career has been with the universities of Umeå and Gothenburg in Sweden, where he was/is professor and chair of the Department of Periodontology, and dean at Gothenburg (1977–1983; 1990–1993), and at the University of Pennsylvania, in the United States, where he was dean of the School of Dentistry between 1983 and 1988.

Lindhe and his coworkers have researched a variety of clinically oriented topics, seeking explanations to clinical phenomena and therapeutic methods. Thus they have analyzed the role of occlusion in periodontal disease, its interaction with gingival inflammation, microbiologic and histologic features of periodontitis, the maintenance phase of therapy, mucogingival surgery as related to gingival recession and case maintenance, regenerative periodontal techniques using guided tissue regeneration, and countless other problems. Lindhe has been especially successful in transmitting his findings to general periodontal audiences. As a result of the findings of his research group and other Scandinavian researchers, a "Scandinavian" approach to periodontal therapy has developed, based on nonsurgical therapy, or restricted surgical indications, scrupulous plaque control, and use of antimicrobial agents.

Lindhe is the editor of the prestigious *Journal of Clinical Periodontology*, which is the official publication of the European Federation of Periodontology that nucleates periodontal societies of Europe and the Middle East. He is also author and editor of the book *Clinical Periodontology and Implant Dentistry*, which has been translated into many languages and is currently in its third edition. Lindhe has earned numerous awards, as well as honorary memberships in many societies and honorary university degrees.

Robert J. Genco was born in Silver Creek, New York, near Buffalo, in 1938, and obtained his dental degree from the State University of New York at Buffalo, in 1963. He completed his training in periodontics and received a PhD in immunology at the University of Pennsylvania in 1967. He is professor and chairman of oral biology at the State University of New York at Buffalo and director of the Buffalo Research Center in Periodontal Disease. Since 1989, Genco has been editor-in-chief of the *Journal of Periodontology*.

Genco's group has conducted extensive research into the immunology and bacteriology of periodontal disease. They helped establish the role of *Porphyromonas gingivalis* as a major cause of periodontal infections and developed clinical methods for detecting this and other bacteria, as well as the role of the neutrophil as a key protective cell. They identified several risk indicators for periodontal disease (diabetes, smoking, stress, and others), studied the relationship between periodontal disease and systemic diseases, providing evidence for the association between periodontal disease and heart disease, stroke, and pulmonary diseases.

Many others have provided outstanding research that leads the field. Among them are Paul N. Baer, Nabil F. Bissada, Romulo L. Cabrini, Juan J. Carraro, Giorgio Cimasoni, Neal Chilton, D. Walter Cohen, Jan Egelberg, Paul Goldhaber, Robert Gottsegen, Daniel Grant, María E. Itoiz, Thorkild Karring, E. Barrie Kenney, Walter Loesche, Melvin Morris, Bernard Moskow, Hubert Newman, Sture Nyman, Timothy O'Leary, Perry Ratcliff, Terry Rees, Morris Ruben, and Knut Selvig. Space does not permit details of their insightful contributions, which can be found in current textbooks in periodontology.

This generation solidified the basic understanding of periodontal pathogenesis, establishing the foundation for the next group, born after 1940, which includes Donald Adams, Gary Armitage, Antonio Bascones, Raul Caffesse, Jack Caton, Marcello Cattabriga, Sebastian Ciancio, David Cochran, Lavinia Flores-de-Jacoby, Gary Greenstein, Vincent Iacono, Marjorie Jeffcoat, Kenneth Kornman, Niklaus Lang, Voja Lekovic, Brian Mealy, Michael Newman, Russell Nisengard, Steven Offenbacher, Bruce Pihlstrom, Alan Polson, Mariano Sanz, Jorgen Slots, Daniel van Steenberghe, Maurizio Tonetti, Arie van Winkelhoff, Jan Wennström, Ray Williams, Joseph Zambon, and many others.

Research in the last two decades of the century has been fruitful, largely because of the conjunction of basic and clinical research. In the words of Roy Page, one of the major protagonists of this progress[25]:

> Scientific consensus has been reached in many areas. In most populations, moderate to severe periodontitis affects a relatively small segment of adults who are at high risk. The microbial etiology is accepted and the identity of the major pathogenic bacterial species is known. The mechanisms through which resistant individuals fend off the microbial chal-

lenge are known, and the immuno-inflammatory pathways activated by bacteria that underlie destruction of the alveolar bone and the connective tissue of the periodontium are reasonably well understood. … Therapeutic modulation of these pathways is now possible, and new treatments based on such modulation are now becoming available. … Concepts and procedures for treatment are generally scientifically based and appropriately applied. Preventive measures are largely successful and widely practiced in industrialized countries. Clearly, control of these ancient chronic diseases is now within our reach.

## References


1. Ash MM. Reflections on Sigurd P. Ramfjord: His contributions to evidence-based periodontics. J Periodontol 2001;72:1124.
2. Cohen DW. Obituary, Henry M. Goldman. J Periodontol 1991;62:589.
3. Glickman I. The experimental basis for the bone factor concept in periodontal disease. J Periodontol 1949;20:7.
4. Glickman I. A change in the aims of dental education. J Dent Educ 1951:109.
5. Glickman I, Shklar G. Modifications of the effect of cortisone upon alveolar bone by the systemic administration of estrogen. J Periodontol 1954;25:231.
6. Glickman I, Smulow J. Alterations in the pathway of gingival inflammation into the underlying tissues induced by excessive occlusal forces. J Periodontol 1962;33:7.
7. Goldman HM. The effect of dietary deprivation and of age on the periodontal tissues of the rat and spider monkey. J Periodontol 1954;25:87.
8. Goldman HM, Cohen DW. The intrabony pocket: Classification and treatment. J Periodontol 1958;29:272.
9. Hassell TM. Obituary, Professor Dr. med., Dr.med.dent., Hans R. Mühlemann 1917–1997. J Periodontol 1998;69:279.
10. Johansen JR. In Memorium (Prof Jens Waerhaug). J Clin Periodontol 1980;7:534.
11. Lang N, Somerman M, Kornman K. Obituary, Sigurd Peder Ramfjord, DDS, PhD. J Periodontol 1997;68:1147.
12. Listgarten MA. Electron microscopic observations on the bacterial flora of acute necrotizing ulcerative gingivitis. J Periodontol 1965;36:328.
13. Listgarten MA, Hellden L. Relative distribution of bacteria at clinically healthy and periodontally diseased sites in humans. J Clin Periodontol 1978;5:115.
14. Listgarten MA, Mao R, Robinson PJ. Periodontal probing and the relationship of the probe tip to periodontal status. J Periodontol 1976;47:511.
15. Löe H. Periodontal diseases: A brief historical perspective. Periodontol 2000 1993;2:7.
16. Löe H. The structure and physiology of the dentogingival junction. In: Miles AEW (ed). Structural and Chemical Organization of Teeth, vol 2. New York: Academic Press, 1967.
17. Löe H, Anerud A, Boysen H, Morrison E. Natural history of periodontal disease in man. Rapid, moderate and no loss of attachment in Sri Lankan laborers. J Clin Periodontol 1986;13:431.
18. Löe H, Theilade E, Jensen SB. Experimental gingivitis in man. J Periodontol 1965;36:177.
19. Lovdal A, Arno A, Waerhaug J. Evidence of clinical manifestations of periodontal disease in light of oral hygiene and calculus formation. J Am Dent Assoc 1958;56:21.
20. McHugh WD. Obituary, Helmut A. Zander. J Periodontol 1992;63:236.
21. Mühlemann HR. Ten years of tooth mobility studies. J Periodontol 1960;31:110.
22. Mühlemann HR, Son S. Gingival sulcus bleeding — a leading symptom in initial gingivitis. Helv Odontol Acta 1971;15:107.
23. Mühlemann HR, Villa P. The marginal line calculus index. Helv Odontol Acta 1967;11:175.
24. Orban BJ, Bathia H, Kollar JA, Wentz FMJ. The epithelial attachment (the attached epithelial cuff). J Periodontol 1956;27:167.
25. Page RC. Milestones in periodontal research and the remaining critical issues. J Periodontal Res 1999;34:331.
26. Page RC, Schroeder HE. Periodontitis in Man and Other Animals. Karger: Basel, 1982.
27. Patur B. Obituary, Irving Glickman. J Periodontol 1972;43:655.
28. Ramfjord SP. Indices for prevalence and incidence of periodontal disease. J Periodontol 1959;30:51.
29. Ramfjord SP. Design of studies or clinical trials to evaluate the effectiveness of agents for the prevention, or treatment, of loss of periodontium. J Periodontal Res 1974;14(suppl):78.

30. Ramfjord SP, Knowles JW, Nissle RR, Shick RA, Burgett FC. Longitudinal study of periodontal therapy. J Periodontol 1973;44:66.
31. Schroeder HE. The Periodontium. Berlin: Springer-Verlag, 1986.
32. Schroeder HE, Listgarten M. Fine structure of the developing epithelial attachment of human teeth. In: Monographs in Developmental Biology, vol 2. Basel: Karger, 1971.
33. Socransky SS, Haffajee AD. Evidence of bacterial etiology: A historical perspective. Periodontol 2000 1994;5:7.
34. Socransky SS, Haffajee AD (eds). Microbiology and immunology of periodontal diseases. Periodontol 2000 1994;5:1–168.
35. Stahl SS, Miller SC, Goldsmith ED. The effects of vertical occlusal trauma on the periodontium of protein deprived young adult rats. J Periodontol 1957;28:87.
36. Stahl SS, Froum SJ, Tarnow D. Human histologic responses to guided tissue regeneration techniques in intrabony lesions. J Clin Periodontol 1990;17:191.
37. Waerhaug J. The gingival pocket. Odontol Tidskr 1952;60(suppl 1).
38. Zander HA. The attachment of calculus to root surfaces. J Periodontol 1953;24:16.
39. Zander HA, Mühlemann HR. The effect of stresses on the periodontal structures. Oral Surg Oral Med Oral Pathol 1956;9:380.

# 25

# After World War II: The Clinicians

The evolution of clinical periodontology involves the practical application of knowledge derived from scientific research and development of new approaches to improve patient care. After World War II, change became the norm. New scientific knowledge and technological discoveries and inventions transformed everyday life in an unprecedented way. Oral health in the United States, as in most developed countries, showed a remarkable and continuous improvement, exemplified by the drastic reduction in unrestored carious teeth and deep pockets and the decline in total edentulousness.[28]

## Diagnosis

At midcentury, the major diagnostic methods were—and continue to be—clinical observation of gingival changes, pocket probing, and radiographic examination. A better understanding of the meaning of pocket probing came after the work of Max Listgarten, Gary Armitage, Jerry Garnick, and others. They determined how deep the probe penetrates when exploring normal or inflamed tissues, the forces used, the influence of the shape of the probe, and the discrepancies in measurements incurred by different examiners.[7,42]

After the 1980s, pressure-sensitive probes, computerized probes, and automated probes were developed, mainly to overcome reproducibility problems, which are inherently important in clinical research but much less so in clinical practice.[42]

Radiographic methods have also in the last quarter of the century seen a number of technological improvements, including xeroradiography, $I_{125}$ absorptiometry, photodensitometric analysis technique, subtraction radiography, computer-assisted subtraction radiography, computer-assisted densitometric image analysis (CADIA), and nuclear medicine systems. All these techniques are still in their experimental and developmental stages and have not been adopted in clinical periodontal practice, but are used in clinical research.[42]

## Nonsurgical Therapy

*Instruments.* The evolution of nonsurgical therapy in the last fifty years has been principally related to the development of new instruments for the removal of calculus, and the use of antimicrobial agents. Instruments most used in the United States have been the Gracey curettes, and these have been supplemented by variations and modifications aimed at better adapting them to special anatomical circumstances such as deep, narrow pockets, furcations, developmental grooves, and line angles. These modified instruments include the extended shank curettes and the mini-bladed curettes, such as the mini-fives and the curvettes.[36] The development of new instruments such as the ultrasonic and sonic instruments, and the air-powder polishing devices such as the Prophy-Jet have been incorporated for use in selected cases.

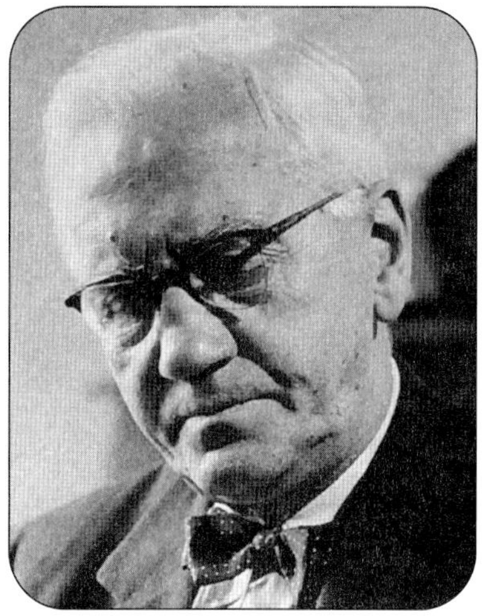

**Fig 75** Sir Alexander Fleming.

Technologic advances such as the use of magnifying systems, including clinical microscopes,[45] and the fiberoptic endoscope, attached to a video camera, which permits the visualization of the subgingival cemental wall of the pocket, have provided means to detect the presence and location of subgingival deposits and guide the operator in their removal.

*Antibiotics.* Antimicrobial agents were used in the nineteenth century as an adjunctive to scaling and root planing. In the twentieth century these agents continued to be a topic of investigation. The pioneering studies of Paul Ehrlich on antimicrobial agents leading in 1909 to the discovery of spirocheticidal drugs for the treatment of syphilis opened a wide field (see Chapter 21). Two decades later, the discovery of penicillin by Alexander Fleming in 1928 and its development for clinical use by Howard Florey and Ernst Chain in the early 1940s, started the antibiotic era in medicine, which of course, included the use of antibiotics in periodontics for several purposes.

Alexander Fleming (1881–1955) (Fig 75) was a Scottish physician and microbiologist who worked at St. Mary's Hospital in London. In the early 1920s he discovered lysozymes and in 1928 he found that a petri dish with a culture of staphylococci accidentally contaminated with a greenish mold had resulted in the disappearance of the bacterial colonies around the contaminated sites. Fleming followed this lead, analyzing in detail the antimicrobial action of the mold, which he identified, with the aid of American mycologist Charles Thom, as *Penicillium notatum.* He presented his findings in a classic paper published in 1929.[13] Fleming's findings, however, were not generally accepted by the medical community, and his attempts to isolate and purify the drug were unsuccessful for lack of funding to obtain the assistance of a biochemist.[6,29]

A few years later (1935), German physician Gerard Domagk (1895–1964) discovered the antibacterial effects of the sulfa drugs. After the outbreak of the Second World War, Australian scientist Howard Florey (1898–1968) and German biochemist Ernst Chain (1906–1979), working at Oxford University, succeeded in isolating and purifying penicillin. Florey's wife, Ethel, also a physician, conducted the initial clinical trials and the industrial production of penicillin started in the United States in 1943. Penicillin was first used in periodontal therapy for the treatment of acute necrotizing gingivitis, by intramuscular injection and locally,[30,44,46,47] and subsequently for the purpose of enhancing the chances of obtaining new attachment and osseous regeneration in infrabony pockets.[10,11]

In 1968 H. I. Bader and Paul Goldhaber[1] found that tetracyclines are excreted in the gingival fluid, and this increased the interest in the use of antibiotics in periodontal therapy. By the end of the century numerous methods had been developed and marketed, placing antimicrobial agents (chlorhexidine, tetracycline, minocycline, doxycycline, metronidazole, etc) in pockets by different controlled-release local delivery systems (capsules, chips, fibers, strips, gels, etc).[24] The concept of local delivery to the periodontal pocket, and the first systems, were developed by Max Goodson, at the Forsyth Dental Infirmary in Boston.[18,19]

## Surgical Therapy

The surgical technique in vogue in the 1950s was the gingivectomy.[16] Development of the surgical pack by A. W. Ward in 1923 had improved the postoperative period. Clarification by Rudolph Kronfeld in 1935 of the character of the osseous lesion, removing the need for osseous surgery, increased the indications of this technique (see Chapter 22). In 1948 Henry Goldman described the gingivoplasty, adding a plastic purpose to the simple removal of the pocket wall.[1] Gradually in the late 1950s and 1960s, indications for the flap operation became clearer and its use more common.

Along with Goldman (see biography in Chapter 24), clinicians John F. Prichard and Saul Schluger guided periodontists all over the world. John F. Prichard (Fig 76) was born in Lancaster, Texas, in 1907, obtained his dental degree from Baylor College of Dentistry, in Dallas, Texas, in 1928, and practiced all his life in Fort Worth, Texas. Prichard was essentially a self-made periodontist, having limited his practice in the mid-1950s after taking many extension courses.[2] Prichard published three periodontics texts, which presented his treatment techniques and practice philosophy and greatly influenced the profession. He was an excellent photographer, and his graphic documentation was a key feature, astonishing readers in the 1950s with his cases of periodontal regeneration.

Prichard was a learned and masterful clinician and surgeon, with a surprising knowledge of the literature. He was a role model for scores of practitioners, including Burton and William Becker, Clifford Ochsenbein, and Gary Maynard. Although he had visiting appointments at various universities, his activities were centered on his private practice. Prichard died on July 29, 1990.

Saul Schluger (Fig 77) was born in Jersey City, New Jersey, on January 9, 1908. He obtained his DDS degree from the University of Louisville in 1931, and, like his close friend John Prichard, was self-trained in periodontics by his extensive readings and a few extension courses. After serving in the army during World War II, Schluger joined the Columbia University faculty and in 1947 was appointed director of its graduate program in periodontics. In 1958 he moved to Seattle, Washington, as professor and director of the periodontal graduate program,[22] which, under his direction, became one of the leading programs in the world, attracting many students who later became prominent clinicians and educators. Among them are Harry Bohannan, William Ammons, Roy Page, and Walter Hall.

Saul Schluger, along with Ralph Yuodelis and Roy Page, authored a leading periodontics text that went through several editions. He earned many honors and awards and occupied important positions in organized dentistry. Schluger died on June 29, 1990.

*Plastic and esthetic surgery.* Techniques for displacing muscular attachments and deepening the mucobuccal fold were developed in the 1930s and 1940s by oral surgeons as a preprosthetic technique, preparatory to the insertion of full dentures. In these cases, maintaining the surgical deepening of the fold was difficult because of the absence of teeth to retain a pack. Different methods, such as the placement of tissue tacks in the bone or even skin grafts, were used to prevent the reunion of the tissues and favor its epithelization.[40]

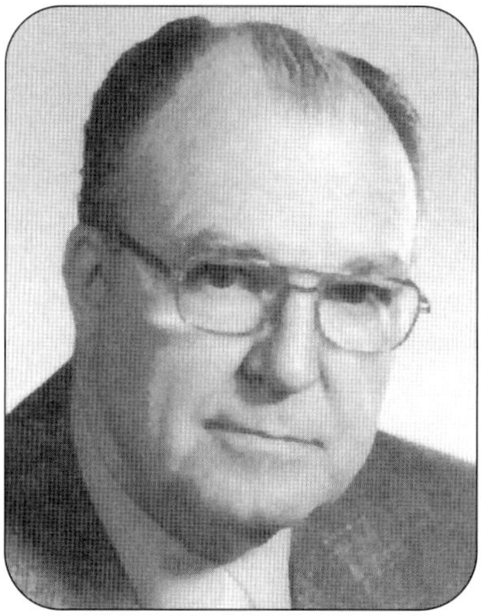

**Fig 76** John F. Prichard.

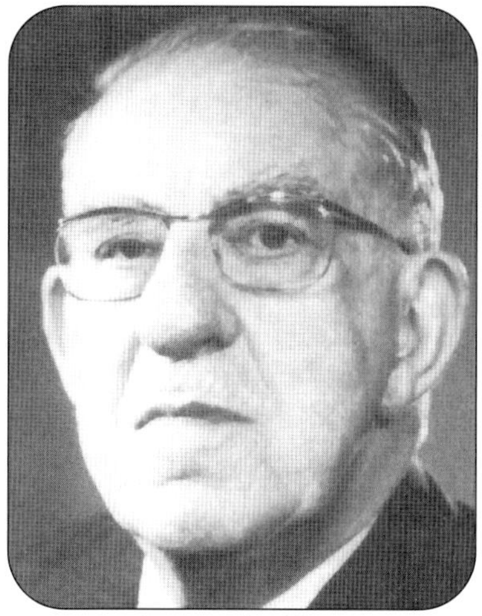

**Fig 77** Saul Schluger.

In the dentate patient, shallow mucobuccal folds were associated with little or no width of attached gingiva, as described by Claude Nabers of Texas, in 1954.[33] An operation called "pushback," was devised consisting of pocket elimination with a gingivectomy, deepening the mucobuccal fold by incision, denudation of the bone by removal of its periosteum, and insertion of a periodontal pack to prevent reunion of the tissues. In 1962, Harry Bohannan,[4,5] student of Saul Schluger and later dean of the School of Dentistry at the University of Kentucky, and others in 1963[9,12] demonstrated that removal of periosteum helps maintain the depth of the fold obtained surgically but causes great marginal bone loss, resulting in a reduced gingival width, as compared to retaining the periosteum in the same procedure.

These and other studies led to the development of the so-called fenestration technique, devised by Earl Robinson, of San Mateo, California, which removed the periosteum only on a thin band at the bottom of the deepened fold.[41] These techniques were replaced by the free gingival graft, initially described by the Swede H. Bjorn, in 1963,[3] and by the apically positioned flap, first presented by Nathan Friedman, of Los Angeles, in 1962,[14] who also introduced the internal bevel incision.[15]

Esthetic results of periodontal surgery gradually became important considerations in the 1970s and beyond, and a number of techniques were developed to solve esthetic problems created by the disease and sometimes uncovered by its treatment. Surgical coverage of denuded roots by means of a laterally displaced pedicle graft was introduced by Harold Grupe and R. F. Warren, of Portland, Oregon.[23] The successful use of free gingival grafts for root coverage was presented by Preston D. Miller, of Memphis, Tennessee, in 1982.[32] The subepithelial connective tissue graft technique was initially detailed by Andres Perez Fernandez, of Madrid,[37] in an obscure Spanish journal, and later by Peter B. Raetzke, of the University of Frankfurt, Germany;[39] the procedure was popularized by Burton Langer and Laureen Langer, of New York.[27] Numerous variations and improvements to these original descriptions can be found in current textbooks.[35] Guided tissue regeneration has also been successfully used for root coverage, as described by Italian researchers Giovanpaolo Pini Prato, Carlo Tinti, Pierpaolo Cortellini, and others.[38] In 1989 the American Academy of Periodontology adopted the name *periodontal plastic surgery* to replace the term *mucogingival surgery*, thus aligning the nomenclature to that used in plastic surgery.

*Reconstructive osseous surgery.* New gingival attachment and reconstruction of the lost marginal periodontium have been goals of periodontal therapy for more than a century. In the second half of the twentieth century numerous techniques, based on different therapeutic principles, have been proposed.[8] Bone grafts from extraoral sites were proposed by Zoltán Hegedüs in 1923 (see Chapter 22), and years later by Robert Schallhorn,[43] but were discarded because of undesirable side effects. Claude Nabers and Timothy O'Leary in 1965,[34] described the use of autogenous grafts, which continue to be used. Also in use are freeze-dried bone allografts (undecalcified and decalcified), proposed in 1976 by periodontal investigators then at the Naval Graduate Dental School in Bethesda, Maryland: James Mellonig, now at the University of Texas, San Antonio, and Gerald Bowers, now at the University of Maryland.[31] Numerous nonbone graft materials (sclera, cartilage, plaster of Paris, plastic materials, calcium phosphate biomaterials, and coral-derived materials) have been investigated but are not in current use.[8]

Early in the twentieth century, clinicians perceived the presence of the junctional and pocket epithelium as a barrier to successful therapy (see Chapter 22). In more recent times various methods have been proposed to eliminate these epithelia and prevent their migration into the healing area. The most successful of these methods has been the so-called guided tissue regeneration described by Jan Gottlow, Sture Nyman, and Jan Lindhe[20,21] of the University of Gothenburg.

Several substances have been used to condition the tooth surface for attachment by connective tissue fibers. More recently the use of growth factors and enamel matrix proteins as inducers of cementum formation has been investigated. Insight into these methods and their proponents can be found in current textbooks.[8]

Constant advancements in surgical techniques led to less invasive procedures and a need for increased surgical skills and greater visual acuity. Thus, microsurgery was developed using clinical microscopes that provide considerable magnification of the operating field.[45] Likewise the development of implant dentistry and its incorporation into the surgical repertoire of the periodontist have added an important dimension to periodontal practice and have meant a revolution in dentistry. The history of implant dentistry is presented in Chapter 26.

Clinical periodontology has continued to progress because of contributions by practitioners who have refined the existing techniques and developed new approaches for surgical solutions to periodontal problems. These clinicians include, among many others, Edward P. Allen, William Ammons, Robert Azzi, William Becker, Jean-Pierre Bernimoulin, Gerald Bowers, Gianfranco Carnevale, Herman Corn, Pierpaolo Cortellini, Connie Drisko, Michael Fritz, Steven Garrett, Marlin Gher, Thomas Han, Kenneth Kalkwarf, Thorkild Karring, William Killoy, Gerald Kramer, Burton Langer, Laureen Langer, Gary Maynard, Pamela McClain, James Mellonig, R. Mengel, Preston D. Miller, Ralf E. Mustchelknauss, Myron Nevins, Sture Nyman, Clifford Ochsenbein, Kent Palcanis, Giovanpaolo Pini Prato, Roberto Pontoriero, Henry Takei, Robert Schallhorn, Jay Seibert, Dennis Tarnow, Carlo Tinti, Jan Wennström, Ulf Wikesjö, Thomas Wilson, and Raymond Yukna.

## References

1. Bader HI, Goldhaber P. The passage of intravenously administered tetracycline into the gingival sulcus of dogs. J Oral Ther Pharmacol 1968;2:324.
2. Becker W, Ochsenbein C. Obituary, John F. Prichard. J Periodontol 1990;61:715.
3. Bjorn H. Free transplantation of gingiva propria. Sver Tandlakarforb Tidn 1963;22:684.
4. Bohannan HM. Studies on the alteration of vestibular depth. I. Complete denudation. J Periodontol 1962;33:120.
5. Bohannan HM. Studies on the alteration of vestibular depth. II. Periosteum retention. J Periodontol 1962;33:354.
6. Carranza FA. Revolucionarios de la Ciencia. Buenos Aires: Vergara, 1998.
7. Carranza FA. Clinical diagnosis. In: Newman MG, Takei HH, Carranza FA (eds). Carranza's Clinical Periodontology, ed 9. Philadelphia: Saunders, 2002.

8. Carranza FA, McLain P, Schallhorn R. Regenerative osseous surgery. In: Newman MG, Takei HH, Carranza FA (eds). Carranza's Clinical Periodontology, ed 9. Philadelphia: Saunders, 2002.
9. Carranza FA, Carraro JJ. Effect of removal of periosteum on postoperative result of mucogingival surgery. J Periodontol 1963;34:223.
10. Carranza FA Sr. Experiencias clínicas sobre reinserción. Ensayos con penicilina. Rev Odontol 1951;39:55.
11. Carranza FA Sr. A technic for reattachment. J Periodontol 1954;25:272.
12. Carraro JJ, Carranza FA, Albano EA, Joly GG. Effect of bone denudation on mucogingival surgery in humans. J Periodontol 1964;35:463.
13. Fleming A. On the antibacterial action of cultures of a penicillium with special reference to their use in the isolation of B influenzae. Br J Exp Pathol 1929;10:226.
14. Friedman N. Mucogingival surgery: The apically repositioned flap. J Periodontol 1962;33:328.
15. Friedman N, Levine HL. Mucogingival surgery: Current status. J Periodontol 1964;35:5.
16. Glickman I. The results obtained with the unembellished gingivectomy in a clinical study in humans. J Periodontol 1956;27:247.
17. Goldman HM. The development of physiologic gingival contours by gingivoplasty. Oral Surg Oral Med Oral Pathol 1950;3:879.
18. Goodson JM. Antimicrobial strategies for treatment of periodontal diseases. Periodontol 2000 1994;5:142.
19. Goodson JM, Haffejee AD, Socransky SS. Periodontal therapy by local delivery of tetracycline. J Clin Periodontol 1979;6:83.
20. Gottlow J, Nyman S, Lindhe J, Karring T. New attachment formation as a result of controlled tissue regeneration. J Clin Periodontol 1984;11:494.
21. Gottlow J, Nyman S, Lindhe J, et al. New attachment formation in human periodontium by guided tissue regeneration. J Clin Periodontol 1986;13:604.
22. Gottsegen R. Obituary, Saul Schluger. J Periodontol 1990;63:661.
23. Grupe HE, Warren RF Jr. Repair of gingival defects by a sliding flap operation. J Periodontol 1956;27:92.
24. Jolkovsky DL, Ciancio SC. Antimicrobial and other chemotherapeutic agents in periodontal therapy. In: Newman MG, Takei HH, Carranza FA (eds). Carranza's Clinical Periodontology, ed 9. Philadelphia: Saunders, 2002.
25. Kazanjian VH. Surgery as an aid to more efficient service with prosthetic dentures. J Am Dent Assoc 1935;22:556.
26. Kazanjian VH. The surgical treatment of abnormalities of the edentulous alveolar processes and the palate. Am J Orthod Oral Surg 1940;26:263.
27. Langer B, Langer L. Subepithelial connective tissue graft technique for root coverage. J Periodontol 1985;56:715.
28. Löe H. Dentistry in the 21st century. In: Simonsen RJ (ed). Dentistry in the 21st Century: A Global Perspective. Chicago: Quintessence, 1991.
29. Maurois A. The Life of Sir Alexander Fleming, Discoverer of Penicillin. Hopkins G (trans). New York: Dutton, 1959.
30. MacGregor AB, Long DA. Use of penicillin pastilles in oral infections. Br Med J 1944;2:686.
31. Mellonig JT, Bowers GM, Bright RW, Lawrence JL. Clinical evaluation of freeze-dried bone allografts in periodontal osseous defects. J Periodontol 1976;47:125.
32. Miller PD. Root coverage using a free soft tissue autograft following citric acid application. Part 1. Technique. Int J Periodontics Restorative Dent 1982;2:65.
33. Nabers CL. Repositioning the attached gingiva. J Periodontol 1954;25:38.
34. Nabers CL, O'Leary TJ. Autogenous bone grafts in the treatment of osseous defects. J Periodontol 1965;36:5.
35. Newman MG, Takei HH, Carranza FA (eds). Carranza's Clinical Periodontology, ed 9. Philadelphia: Saunders, 2002.
36. Pattison A, Pattison G. Periodontal instrumentation. In: Newman MG, Takei HH, Carranza FA (eds). Carranza's Clinical Periodontology, ed 9. Philadelphia: Saunders, 2002.
37. Perez Fernandez A. Injerto submucoso libre de encia. Una nueva perspectiva. Bol Inf Dent 1982;42:63.
38. Pini Prato G, Tinti C, Vincenzi G, et al. Guided tissue regeneration versus mucogingival surgery in the treatment of human buccal gingival recession. J Periodontol 1982;63:919.
39. Raetzke PB. Covering localized areas of root exposure employing the "envelope" technique. J Periodontol 1985;53:397.
40. Ries Centeno GA. Cirugia Bucal, ed 9. Buenos Aires: El Ateneo, 1987.
41. Robinson RE. Periosteal fenestration in mucogingival surgery. J West Soc Periodontol Abstr 1961;9:107.

42. Sanz M, Newman MG. Advanced diagnostic techniques. In: Newman MG, Takei HH, Carranza FA (eds). Carranza's Clinical Periodontology, ed 9. Philadelphia: Saunders, 2002.
43. Schallhorn RG. The use of autogenous hip marrow implants for bony crater defects. J Periodontol 1968;39:145.
44. Schuessler CF, Fairchild JM, Stransky IM. Penicillin in the treatment of Vincent's infection. J Am Dent Assoc 1945;32:551.
45. Shanelec DA, Tibbetts LS. Recent advances in surgical technology. In: Newman MG, Takei HH, Carranza FA (eds). Carranza's Clinical Periodontology, ed 9. Philadelphia: Saunders, 2002.
46. Strock AE. The treatment of acute ulcerative gingivostomatitis (Vincent's infection) with penicillin. N Y J Dent 1945;15:263.
47. Sweeney JS, Morginson WJ, Robinson RW, Kilpatrick EM. Therapeutic effectiveness of penicillin in treatment of Vincent's stomatitis and its failure to influence favorably certain other medical conditions. J Lab Clin Med 1945;30:132.

# 26

# Implant Dentistry

The replacement of human teeth by implants placed in the alveolar process has been attempted for more than two thousand years, but only recently have dentists and patients accepted it.

The French anthropologists Eric Crubézy, Pascal Mureil, Louis Girard, and Jean-Pierre Bernadou, have reported finding a wrought iron dental implant in the skull of a 30-year-old man, found at a Gallo-Roman necropolis at Chantambre, in Essone, France.[9] The skull was dated by associated pottery and radiocarbon to the end of the first century or beginning of the second century AD. The metal root was in the socket of a right, maxillary second premolar and, analyzed by X-ray microanalysis and scanning electron microscopy of an apical fragment, was found to be composed of iron and oxygen with some areas containing traces of silicon and calcium. The authors believe that the metal was shaped by a hot-hammering and folding process, using the original tooth as a model.[9] The radiograph of the area showed a perfect fit between the alveolar bone and the metallic implant, without peri-implant radiolucent areas, which to the authors suggests osseointegration.[9] The possibility of the implant having been placed post-mortem cannot however be discarded.

Dental historian Bernard Weinberger[40,41] describes a true dental implant in a pre-Columbian human skull found at Copan, Honduras, by Robert Rollins Andrews.[1] A fine dark stone, shaped like the natural tooth, was neatly fitted in the socket of the mandibular left lateral incisor. It had thick calculus deposits on it, indicating it had been worn for some time.[1,41] Malvin E. Ring's book shows a mandible of Mayan origin, dated at about 600 AD (Fig 78), found by Dr. and Mrs. Wilson Popenoe in Honduras in 1931, with three pieces of shell in place of three missing mandibular incisors.[31] Ring mentions that Dr. Amadeo Bobbio, of São Paulo, Brazil, found radiographically compact bone around the implants, thus confirming that they had been placed during the life of the individual.[31] The specimen is held by the Peabody Museum of Archeology and Ethnology of Harvard University, in Cambridge, Massachusetts.

Transplantation of teeth from one subject to another, or from one alveolus to another in the same subject, has been practiced for centuries. Morse[28] notes that archeological findings evince transplantation of teeth by Egyptians, Arabs, Greeks, Romans, Etruscans, and Chinese. Weinberger[40,41] relates that Marshall Henry Saville in his explorations of North Ecuador at the turn of the twentieth century, found skulls of pre-Inca, South American Indians with evidence of transplantation of teeth.

In the sixteenth century, Ambroise Paré (1509–1590) (see Chapter 8) pointed to a case of successful tooth transplantation (cited by Weinberger[40]). In the eighteenth century, John Hunter (1728–1793) (see Chapter 10), dedicated a chapter of *The Natural History of the Human Teeth* (Part I) to transplantation.[19] Entitled "Of transplanting of teeth," the chapter demonstrates that in spite of the differences in shape and size of the teeth from one person to another,

> we can actually transplant a Tooth from one person to another, without great difficulty, nature assisting the operation, if it is done in such a way that she can assist; with respect either to size or shape, is by having the fang of the transplanted Tooth rather smaller than the socket. The socket in this case grows to the Tooth.

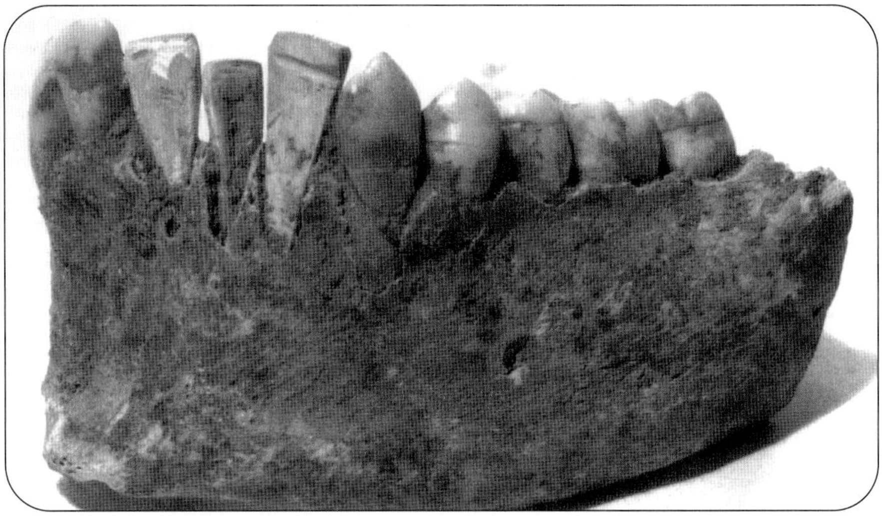

**Fig 78** Mayan mandible from sixth century AD, with three implanted pieces of shell in place of three mandibular incisors.

In Part II of the same treatise, Hunter adds that only single-rooted teeth should be transplanted because of the difficulty of finding molars that would fit the empty alveolus. Hunter's teachings gained many followers, and transplantation of teeth was performed frequently, although with scant success. Thomas Berdmore (1740–1785) advocated the extraction of abscessed teeth, cleaning and filling them and subsequently, reimplanting them in the socket, but he opposed transplantation.[40] According to Weinberger,[40] the reimplantation and transplantation of teeth was introduced in the United States by Jean Pierre Le Mayeur (1781–1806).

Josiah Flagg (1763–1816), of Boston, advertised in 1796 that he "transplants both live and dead teeth with greater convenience, and gives less pain than heretofore practiced in Europe and America." Flagg offers "cash for handsome and healthy live teeth," to be used to replace destroyed incisors in the mouth of rich patients.

In 1917 transplantation of impacted canines to an upright aligned position was first attempted by Swedish practitioner Leonard Widman.[42] Miller transplanted third molars to first molar positions in 1950.[27,33]

Attempts at replacing lost teeth by implantation of foreign substances also was tried repeatedly. Early in the nineteenth century (1809), Italian researcher M. Maggiolo, in a book entitled *Manual of Dental Art* (English translation of Italian title),[21,25] presents an elaborate technique to replace destroyed roots with an "artificial root made of gold, which should be strong enough to support a pivot tooth as solid as if it had been placed on a natural tooth."

He then describes the artificial root as formed by a solid central cylinder with a horizontal platform in its apical part, and, in the coronal end, four extensions bent "to form a sphere," to hold the crown. All parts are made of 18-karat gold and soldered together. Maggiolo explains that bone will grow into the socket, solidifying the position of the implant in just a few days. The pivot with the crown is to be placed no sooner than one month after the implant surgery. He also explains the importance of carefully extracting the tooth or roots so as not to fracture the socket walls, and claims he "almost always obtained results that were as satisfactory to me as to the persons on whom I have operated."

Edward Kirk credits numerous colleagues who presented implant systems in the United States.[21] They include S. M. Harris, of Grass Valley, California, in 1887; J. M. Edmunds, of New York, in 1889; W. G. A. Bonwill, of Philadelphia, in 1895. Also N. N. Znamensky, the

Russian professor that a few years later described in amazing detail the histopathology of the periodontal pocket, reported in 1891 on the implantation of porcelain teeth.[44] Isaih Lew,[23] of New York, cites J. W. Edwards in 1885[12] and Schnell in 1905, as others who, at the turn of the century, attempted to implant foreign bodies to replace lost teeth.

In 1901, R. E. Payne, of New York, presented a clinical demonstration at the Third International Dental Congress, in which he extracted some root remnants of the maxillary left first premolar in a 25-year-old woman. He then enlarged the socket with a trephine, which gave the socket a cylindrical shape, and then introduced by pressure a silver capsule. Into this capsule he placed a porcelain tooth, crown and root, fixing it with gutta-percha. After a few weeks he indicated the porcelain tooth could be removed and set permanently with cement.[30]

The Wichita, Kansas, dentist, E. J. Greenfield, presented in 1913 a carefully documented implantation system as follows:[15]

> The artificial root used for this process is a hollow, latticed cylinder of iridioplatinum, No. 24 gage, soldered with 24-karat gold. It is impervious to acids, and does not injure the tissue which grows about it. The disk-shaped cast base with groove or slot in which the crown attachment is inserted, is made of 22-karat gold, and is soldered to the metal frame of the root.
>
> Special machinery is necessary for cutting and shaping these roots. Absolute accuracy is essential, for the artificial root must fit exactly the circular incision or socket made for it in the jaw-bone of the patient.
>
> These roots are made in three different sizes or diameters, 3/16, 5/16 and 7/16 of an inch respectively, and are 1/2 inch in length.

Greenfield details implant selection, depending on the root to be replaced and the shape of the ridge, and stresses the importance of proper sterilization of instruments and material to be implanted. The surgical technique first calls for a tubular knife mounted in the dental engine to remove the gingiva, then a trephine with a guiding center rod to guide the initial penetration. The author recommends the technique not only for isolated teeth, but also in edentulous jaws and for construction of fixed bridges. In spite of its sound conceptual foundation, Greenfield's system was not successful to carry the extensive gold reconstruction it anchored.

Steflick and McKinney[35] look at attempts by Leger-Dorez in the 1920s, Tomkins in 1925, Brill in 1936, and Adams in 1937 to develop artificial tooth replacements, some of which hint at the designs that would come in the latter third of the century. None of these techniques, however, was successful and the dental profession did not accept replacement of lost teeth with implants.

In 1924, Zierold investigated the bone response to implantation of various metals,[43] none of which was found to be completely inert and biocompatible. In 1937, Venable, Stuck, and Beach[38] showed that an electrolytic reaction takes place when most metals come in contact with body fluids. The development of Vitallium in the late 1930s, by the Austenal Laboratories of New York, offered hope of a biocompatible material that could be used for tooth implants. Composed of 85% cobalt, 10% chromium, and 5% molybdenum, trials were immediately performed by orthopedic surgeons for the surgical repair of bone and by dentists for tooth replacement.

In 1939, Alvin Edward Strock, of the Harvard Medical School Surgical Laboratory and the Dental Service of Peter Bent Brigham Hospital, in Boston, suggested a method for the replacement of missing teeth by direct implantation of a metal support into the alveolus, using Vitallium screws placed into sockets of recently extracted teeth.[36] Strock presented two human cases, in both of which the implants were firm after six months, and an experimental clinical study in two dogs.[36] Fifty years later (1986) Strock related his first implant experience as follows:

> In those days, there was no protocol necessary for experimental surgery. I watched out in the dental clinic for a suitable case, and located one with a diseased mandibular incisor with an apical lesion. ... The Venable Vitallium screw was placed immediately after extraction, using a celluloid crown form on the screw head as a functional crown.

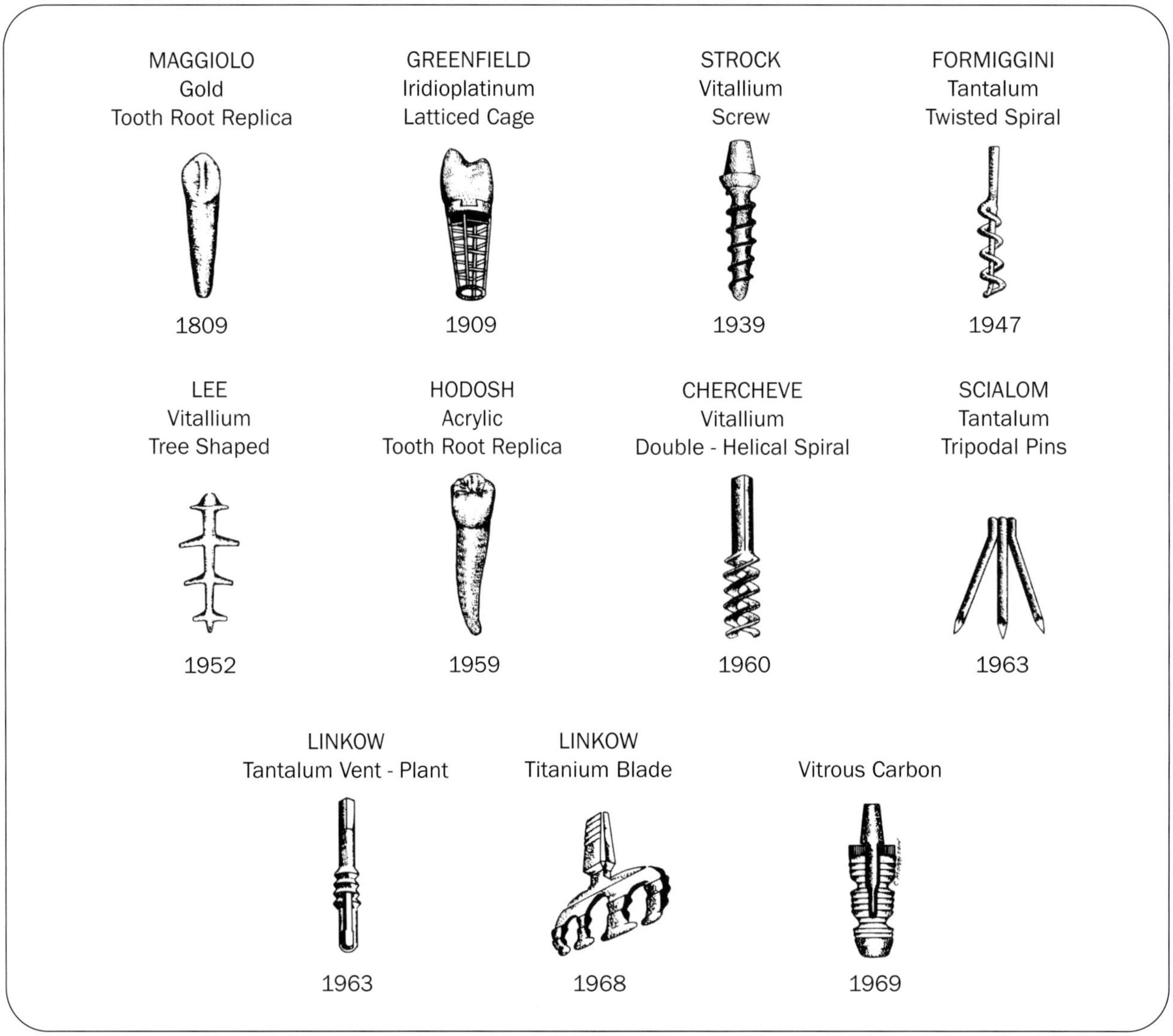


**Fig 79** The evolution of endosseous implants showing variations in design and materials from the early attempts.

> War then came on—our work was interrupted. When I returned, I was fortunate to be able to locate my first case. I wondered if exfoliation of the implant occurred in the years of my absence—but no, all was intact! Patient E.B. was followed for a total of 15 years, until 1953, when he was unfortunately killed in an auto crash, far from Boston.[11,37]

In the late 1940s, the Italian researcher Manlio Formiggini began to experiment with stainless steel and tantalum implants, developing a spiral-shaped implant.[6] Figure 79 shows some types of implants that were subsequently developed.

The tripodal pin implant of Jacques Scialom explored a different concept, as did the blade-vent implant developed by Leonard Linkow, of New York, and Rafael Cherchève, of Paris, in the late 1960s.[24] The blade-vent model is a thin, wedge-shaped Vitallium implant, of many different sizes and shapes, held in place by its mesiodistal dimension rather than its depth.

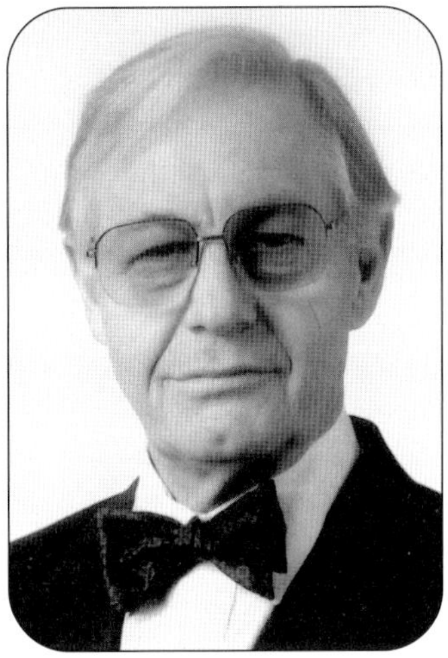

Fig 80 P.-I. Brånemark.

The other basic type is the subperiosteal implant, which consists of a Vitallium cast framework inserted over the cortical bone and under the periosteum. Described initially in Sweden by Dahl in 1941, and in the United States by N. I. Goldberg, and Aaron Gershkoff, of Boston University, in the late 1940s, it required two surgical interventions: one to obtain an impression of the exposed bone, and another to install the framework.[7,14] Lew, Berman, Marziani, Linkow, Weber, Cranin, and others presented variations of this approach.[34]

In 1959, Milton Hodosh, of Providence, Rhode Island, working at Tufts University in Boston, described a new concept in implant dentistry, using polymer replicas of the extracted tooth placed into the extraction socket. The periodontal tissues would gradually adapt to the implant, showing microscopically a firm tissue attachment to the roots of the implant and maintenance of the gingival attachment and periodontal bone.[17,18]

All the above mentioned techniques were developed by the tenacious and indefatigable work of one or more clinical and basic researchers. But none gained wide usage because of a scarcity of documented case series to clearly establish the success rates and ascertain the causes of failure. Although the subperiosteal implant and the blade-vent implant were more favorably received than other techniques, none reached a reasonable degree of acceptance by clinicians and were not generally taught at major universities. Eventually these techniques were superseded by the findings of Swedish orthopedic surgeon Per-Ingvar Brånemark (Fig 80), using titanium screw-shaped intra-osseous implants. Titanium was chosen because of its inertness as shown by Laing et al.[22]

Brånemark began his research in 1952, at the Laboratory for Vital Microscopy, in the Department of Anatomy of the University of Lund, in Sweden. In 1960 he moved to the Laboratory for Experimental Biology at the University of Göteborg and in 1978 to the Institute for Applied Biotechnology, in Göteborg, Sweden.

Brånemark's research started with vital microscopy studies of bone marrow in rabbit's fibula, directed particularly to analyze the revascularization phenomena and the microvascular structure in tissue injury and repair.[4] To observe these vascular changes, Brånemark implanted in the bone metallic chambers containing an optical system for transillumination. Some were made out of tantalum and others of titanium.

These studies showed that, while the tantalum chambers could be easily removed after the experiment, the titanium chamber became integrated with the surrounding bone and could not be removed after healing.[4] This lead to the investigation of the role of titanium fixtures in the repair of large mandibular and tibial defects in dogs. Integration was found to occur in jaw bone–anchored implants when loading was delayed, and the surgical technique was scrupulously performed in the absence of contamination and with gentle preparation of the site.

Brånemark and coworkers[3,4] demonstrated in dogs and in humans that the implants achieved osseointegration, which they defined as the absence of interposed tissue between fixture and bone. Other investigators have described, at the ultramicroscopical level, the existence of a thin, amorphous cell-free layer (20 to 1000 nm thick) interposed between the implant and the bone.[32]

The system developed by Brånemark and coworkers was marketed by Biotes (later renamed Nobelpharma, and then Nobel Biocare) and is based on the use of commercially pure titanium implants with a two-stage surgical procedure. The first intervention is performed to place the implant in the bone, covering it with the flap to isolate the healing area from the possibility of infection until the biological union has been established. The initial surgical procedure must follow a very strict operative protocol to avoid infection and overheating of the bone. The second procedure, performed three to six months later, uncovers the implant and is followed by the construction of the prosthetic suprastructure.

The Brånemark system was the first, in 1986, to be provisionally approved by the American Dental Association. Numerous variations of the Brånemark concept have appeared in the last two decades, including the IMZ system developed by Alex Kirsch, of Stuttgart, Germany; the CoreVent system of G. A. Niznick, of Los Angeles; and the International Team of Implantologists, led by Swiss researcher A. Schroeder, which developed the plasma-sprayed titanium surface implants. Numerous technical variations were also developed, such as techniques for the surgical placement of implants, techniques to improve the quality and quantity of bone in the recipient sites, changes in the implant surface to improve the chances of osseointegration, and simplification of the surgical technique to a one-stage procedure. Current books review these techniques in detail.[29,34]

Implantology has become a widely used technique that has revolutionized the practice of dentistry. Concepts of prognosis and treatment planning are being revised, with the new option of implant placement appearing often as more reasonable and safe than the heroic attempts to save teeth with severe endodontic or periodontal problems. Prosthetic therapy is also changing with the new possibility of using implants to replace lost isolated teeth rather than the conventional bridges, and also as bridge abutments or to improve the stability and comfort of full dentures. General dentists are increasingly involved with implants, periodontists and oral surgeons with their surgical placement, and prosthodontists with the construction of the suprastructure.

Throughout the world, numerous dental societies and journals of implant dentistry have sprung up in the last few decades. The subject is taught in depth in graduate level programs in periodontics, oral surgery, and prosthetics, and in special continuing education courses.

## References


1. Andrews RR. Evidence of prehistoric dentistry in Central America. Proc Pan Am Med Cong 1893;2:1872. Cited by: Weinberger BW. An Introduction to the History of Dentistry, vol 1. St. Louis: Mosby, 1948.
2. Babbush CA. Endo-osseous blade-vent implants: A research review. J Oral Surg 1972;30:168.
3. Brånemark PI, Adell R, Breine U, et al. Intraosseous anchorage of dental prostheses. I. Experimental studies. Scand J Plast Reconstr Surg 1969;3:81.
4. Brånemark PI, Zarb GA, Albrektsson T (eds). Tissue Integrated Prostheses. Chicago: Quintessence, 1985.
5. Carrels WB. End results in 100 fractures treated by internal removable fixation. J Bone Joint Surg 1936;18:408.
6. Cherchève R. Endosseous implantology. In: Cranin AN (ed). Oral Implantology. Springfield, IL: Charles C. Thomas, 1970.
7. Cranin AN (ed). Oral Implantology. Springfield, IL: Charles C. Thomas, 1970.
8. Cranin AN, Cranin SI. The intramucosal insert: A method of maxillary denture stabilization. J Am Dent Assoc 1958;57:188.
9. Crubézy E, Mureil P, Girard L, Bernadou J-P. False teeth of the Roman world. Nature 1998;391:29.

10. Dahl G. Subperiosteal implants and superplants. Dent Abstr 1957;2:685. Cited by: Cranin AN, Cranin SI. The intramucosal insert: A method of maxillary denture stabilization. J Am Dent Assoc 1958;57:188.
11. Dahle E. Transplantation to osseointegration: A chronology of dental implants. Bull Hist Dent 1990;38:19.
12. Edwards JW. Implantation of metallic capsules. Dent Off Lab 1889;3:84.
13. Fong CC, Agnew RG. Transplantation of teeth: Clinical and experimental studies. J Am Dent Assoc 1958;56:77.
14. Goldberg N, Gershkoff A. The implant lower denture. Dent Dig 1949;55:490.
15. Greenfield E. Implantation of artificial crowns and bridge abutments. Dent Cosmos 1913;55:364.
16. Hagy DM, Richards LW. Dental implants: Fact and fantasies. In: Steiner RB, Thompson RD. Oral Surgery and Anesthesia. Philadelphia: Saunders, 1977.
17. Hodosh M, Montagna W, Povar M, Shklar G. Implants of acrylic teeth in human beings and experimental animals. Oral Surg Oral Med Oral Pathol 1964;18:569.
18. Hodosh M, Povar M, Shklar G. Periodontal tissue acceptance of plastic tooth implants in primates. J Am Dent Assoc 1965;70:362.
19. Hunter J. The Natural History of the Human Teeth, ed 2. London: Johnson, 1778.
20. Jovanovic S. Clinical aspects of dental implants. In: Newman MG, Takei HH, Carranza FA (eds). Carranza's Clinical Periodontology, ed 9. Philadelphia: Saunders, 2002.
21. Kirk EC. Discussion of Dr. E. Greenfield's paper. Dent Cosmos 1913;55:432.
22. Laing PG, Ferguson AB Jr, Hodge ES. Tissue reaction in rabbit muscle exposed to metallic implant. J Biomed Mater Res 1967;1:135.
23. Lew I. Progress in implant dentistry: An evaluation. J Am Dent Assoc 1959;59:475.
24. Linkow LJ, Cherchève R. Theory and Techniques of Oral Implantology. St. Louis: Mosby, 1970.
25. Maggiolo M. Manual of Dental Art, 1809. Cited by: Kirk EC. Discussion of Dr. E. Greenfield's paper. Dent Cosmos 1913;55:432.
26. Matthews SA. Simple wire pin skeletal apparatus. J Bone Joint Surg 1931;13:595.
27. Miller HM. Tooth transplantation. J Oral Surg 1951;9:68.
28. Morse DR. Plantation procedures: History, immunology and clinical considerations. J Oral Implantol 1977;7:176.
29. Jovanovic S (assoc ed). Chapters 68–73: Oral implantology. In: Newman MG, Takei HH, Carranza FA (eds). Carranza's Clinical Periodontology, ed 9. Philadelphia: Saunders, 2002.
30. Payne RE. Implantation of silver capsule. Dent Cosmos 1901;43:1401.
31. Ring ME. Dentistry: An Illustrated History. St. Louis: Mosby-Year Book, 1985. Reprinted, New York: Harry N. Abrams, 1992.
32. Schroeder A, Sutter F, Krekeler G. Orale implantologie, allegemeine grundlagen und ITI-Hohlzylindersystem. Stuttgart: Thieme, 1988.
33. Shulman LB. Allogeneic tooth transplantation. J Oral Surg 1972;30:395.
34. Spickermann H. Implantology. New York: Thieme Medical, 1995.
35. Steflick DE, McKinney RV. History of implantology. In: McKinney RV (ed). Endosteal Dental Implants. St. Louis: Mosby-Year Book, 1991.
36. Strock AE. Experimental work on a method for the replacement of missing teeth by direct implantation of a metal support into the alveolus. Am J Orth Oral Surg 1939;25:467.
37. Strock AE. Follow-up report on a method for the replacement of missing teeth by direct implantation of a metal support in the alveolus. J Oral Implantol 1986;12:627.
38. Venable CS, Stuck WG, Beach A. Effects on bone of the presence of metals, based upon electrolysis: Experimental study. Ann Surg 1937;105:917.
39. Younger WJ. Some of the latest phases in implantation, etc. Dent Cosmos 1893;35:102.
40. Weinberger BW. An Introduction to the History of Dentistry, vol I. St. Louis: Mosby, 1948.
41. Weinberger BW. Ancient dentistry in the Old and New World. Ann Med Hist 1934;6:274.
42. Widman L. Om transplantation av retinerade horntander. Sven Tandlak Tikskr 1917;10:29.
43. Zierold AA. Reaction of bone to various metals. Arch Surg 1924;9:365.
44. Znamensky N. The implantation of artificial teeth. Br J Med Sci 1891;34:314.

# 27

# Organized Periodontics

## American Academy of Periodontology

Around the turn of the century many dental practitioners in the United States enthusiastically supported what they called *oral prophylaxis* for the treatment of periodontal disease. Today it would probably be referred to as *scaling and root planing* and *plaque control.*

Two individuals were responsible for stimulating their colleagues' interest in this type of therapy. They were David D. Smith and Edward B. Spalding.[8] David D. Smith was born in 1839, in Green County, New York, and died in 1920. After serving in the Union Army during the Civil War, Smith apprenticed with a dentist in Cambridge, Massachusetts, and later enrolled in the Philadelphia Dental College, where he received his dental degree in 1867. In 1878 he received the MD from Jefferson Medical College. He was professor of mechanical dentistry and in 1880, dean of the Philadelphia Dental College.[12] Smith published many articles on "oral prophylaxis," which he defined as

> the careful and complete removal of all calcic deposits, inspissated secretions, bacterial plaques and all accretions that gather on the surfaces of the teeth and between them, especially at the gum margins, followed by throrough polishing of all tooth surfaces by hand methods [transcribed from Merritt[8]].

While Smith was a skillful dentist who performed impeccable restorative work, he was not well liked, owing to his authoritarian, dogmatic, and aloof nature. However he commanded a good deal of respect, and many practitioners visited his office to learn his methods. One of these was Edward Spalding, of Detroit, Michigan.

Edward B. Spalding was born in Eagle Rock, Michigan, in 1868 and graduated from the University of Michigan School of Dentistry in 1892. He practiced in the Detroit and Birmingham areas and died on November 2, 1960.[13] Spalding was a likable fellow and a great admirer of Smith's work. Merritt credits him with releasing, through Robert McBride in the United States and N. S. Jenkins in Germany, Smith's groundbreaking findings.

Spalding gained Smith's permission to invite several dentists to observe his techniques and the excellent results he obtained with his prophylactic technique. In 1904 Spalding persuaded a young, recent graduate, Grace Rogers (Fig 81), to spend a year in postgraduate work at the University of Michigan, and a year later to open, in Detroit, a practice devoted to "oral prophylaxis."

Another dentist, Gillette Hayden (1880–1929) (Fig 82), a graduate of the Ohio Medical University College of Dentistry (today Ohio State University), practiced in Columbus, Ohio. Since early in her career, she was interested in periodontics. For three years Gillette was an associate of McBride and Jenkins, who ran in Dresden, Germany, a practice of what was then known as oral prophylaxis. Upon her return she visited Spalding and Rogers' office in Detroit, and became a convert to Smith's method. (Hayden was the great-granddaughter of Horace H. Hayden, cofounder [1839] with Chapin A. Harris, of the world's first dental school, the Baltimore College of Dental Surgery.)

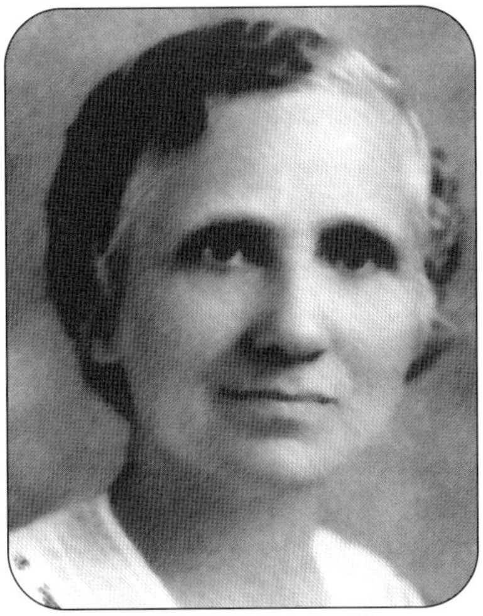
**Fig 81** Grace Rogers Spalding.

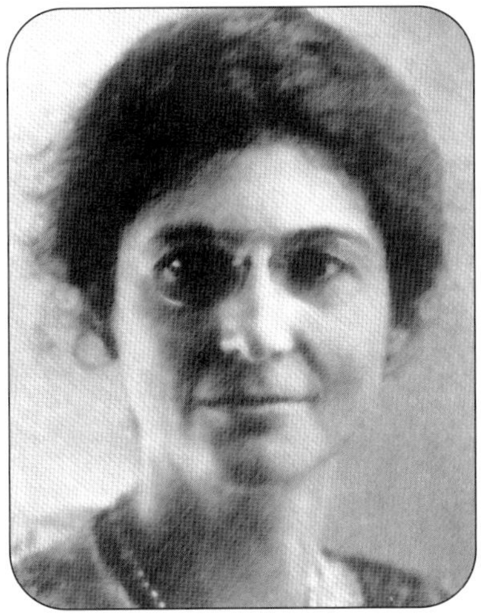
**Fig 82** Gillette Hayden.

Gillette Hayden and Grace Rogers (Rogers had by then married Edward Spalding) conceived the idea of a society to promote and divulge the knowledge on "oral prophylaxis." For this purpose, they met in 1913 and 1914, at dental meetings in Kansas City and in Toledo, Ohio, and with the support of many followers of Smith's, formed an organizing committee, with Hayden as chair and Grace Spalding as secretary. On May 23, 1914, an organizational meeting held in Cleveland, Ohio, created the American Academy of Oral Prophylaxis and Periodontology.

Another person involved in the creation of the American Academy of Oral Prophylaxis and Periodontology was John Oppie McCall, then of Buffalo, and later of New York. (See Chapter 28 for McCall's biography and portrait.) McCall had graduated from the University of Buffalo in 1904 and, as all recent graduates, was at a loss to treat the many patients with periodontal disease that sought his care. In 1906 he met C. M. Carr, who had designed a set of instruments and taught him how to use them.[1]

From Carr, McCall learned of other groups that were interested in the subject and had created "C. M. Carr Clubs." McCall was then commissioned to contact all these clubs, and a meeting took place in Cleveland in 1914.[1]

Arthur Merritt credits the following individuals as the original organizing group of the Academy:[7] Gillette Hayden, Columbus, Ohio; Grace Rogers Spalding, Detroit, Michigan; John Oppie McCall, Buffalo, New York; M. Gearhart, Washington, DC; J. W. Jungman, Cleveland, Ohio; Austin F. James, Chicago, Illinois; and Andrew J. McDonagh, Toronto, Canada. Austin F. James (1871–1952) was elected president; McDonagh, vice president; Charles Wood, secretary; and Mary Alleyne; treasurer.

A second organizational meeting was held in Rochester, New York, on July 10, and the first annual meeting in Washington, DC, took place on November 5 through 7, 1914. Seventeen people attended. Hayden replaced Wood as secretary.

The second annual meeting took place in Detroit, on September 20 through 22, 1915. Hayden was elected as the new president. In 1919 the name of the academy was shortened to American Academy of Periodontology (AAP). The academy has since had annual meetings, with the exception of the years 1942 to 1945, because of World War II.

The *Journal of Periodontology* started publication in 1930, with two issues a year. It became a quarterly in 1946, a bimonthly in 1963, and has been a monthly publication since 1969. The journal has been dedicated to the memory of Gillette Hayden, who died on March 27, 1929. The following have been editors of the *Journal of Periodontology*: Grace Rogers Spalding

(1933–1950), Maynard K. Hine (1951–1965), Henry M. Goldman (1966–1980), Timothy O'Leary and William C. Hurt (coeditors, 1966–1988), and Robert J. Genco (1988–present). In 1996 the *Journal of Periodontology* started another publication, called *Annals of Periodontology*, which is devoted to conferences, workshops, and symposia.

The AAP has sponsored and published the proceedings of the World Workshops in Periodontics, held in Ann Arbor, Michigan, in 1966; the World Workshop in Clinical Periodontics, held in Princeton, New Jersey, in 1989; and the World Workshop in Periodontics in Landsdowne, Virginia, in 1996.

*American Board of Periodontology.* The American Board of Periodontology was organized in 1939, following a recommendation of AAP President Edward Spalding in 1937. Its first meeting was held in Milwaukee, Wisconsin, under the chairmanship of Arthur Merritt. The first members of the Board were Dickson Bell, of San Francisco; M. Monte Bettman, of Portland, Oregon; A. W. Bryan, of Iowa City, Iowa; Austin F. James, of Chicago; Olin Kirkland, of Montgomery, Alabama; Harold J. Leonard, of New York City; and Arthur H. Merritt, of New York City. Merritt was chairman, Kirkland, vice chairman, and Leonard, secretary. The Board was approved by the ADA in 1948.[7]

*AAP Foundation.* In 1993, the American Academy of Periodontology established a charitable organization, the AAP Foundation. The Foundation was led by past president Charles Finley and a Board of Directors that included Erwin Barrington, William James, Robert Ferris, Donald Adams, Richard Bradley, Sebastian Ciancio, Kenneth Kornman, Michael Newman, R. Earl Robinson, Leonard Tibbetts, Bud Tarrson, and Alice de Forest. This group developed a mission statement, reaffirmed in 2000, to "improve the periodontal health of the public by increasing public and professional awareness of periodontal diseases, stimulating and supporting clinical research and the generation of new knowledge and enhancing educational programs and opportunities in periodontology."

*American Society of Periodontists.* The American Academy of Periodontology, at the time of its organization and after considerable discussion, decided to accept as members those "especially interested" in periodontics, not requiring that they limit their practice to this field of dentistry. The debate continued, however, for many years, and after the creation of the American Board of Periodontics in 1939, and its approval by the American Dental Association in 1948, it intensified. In 1961 the American Society of Periodontists (ASP) was created limiting its membership to individuals that practiced periodontics exclusively. Their first meeting was in Seattle, July 5–7, 1962, and the second in Denver, May 5–8, 1963.[7]

The ASP created its own journal, called *Periodontics*, under the editorship of Henry M. Goldman. Shortly after the creation of the ASP, it became clear that one organization would better serve the needs of the profession and the public. Many meetings were held between members of both organizations to decide on terms of a merger. Joint meetings were held by Maynard K. Hine, Donald Kerr, and Charles Williams, representing the Academy, and D. Walter Cohen, William Hiatt, and Saul Schluger, representing the Society. Finally the merger took place in October 1967, with a joint meeting in Washington, DC.[7]

## U.S. State and Regional Societies

There are many state and regional societies of periodontology in the United States. Among them the Western Society of Periodontology, that nucleates the states of California, Oregon, Washington, Nevada, Arizona, and Utah. It publishes, since 1953, the quarterly *Journal of the Western Society of Periodontology (Periodontal Abstracts).* The Northeastern Society of Periodontology includes all the New England states, plus New York, New Jersey, Pennsylvania, Maryland, and the District of Columbia.

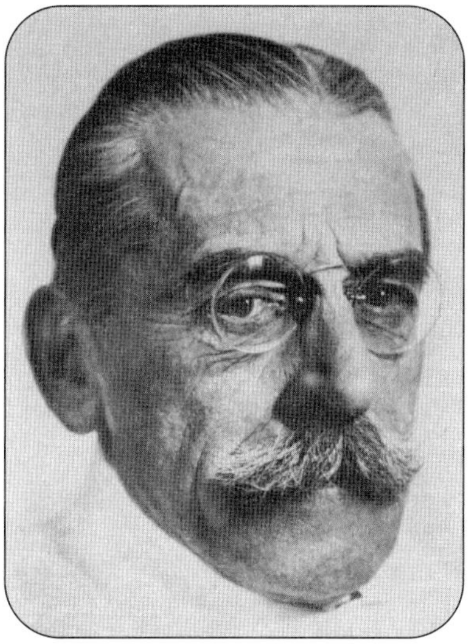

**Fig 83** Otto Loos.

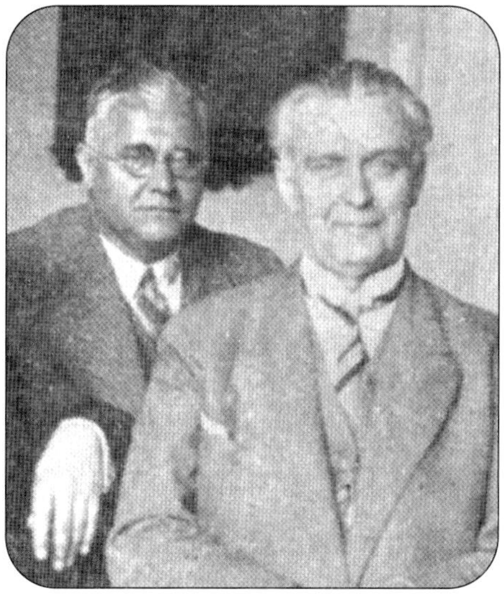

**Fig 84** Oskar Weski *(left)* and René Jaccard.

## ARPA International

In the years 1922 through 1924, several prominent periodontal clinicians and researchers met in Berlin to create a society devoted to the study of periodontal problems. Among several others this group included Oskar Weski, Robert Neumann, Bernhard Gottlieb, A. Kantorowicz, and Harry Sicher. The society was created in 1925 as a German institution (*Deutsche Gesellschaft für Parodontologie*). This was the German ARPA, whose name derives from the initials of its name *Arbeitsgemeinenschaft für Parodontosenforschung*. It was first presided by Otto Loos (Fig 83), with Oskar Weski (Fig 84) as general secretary, both of whom remained in their positions until 1935. In 1929 the society started the publication of the journal *Paradentium*.

The international ARPA was founded on May 30, 1932. Founding members of ARPA International were German researchers Oskar Weski (1879–1952) and Otto Loos (1871–1936), the French scientist Chactas Hulin (1888–1977), the Swiss investigator Arthur-Jean Held (b. 1905), and René Jaccard (1885–1960) (Fig 84), who became its first president.[4,5,11] The purpose was to create an international organization devoted to study and research in periodontology. ARPA had branches in North and South America and other parts of the world, although it was essentially a European organization. In the 1930s, as Adolf Hitler and the Nazi Party tightened their rule in Germany and Austria, several prominent periodontists emigrated to the United States and other countries. This group included Gottlieb, Orban, Sicher, Türkheim, Munzesheimer, Waldsachs, and Kantorowicz.[10]

The initial meeting of International ARPA took place in the city of Frankfurt in 1932. Many meetings followed in other European cities (Paris 1933, Como 1934, Budapest 1935, Vienna 1936, Copenhagen 1937, Prague 1938, Berlin 1939, Groningen 1949, Madrid 1951, Geneve 1953, Venice 1955, Paris 1958, Vienna 1960, Athens 1963, Berlin 1966, and Basel 1969). The International ARPA was dissolved in 1974.[4,5,11]

ARPA adopted the concept of the *paradentium*, created by Oskar Weski in 1921,[13] which included an organ composed of gingiva, alveolar bone, periodontal ligament, and cementum. Embryologic and pathologic reasoning supported the inclusion of the cementum in this concept, as suggested by Weski. The concept of paradentium was adopted throughout Europe and

Latin America.[5] In 1924 the American Dental Association (ADA) accepted the idea with two modifications. It changed the name to *parodontium*, and excluded the cementum from its components. In 1933 ARPA accepted the name *paradentium*. In 1937, the ADA and the AAP agreed on the name *periodontium*, and finally agreed, in 1939, to include in it the cementum.[2,5]

## European Federation of Periodontology

In 1974 the periodontal societies of Germany, Great Britain, Holland, France, Switzerland, and the Scandinavian countries founded the *Journal of Clinical Periodontology*. Its first editor was the Swiss investigator and educator Hans Mühlemann, and he was succeeded a few years later by the Swedish researcher Jan Lindhe. This joint effort was the unifying base that crystallized a few years later in the creation of a continental periodontal institution.

In August 1987 plans for a European society were started by Hans Rodenburg, Daniel van Steenberghe, and Peter Floyd, with support of the societies in Belgium, Great Britain, the Netherlands, Spain, France, and Switzerland. In a meeting in Santa Margherita in 1989, with additional representatives from Germany, Italy, Portugal, and the Scandinavian countries, a federation was proposed. The organization was formalized in a subsequent meeting in Maastricht, both chaired by U. van der Velde of the Netherlands.[9] The first president of the European Federation of Periodontology (EFP) was Lavin Flores-de-Jacoby, of Marburg, Germany. The EFP meetings are called EuroPerio and are held every three years. They have convened in Paris (1994), Florence (1997), and Geneva (2000). The EFP has also established the European guidelines for undergraduate pre- and postdoctoral periodontal education.[9,10]

At present the member societies of the European Federation of Periodontology are from Belgium, Denmark, Finland, France, Germany, Great Britain, Greece, Ireland, Italy, the Netherlands, Norway, Portugal, Spain, Sweden, Switzerland, and Turkey. Associate members are the societies in Austria, the Czeck Republic, Hungary, Israel, Poland, and Slovenia.[9]

## References


1. American Academy of Periodontology. Nomenclature in periodontia. J Dent Educ 1941;5:291.
2. A pioneer looks back. American Academy of Periodontology Newsletter 1974;9(1).
3. Bánóczy J. The evolution of dental education: A European perspective. J Dent Educ 1993;57:634.
4. Bertzbach K. Geschichte der Arbeitsgemeinschaft für Paradentose-Forschung (ARPA) un der Deutschen Gesselschaft für Parodontologie (DGP) 1924–1974. Koln: Deutsche Gesselschaft Parodontologie, 1982.
5. Febres Cordero F. Vocabulary in periodontology. Part I: The concept of "paradentium." Periodontics 1966;4:137.
6. Held AJ. Chactas Hulin (1888–1977). Bull Hist Dent 1993;41:73.
7. Hine MK. History of the American Academy of Periodontology, 1945–1989. Chicago: American Academy of Periodontology, 1989.
8. Merritt AH. History of the American Academy of Periodontology. J Periodontol 1947;18:121.
9. Meyle J, Hillam D. History of the European Federation of Periodontology. Available at: www.efp.net/info_index.html. Accessed July 2002.
10. Mustchelknauss RE. 65 Jahre ARPA/DGP Entwicklung der Parodontologie in der Bundesrepublik Deutschland. Parodontologie 1991;2:107.
11. Mustchelknauss RE. Geschichte der Parodontologie unter besonderer Berücksichtigung der Verhältnisse in Deutschland. In: Mustchelknauss RE (ed). Lehrbuch der klinische Paradontologie. Berlin: Quintessenz, 2000.
12. Obituary, David D. Smith. Dent Cosmos 1920;62:911.
13. Obituary, Edward Bartlett Spalding. J Periodontol 1960;31:418.
14. Weski O. Röntgenologisch-anatomische Studien aus dem Gebiet der Kieferpathologie. Vjschr Zahnheilk 1921;37:1 and 1922;38:1.

# 28

# Periodontal Education

Dental education has evolved in the last two centuries, from a period of apprenticeship to a full-fledged, recognized field of university study with a sound basis of scientific research and technological advances. A brief discussion of the history of dental education in the United States appears relevant, particularly with relation to medicine, since this may have influenced the teaching of periodontics.

## United States

Formal dental education began in the United States with the creation of the Baltimore College of Dental Surgery in 1839, by Horace H. Hayden (1769–1844) and Chapin A. Harris (1806–1860). It was initially Hayden's plan to have the school become a department within the University of Maryland, with students taking the first year of study with the medical students and the second year concentrating on dentistry. But the university rejected his plan.

Why the University of Maryland rejected Hayden's plan is not clear. It has been assumed that they considered dentistry unworthy of university status. This does not seem consistent with the fact that within a year Hayden was awarded an honorary Doctor of Medicine degree and that the university did not prevent the Maryland legislature from approving the charter for a dental school.[6] According to Waite, Hayden's plan was refused by the university because one of his collaborators, Baxley, a physician and former faculty member at the University of Maryland, had recently been dismissed and the medical faculty rejected the plan so he would not be readmitted.[6] Hayden then called on Harris, and together they founded the Baltimore College of Dental Surgery, as an independent institution. Eighty four years later, in 1923, the University of Maryland incorporated the dental school.[2]

Several other dental schools opened in the following years, as independent institutions: the Ohio College of Dental Surgery in 1845; the New York College, in Syracuse, in 1852; and the Philadelphia College, also in 1852.[2,4] Although these schools were independent, the faculty and the preceptors attached to them were all university-trained physicians or dentists. At that time, most medical schools were independent, and clinical teaching was carried out under the preceptor system.

Self-trained or purely preceptor-trained dentists were not accepted as members of the dental societies, but they could attend dental conventions by paying the inscription fee ($5).[6] Conventions became frequent areas of angry arguments and bitter controversies between medical dentists and "craftsmen" dentists. One such debate was the "amalgam war" which the craftsmen defended because of the ease of manipulation of material, while the medical dentists opposed because of the danger of mercurial poisoning.[6] This controversy occurred around the middle of the century.

The antagonism between the two groups increased because the nonmedical dentists soon developed methods and medicines that they patented, and this was considered by the professionals to be quackery and unprofessional conduct. As a consequence the medical profession accused dentistry of commercialism.[6] In addition to this, medicine was then opposed to specialization; all physicians had to be generalists, and even limited practice was seen as inferior. No specialties were recognized, and dentistry was therefore rejected.

Independent proprietary schools favored teaching the technical and mechanical aspects of dentistry while dropping or reducing their instruction in basic medical sciences. Periodontology requires local techniques for therapy and basic science knowledge for the understanding of tissue changes and etiologic factors. The strong technical approach of American dentistry, and its consideration of local causes of dental diseases, permitted the development of effective periodontal therapies. Refined scaling technique, improving on Fauchard's legacy by Riggs and his followers, developed in the United States and is the basic technique to this day. The development of pathology and bacteriology in Europe, by Rudolf Virchow and Robert Koch, led the periodontal studies in these areas, with W. D. Miller and N. N. Znamensky.

The schism began to heal when the first university-affiliated dental schools were founded. But healing was slow. The first dental school created as part of a university was Harvard's, in 1867. Nathan Cooley Keep, dean of the Harvard school, was a strong force, attempting to return to the teaching of basic medical sciences and regaining the confidence and respect of the medical profession. In 1875 the University of Michigan approved a dental school under the leadership of Jonathan Taft. Soon after, the University of Pennsylvania established a dental school, soon to be endowed by Thomas W. Evans, an American dentist who practiced in Paris and had been a close friend of Napoleon III.[1] The university schools provided a stronger basic science and medical foundation for teaching dental therapies.

In 1884 the National Association of Dental Faculties was created, and this brought some order into the educational institutions of the country.[4] By the end of the nineteenth century there were fifty-two dental schools in the United States, thirty-two of which were part of universities. The number of proprietary schools increased in the latter part of the nineteenth century but in the twentieth century it rapidly declined as the states required licensure examinations. These exams could be taken only by graduates of "reputable" schools, a term not defined but that in practice meant nonproprietary school. Special reports, such as the Flexner report, in 1910, and the Gies report, in 1926, dealt with medical and dental education, respectively. The Gies report recommended that the dental schools deserved earnest attention by the universities, not as profit centers channeling funds to the medical schools, but as an autonomous specialty of medicine. Gies urged recruitment of well-qualified, full-time faculty, a liberal preprofessional education, and that the three-year dental program be increased to four years by an increased "correlation" with clinical medicine. The latter recommendation was not followed and a four-year curriculum gained acceptance only after a 1934 recommendation by the American Dental Association (ADA).[2]

Subsequent reports, including the Blauch report (AADS) in 1935; the Council on Dental Education (CDE) of the ADA in 1941; the Horner report (CDE) in 1947; the Hollinshead report (W. K. Kellogg Foundation) in 1961; the ADA reports of 1977 and 1980; and the Fields report (Institute of Medicine) in 1995, document the evolution of the dental curriculum and the struggle of educators and practitioners to set higher standards for dental schools and improve the stature of the profession.[2]

Specialties were recognized by the ADA as follows: oral and maxillofacial surgery, orthodontics, pediatric dentistry, periodontics, and prosthodontics in 1947; oral pathology in 1949; dental public health in 1950; and endodontics in 1963.

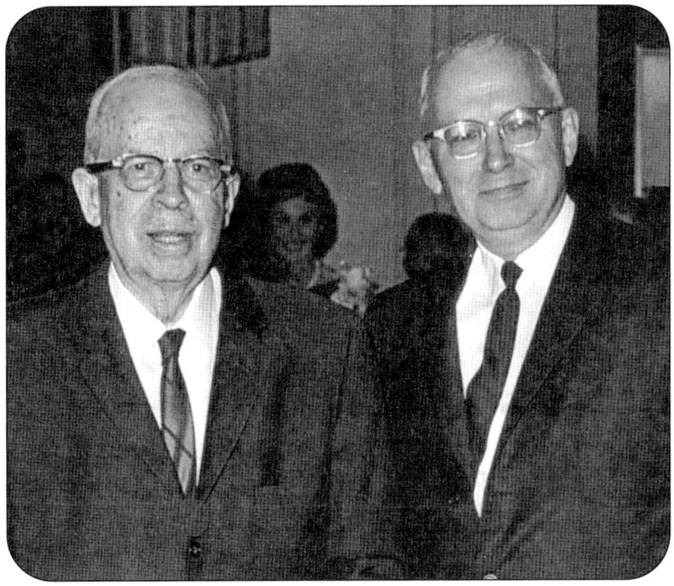

**Fig 85** John Oppie McCall *(left)* and Maynard Hine.

## Europe

In Europe dental institutes and schools also started to appear in the mid-nineteenth century. In Germany, Eduard Albrecht founded the first dental school in Berlin in 1855. In England the London School of Dentistry opened in 1859. In France *l'Ecole Dentaire de Paris* started in 1880, under the leadership of Charles Godon. In Switzerland the first school appeared in 1881, in Sweden in 1888, and in Austria in 1890.[4]

In northern Europe dental schools generally followed the independent model, while in other European countries (France, Spain, Italy, Austria) dentistry was part of the medical school curriculum; graduates obtained the MD first and then undertook dentistry as a medical specialty. This persisted until the 1980s when directives of the European Economic Community forced a change in the policy.[2]

## Training in Periodontics

Periodontal teaching in dental schools had a slow start and ranked well below the restorative sciences with respect to the time devoted to it.[3] The Horner report of 1946 indicates that the teaching of periodontics occupied 2.1 percent of the entire dental curriculum, less than the time allotted to dental materials, and ten times less than restorative dentistry (prosthodontics and operative dentistry).[5] Although the situation has improved, in many schools, allotted time is still insufficient to cover even the basic diagnostic understanding and therapeutic skills required to treat common periodontal problems. Irving Glickman's 1951 article "A change in the aims of dental education,"[5] elucidates a problem still relevant in many schools.

The first independent full-fledged department of periodontics in an American dental school was created at the New York University College of Dentistry in 1926. The first chairperson of this department was John Oppie McCall (1879–1978), of Buffalo.

John Oppie McCall (Fig 85) had a long and distinguished career as a periodontist and dental educator. He was an advocate of the "nonsurgical" treatment of periodontal disease, and of the role of trauma from occlusion in the etiology of periodontal disease. He was a founder, and president, of the American Academy of Periodontology.

Born in Geneva, New York, in 1879 as John Oppie, he was adopted, after the death of his parents by his maternal uncle, Dr. Charles W. McCall, whose last name he took, thus becoming John Oppie McCall (his mother's maiden name). He attended Rutgers and Yale University, and obtained his dental degree from the University of Buffalo in 1904. McCall started his practice in Binghampton, New York, and in 1910 moved to Buffalo, where he limited his practice to periodontics and taught at the University of Buffalo. In addition, from 1916 to 1923, he traveled to New York to teach periodontia at Columbia University. He moved to New York in 1924 and became the first chairman of the newly created Department of Periodontia at New York University. McCall was succeeded as chair by Samuel Charles Miller, of New York (1904–1958). McCall authored many articles and several books, including the *Textbook of Clinical Periodontia*, with Paul R. Stillman. McCall earned many awards. He died in 1987, at 98 years old.

Many periodontists have been deans of their dental schools and some have reached higher positions in university administration. Among them are Maynard K. Hine (1907–1997) (Fig 85) was dean of the University of Indiana School of Dentistry. After the merger of Indiana and Purdue Universities he became the first chancellor of Indiana University–Purdue University Indianapolis (IUPUI); Henry M. Goldman (1911–1991) was the founding dean of Boston University School of Dentistry, later named after him; D. Walter Cohen (b. 1926) was dean of the University of Pennsylvania School of Dentistry and later became president of the Medical College of Pennsylvania, and chancellor of the M. C. P. Hahnemann University School of Medicine; Harald Löe (b. 1926) was dean of the University of Connecticut School of Dentistry, and later became director of the National Institute of Dental Research; Paul Goldhaber (b. 1924) was dean of Harvard University School of Dental Medicine from 1968 to 1992; Harry Bohannan (b. 1927) was dean at University of Kentucky College of Dentistry (1968–1974); Jan Lindhe (b. 1935) was dean of the University of Gothenburg Dental School (1977–1983 and 1990–1993), and of the University of Pennsylvania School of Dental Medicine (1983–1988); Paul B. Robertson was dean of the University of Washington Dental School, in Seattle, from 1992 to 2001. There is a long list of other periodontists who became deans of dental schools in the U.S. and abroad.

*Periodontal graduate programs.* The American Board of Periodontology was organized in 1939, following a recommendation by American Academy of Periodontology President, Edward Spalding in 1937. The Board was approved by the American Dental Association in 1948.

Graduate programs in periodontics started in the late 1940s at Michigan University, Ann Arbor; Columbia University, New York; and Tufts University, Boston. Several other universities started similar programs shortly thereafter. They were one-year programs, and expanded to two-year programs in the late 1950s.

Around 1990, the explosion of knowledge in periodontics and related fields, including the addition of implant dentistry, conscious sedation, and other areas to the curriculum, made it necessary to expand the graduate courses to three years. In the United States there are more than fifty periodontal graduate programs, based in universities and hospitals.

## References


1. Carson G. The Dentist and the Empress. Boston: Houghton Mifflin, 1983.
2. Field MJ (ed). Dental Education at the Crossroads. Washington, DC: National Academy Press, 1995.
3. Glickman I. A change in the aims of dental education. J Dent Educ 1951;15:109.
4. Hoffman-Axthelm W. History of Dentistry. Chicago: Quintessence, 1981.
5. Horner HH. Dental Education Today. Chicago: University of Chicago Press, 1946.
6. Waite FC. The background of modern American dentistry. J Dent Educ 1937;1:91.

# 29

# Dental Hygiene

Dental hygiene has become a significant discipline allied to periodontology. The dental hygienist is the major dental auxiliary and is licensed to carry out a number of specific procedures on patients, including removal by scaling of supragingival and subgingival hard and soft deposits, polishing the teeth, and providing home care instruction.[17]

The importance of cleanliness of the teeth has been recognized since the earliest days of civilization (see Chapter 21). Early in the twentieth century many dentists realized the importance of the so-called oral prophylaxis performed at regular intervals to mantain patients' oral health. Among them was David D. Smith (1839–1920), a skillful dentist whose expertise in restorative dentistry won him considerable respect (See Chapter 27 for Smith's biography). Smith demonstrated his techniques and had many dentists visit his office, impressing them with his system of periodic oral prophylaxis, and home care instruction.[10]

From the last decades of the nineteenth century, interest was shown in dental assistants to perform some of the nonsurgical tasks carried out by dentists. C. M. Wright in 1902[18] published the first suggestion to train "women of education and refinement, who are seeking a field of work of an honorable and useful kind and among people of culture."

Wright suggested training them in dental schools for one year, including clinical training and instruction in anatomy, pathology, and physiology of the teeth. Other dentists who advocated this include Sidney J. Rauh (1873–1935), and M. L. Rhein of New York.[13,14] In a paper published in 1903, Rhein proposed the training of women as dental nurses to perform this treatment, under supervision of the dentist.[9] Rhein stressed three important reasons for the introduction of dental nurses:

> (1) it will tend materially toward the public good,
> (2) it will open to womankind a new vocation second to none in desirability, and
> (3) it will materially aid the stomatologist in the quality of his results.[14]

In the first decade of the century, several dentists attempted to change the legislation of various states to allow hygienists as dental auxiliaries. C. M. Wright in Ohio, Albert H. Stevenson in New York, and H. S. Seip in Pennsylvania attempted such change. Arthur Merritt of New York and others supported these attempts.[11]

This idea of creating a dental hygiene school was taken up by Alfred C. Fones. Fones (Fig 86) was born in Bridgeport, Connecticut, on December 17, 1869, and graduated from the New York College of Dentistry in 1890. Alfred Fones was a prominent dentist in his state and nationally, earning numerous awards for his achievements. He practiced in Bridgeport until his death on March 17, 1938.[12]

After listening to a lecture by David Smith in Philadelphia in 1899, Fones started to use Smith's preventive techniques.[6] In 1906, Fones hired a dental assistant, Irene Newman (Fig 87), and meticulously taught her how to scale teeth. He began with teaching her dental anatomy, scaling on extracted teeth, and how to remove stain from the teeth. Newman then started polishing children's teeth. Eventually she scaled teeth on patients with periodontal disease. Irene Newman can be considered the first dental hygienist.[15]

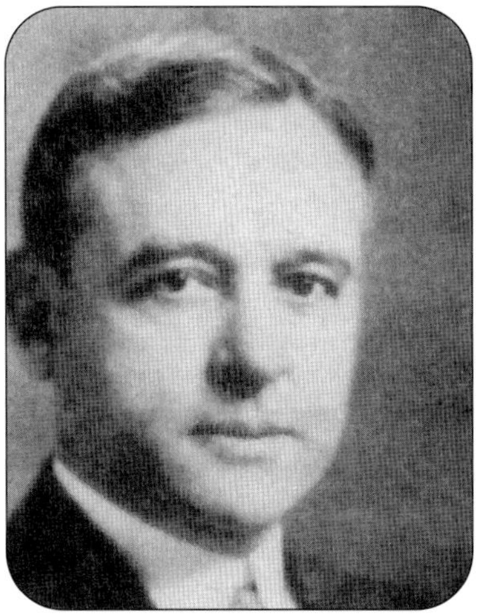
**Fig 86** Alfred C. Fones.

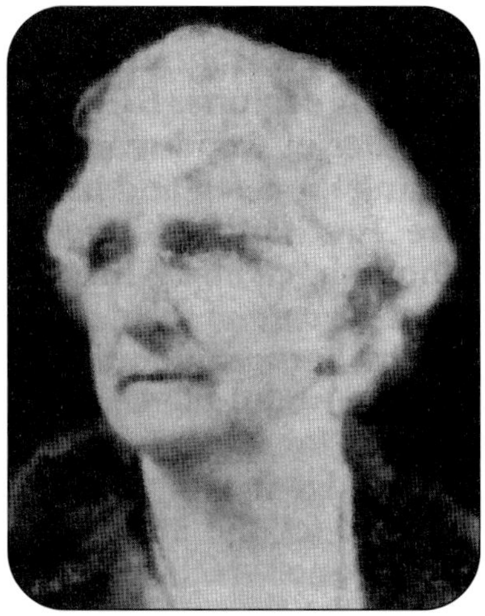
**Fig 87** Irene Newman.

In spite of the opposition of dentists, Fones founded in 1913 the Fones Clinic for Dental Hygienists, in Bridgeport, graduating the first class of 27 students, all female, in June 1914. He gathered an impressive faculty for this school, including the dental school deans of Pennsylvania and Harvard, seven professors from Yale University, two from Columbia, as well as three New York specialists.[8] Fones edited the lectures presented by the faculty and compiled them into a textbook—the first textbook for dental hygienists.[7] All the graduates of the first class entered the Bridgeport school system, and the caries rate of the attending children dropped a spectacular 75 percent.[15]

Several other dental hygiene schools opened in the years following Fones' dental hygiene school. C. M. Wright, who had long urged the Ohio College of Dental Surgery to start such a course, finally succeeded.[2] Eleven programs started between 1913 and 1923. The Fones school closed in 1917.

M. L. Rhein and Louise C. Ball, both dentists, opened in 1916 the New York School of Dental Hygiene, under a grant from the Rockefeller Foundation. The following year this school affiliated with Columbia University. Robin Adair (1878–1929), a dentist and physician of Atlanta, Georgia, was another pioneer in dental hygiene. In 1928 he opened a dental hygiene school in Atlanta, but died a year later in an automobile accident.[4]

Some children's dental clinics funded by philantropic foundations also included schools of dental hygiene, such as the Guggenheim Clinic in New York City, the Eastman Dental Clinic in Rochester, New York, and the Forsyth Infirmary, in Boston. Tufts University and Harvard University Dental Schools also developed dental hygiene courses, and other dental schools followed.

Dental hygiene practice was regulated by law in the state of Connecticut in 1915, then by New York, Massachusetts, and Maine in 1917. In 1922 the American Dental Association (ADA) drafted a model law, regulating the practice of dental hygiene, that could be followed by state boards. The ADA suggested a curriculum that included teaching of the basic dental sciences and clinical training in dental hygiene. It stated that hygienists would remove deposits on the teeth but not perform invasive operations on the teeth or other oral tissues.

The American Dental Hygienists Association (ADHA) was founded in 1923, under the sponsorship of the American Dental Association, and in 1927 began the publication of a journal to keep hygienists informed of developments in their profession.

In the 1970s several schools started, on a trial basis, to teach expanded dental hygiene functions, which included administration of local anesthesia, subgingival scaling and root planing, and some operative dentistry procedures. This expanded-duties practice spread rapidly throughout the country. Additionally, attempts to allow the hygienists independent practice started around 1944. After many vicissitudes, this caused a split between the ADA and the ADHA in 1978. In the 1980s, efforts were renewed to allow hygienists to conduct independent practice, but they succeeded only in the state of Colorado, where hygienists are permitted a limited independent practice that does not include taking radiographs or giving local anesthesia.[4]

In recent years dental hygienists have participated in many research programs with their dental mentors. Education of hygiene students has increased and graduate programs leading to MS degrees have been developed. In 1989 it was estimated that there were, in the United States, 98,000 licensed hygienists, of which 71,540 were actively practicing—typically in offices of general dentists, periodontists, nursing homes, and universities.[5]

The role of the hygienist varies greatly from country to country. From governments that do not permit dental auxiliaries to perform any intraoral tasks to those such as New Zealand, where expanded-duty dental nurses carry out many dental operative procedures in children, thus improving the overall dental health of the population.

## References


1. Brown LP. The greatest dental family. Dent Cosmos 1923;65:251.
2. Bulletin of Ohio College of Dental Surgery, Cincinnati, OH. Sessions 1910-1911 and 1913-1914. Cited by: Motley W. The movement for independent practice of dental hygienists: From evolution to revolution. Bull Hist Dent 1988;36(2):108.
3. Bunting R. Oral Hygiene. Philadelphia: Lea & Febiger, 1957.
4. Fales MH. History of periodontology and the role of the dental hygienist. In: Perry DA, Beemsterboer PH, Taggart EJ (eds). Periodontology for the Dental Hygienist. Philadelphia: Saunders, 1996.
5. Field MJ (ed). Dental Education at the Crossroads. Washington, DC: National Academy Press, 1995.
6. Fones AC. The necessity for training a prophylactic assistant. Dent Cosmos 1912;54:264.
7. Fones AC. Mouth Hygiene: A Textbook for Dental Hygienists. Philadelphia: Lea & Febiger, 1916.
8. Fones AC. The origin and history of the dental hygiene movement. J Am Dent Assoc 1926;13:1809.
9. Lufkin AW. A History of Dentistry, ed 2. Philadelphia: Lea & Febiger, 1948.
10. Merritt AH. Biographical sketches (from a symposium on "The Historical Background of Periodontology"). J Periodontol 1939;10:7.
11. Motley W. The movement for independent practice of dental hygienists: From evolution to revolution. Bull Hist Dent 1988;36(2):108.
12. Obituary, Alfred C. Fones. J Am Dent Assoc 1938;67:798.
13. Rhein ML. Oral hygiene. N Engl J Dent 1884;3:356.
14. Rhein ML. The trained dental nurse. Dent Cosmos 1903;45:628.
15. Ring ME. Dentistry: An Illustrated History. St. Louis: Mosby-Year Book, 1985. Reprinted, New York: Harry N. Abrams, 1992.
16. Wheeler HL. The history of the dental hygiene movement. Dent Cosmos 1911;53:327.
17. Wilkins EM, McCullough PA. Clinical Practice of the Dental Hygienist. Philadelphia: Lea & Febiger, 1962.
18. Wright CM. A plea for a subspecialty in dentistry. Int Dent J 1902;23:235.

# 30

# The Future of Periodontology

The preceding chapters of this book have told the remarkable stories of people, events, and discoveries that over the centuries have brought us to modern periodontology. When one realizes just how extraordinary the journey has been and where we are today, it is exciting to imagine the vast number of possibilities for tomorrow's specialty of periodontology.

In looking at the new century and in trying to predict what the future may hold, it is helpful to look at the recent twentieth century and to note clues from the nineteenth century that would have foreshadowed what occurred.[19] In Part IV of this book, several key events in medicine and dentistry are detailed that, in retrospect, signaled the course of change in periodontology in the twentieth century and led to the development of a mechanical-surgical model and a medical model of periodontal treatment. It is helpful to review some of the important steps that brought us to the present.

The extraordinary advances in the mechanical-surgical model for treating periodontal disease must surely be traced first to the discovery of anesthesia in 1845, followed by the discovery of local anesthesia (Chapter 12). In addition, the discovery of X rays in 1895 quickly allowed clinicians to visualize the extent and severity of bone loss around teeth and opened up the world of diagnosis (Chapter 14). With these three seminal discoveries in hand at the end of the nineteenth century, twentieth-century pioneers in dentistry were ready to begin treating periodontal disease through mechanical-surgical intervention.

The mechanical-surgical model of periodontal disease treatment would see impressive advances throughout the twentieth century. Scaling and root planing, and root debridement would eventually become the standard of care (Chapters 15 and 21). Surgical techniques were also performed, and the contributions of Robert Neumann and Leonard Widman to the development of the flap technique mark an important technical breakthrough (Chapter 22). The flap technique entailed reshaping of alveolar bone to foster a more physiologic healing of the tissues. Subsequently other pioneer surgeons started experimenting with various grafting materials, such as bone powder, to rebuild lost bone and periodontal attachment structures. Other clinicians would begin to cover exposed roots with free gingival grafts and coronally repositioned flaps, starting a century of progress in esthetic periodontal surgery. Last but not least, dentists began to design pre-formed "dental implants" that could be used to replace missing teeth. The interest in implants existed for centuries, but the twentieth century saw these efforts come to fruition through the work of pioneers such as Alvin Strock, in Boston, who showed a successful long-standing case (Chapter 26).

Important discoveries in the nineteenth century, also, would lead to the development of the medical model of periodontal treatment. Certainly the introduction of the germ theory of disease by Louis Pasteur and Robert Koch was a major turning point for modern periodontology (Chapter 13). With the introduction of the germ theory, dentistry began to study whether bacteria were causative agents for periodontal disease and caries. Paul Ehrlich, a young physician trained in the theory and practice of staining animal tissues for histology, worked with Robert Koch at the newly established Institute for Infectious Diseases in Berlin. Ehrlich soon began to test the effects of various dyes on bacteria. This work ultimately led him to the discovery that the 606th arsenical compound he had tested was effective against the spirochete that caused syphilis (Chapter 21). This seminal discovery was another turning point for medicine and dentistry. Suddenly it was revealed that certain pathogenic germs could be killed with chemical substances. Clearly this was the advent of the use of antimicrobials in dentistry and medicine.

Not long after the introduction of the germ theory of disease, American scientist Willoughby D. Miller, a graduate of the first class of the University of Pennsylvania Dental School and a professor at the University of Berlin (Chapter 13), was convinced that oral bacteria and oral infectious disease such as periodontal disease caused most of humankind's systemic illnesses. While giving a lecture in London, Miller convinced William Hunter, an attending physician at the London Fever Hospital who was in the audience, that oral disease could explain most systemic illnesses. It would be but a short time until the writings of Miller and Hunter would introduce the era of "focal infection," an era in which periodontal disease would be considered causative of most systemic conditions (Chapter 23).[7,8,12]

Another landmark event in the nineteenth century that would usher in an era of progress in the medical model of periodontal disease treatment was the discovery that the component in the bark of the willow tree that reduced fever could be synthesized. Thus acetylsalicylic acid (aspirin) was introduced for the treatment of fever and pain (inflammation) in 1899 (Chapter 22).

It is extraordinary to now look back at these important discoveries of the nineteenth century and see how they became a springboard for the advances of the subsequent century. With the knowledge that germs cause periodontal disease, dentistry started the twentieth century with antibacterial approaches, including for a brief time the use of vaccines[2] (Chapter 19). Lawrence and Lambert, using the essential oils to treat wounds in the Boer War, introduced an antiseptic mouthrinse, naming it after one of the fathers of antisepsis, Joseph Lister.

The seminal breakthrough which led to the medical model of periodontal disease treatment was the discovery of penicillin by Alexander Fleming in 1928, and its purification and development for clinical use by Howard Florey and Ernst Chain in the early 1940s. It would not be long before dentistry and medicine would venture into the new world of antibiotics for the treatment of bacterial infections (Chapters 21 and 25). Alvin Strock would be the first dentist to report the use of penicillin (topically applied as a rinse) for the treatment of periodontal disease.[17] In 1945 Carlos Schuessler would report that penicillin administered by mouth was a successful treatment of periodontal disease.[16] Thus as Alexander Fleming was being awarded the Nobel Prize (1945) for his discovery of penicillin, Strock and Schuessler were introducing penicillin and, thus, antibiotics as a medical approach for the treatment of periodontal disease.[6,9]

Thirty-four years later, Max Goodson and his colleagues Jan Lindhe and Sigmund Socransky, introduced the concept of treating periodontal disease by locally delivering antibiotics to the periodontal pocket. Their two landmark publications in 1979[6,10] initiated a quarter century of impressive advances in the use of locally delivered antimicrobial agents for the medical model management of periodontal disease.

The twentieth century also saw the introduction of "host modulation" as a medical approach to periodontal treatment. The synthesis of aspirin in 1894 would ultimately lead to the discovery by Sune Bergstrom, Bengt Samuelsson, and John Vane in 1971 that the mechanism of action of aspirin-like drugs was their inhibition of the formation of prostaglandins.[18] A year later Max Goodson reported that prostaglandins were in fact important mediators of bone resorption in periodontitis,[5] and subsequently Paul Goldhaber proposed that aspirin and aspirin-like drugs might be used to block periodontal disease progression.[3] In 1979, Jan Lindhe and his colleagues first introduced the concept of host modulation as another component of the medical model of periodontal disease management. In a landmark paper these investigators reported that it was in fact possible to block periodontal disease bone loss in an animal model using the aspirin-like drug, indomethacin.[14]

The concept that blocking or altering destructive host pathways with pharmacological agents can be a medical approach for treating periodontal disease has had a remarkable development over the last quarter of the twentieth century. Clinical trials of aspirin-like drugs, of inhibitors of collagenase and of inhibitors of osteoclasts (bisphosphonates) have ably shown that it is possible to treat periodontal disease medically by blocking specific host responses.[15]

The late twentieth century also brought the introduction of biological mediators for wound healing and repair in general, and this was rapidly transferred to bone and periodontal regeneration. Marshall Urist discovered in 1965 that new bone could be formed at nonmineralizing sites by implanting in them demineralized "bone powder." Soon it was discovered that the important elements within the bone powder that induced bone formation were proteins called *bone morphogenetic proteins*, or BMPs. Following that landmark discovery, dental and medical investigators found a variety of proteins such as polypeptide growth factors and enamel matrix related proteins that could enhance both hard and soft tissue wound healing, fostering repair and regeneration of bone and periodontal tissues.[1,9]

Last but not least, near the end of the twentieth century it again became apparent that in preventing and treating periodontal disease there is more at stake than just saving teeth. Kimmo Matilla's report in 1989 reintroduced the possibility that periodontal disease could represent a risk for systemic conditions such as heart attack and stroke.[11] A decade of subsequent research has brought compelling findings from investigators worldwide that untreated periodontitis is a risk factor for cardiovascular disease; pre-term, low-birth-weight infants; diabetes; and respiratory disease.

And so, we come to the present, anxious to look into and be ready for the future of periodontology. It is immediately apparent that throughout the twentieth century, two separate, but very connected, models of periodontal disease management evolved: the medical model and the surgical model. It is also apparent that the progress made in these two models has been phenomenal.

One might thus ask the question, Is one model superior or preferred to the other? The answer is clearly *no*. Rather, periodontology has come to today with two management tracks: a medical track and a surgical track. This is not surprising. Many other specialties have arrived at the same point. For example, obstetrics and gynecology uses advanced surgical techniques to treat a wide range of conditions, from childbirth to removal of diseased tissues. At the same time it uses many medical approaches to prevent and treat disease.

The first step in the future of periodontology must be to rename it as the specialty of *periodontal surgery and medicine*. Simple renaming will more accurately define the specialty and reflect how it has evolved in the management of periodontal diseases and related conditions. The new name should open wide the gates for an unprecedented future of advances.

We must then begin to understand and define what is meant by "periodontal surgery and medicine." A look at each separately may be helpful. Periodontal medicine implies that the specialty must advance by pursuit of the medical management of disease (both primary and recurring disease), by continuing to explore how periodontal disease contributes to systemic conditions, and by extending our understanding of how systemic conditions affect the periodontium. It is exciting to envision what the future may hold for the development of this track of periodontology.

It can be expected that new medicines for treating periodontal disease will emerge on a steady basis. Antibiotics for patient management have been available for only half a century. Much can be done to improve currently available antibiotics and antimicrobials for altering or eliminating bacteria responsible for disease causation. In looking at another approach, the surface is barely scratched with the concept of modulating destructive host responses as a means of treating disease. The use of prostaglandin inhibitors, collagenase inhibitors, and osteoclast inhibitors is a worthy start. But stay tuned: as our understanding of disease causation, susceptibility, and pathogenesis improves, clues will emerge for the medical treatment of the disease.

Researchers have not yet begun to explore how pharmacogenomics will help with the medical treatment of periodontal disease. Soon drugs are likely to be created based on the proteins, enzymes, and RNA molecules associated with genes and diseases. This will foster drug discovery and the introduction of drugs targeted to specific diseases such as periodontitis.

We are also at the point of unlocking the secrets of how periodontal infection and inflammation can confer risk to the whole body and contribute to systemic conditions. Valuable clues about a relationship have been gleaned from large, but flawed, epidemiologic data sets. Now, mechanisms whereby periodontal disease could contribute to systemic disease are being explored. Perhaps more importantly, we are gaining insight into the impact of treating periodontal disease as a way to reduce the risk of systemic disease. Initial findings from intervention studies in pregnant women indicate that treating periodontitis can reduce the incidence of pre-term, low-birth-weight babies by 70 percent (M. Jeffcoat, personal communication, 2002). This finding is extraordinary and indicates that there is much to be done in the coming years to understand the periodontitis-systemic health connection. Understanding of this relationship will enhance comprehension of periodontitis as a risk factor, disease susceptibility in patients with periodontal disease, and prevention and treatment of systemic complications.

It is also exciting to envision where the specialty will go as the periodontal surgery model of disease management is developed. The concept of using biological mediators for periodontal regeneration has only been around for about fifteen years, and the emerging field of tissue engineering holds tremendous promise for periodontal surgery. We are just beginning to learn how to engineer or regenerate new tissue from preexisting tissue. Since the success with guided tissue and bone regeneration demonstrated that it is possible to gain new attachment, major leaps forward can be expected as we learn to engineer a patient's individual cells to build attachment apparatus structures and basal and alveolar bone. It is likely that in the near future the major indication of periodontal flap surgery will not be debridement, but regeneration and repair.

Around 1990, "the replacement of missing teeth with substitutes" was added to the definition of periodontics. Thus began an extraordinary decade of incorporating dental implants into the specialty. Initially there was much scrambling as clinicians learned advanced surgical techniques to facilitate implant placement, and as training programs incorporated implants into the curriculum. Now it is difficult to remember a time when we did not replace missing teeth with implants. The future is clearly exciting as we move from learning how to surgically place implants to leading the field. Our periodontal surgery track will greatly advance implant dentistry. Computer-assisted imaging techniques will facilitate whole-mouth imaging; robotics will assure accurately and easily placed implants where needed. Tissue engineering advances will be on board to foster the replacement or addition of bone as necessary. And certainly the direction of implant design and technology cannot be ignored. Considering only the dental implant component of our specialty, it will be a scramble to keep up with the advances of the future.

This chapter would be incomplete if we did not mention how periodontal medicine and periodontal surgery will affect education and patient care. Graduate training programs will have to become innovative to include all that must be taught in a finite time. State-of-the-art learning methodologies, including the concept of distance learning, will be employed.

At what point will young specialists be required to subspecialize in either periodontal medicine or periodontal surgery? Will a subset of periodontists be required to have the MD degree? Periodontal educators and educational institutions have a daunting, but exciting, task ahead.

Finally, how can we assure that all persons have access to periodontal care? Surely the future will see more people worldwide receiving professional assistance for prevention of, and treatment for, periodontal disease so that all persons can enjoy better health. What a phenomenal moment in time has come to periodontics as a specialty of dentistry and medicine. We can look back with pride and satisfaction at the extraordinary evolution of periodontics, and we can look forward with excitement, and perhaps a little awe, to where we are about to go. Let's enjoy the future.

## References


1. Giannobile W. Periodontal tissue regeneration by polypeptide growth factors and gene transfer. In: Lynch S, Genco R, Marx R (eds). Tissue Engineering. Chicago: Quintessence, 1999.
2. Goldenberg L. Stock vaccines in the treatment of pyorrhea alveolaris. Br Dent J 1928;72:85.
3. Goldhaber P, Rabadjija L, Beyer WR, Kornhauser A. Bone resorption in tissue culture and its relevance to periodontal disease. J Am Dent Assoc 1973;87:1027.
4. Golub LM, Ramamurthy N, McNamara TF, et al. Tetracyclines inhibit tissue collagenase activity—A new mechanism in the treatment of periodontal disease. J Periodontal Res 1984;19:651.
5. Goodson JM. Prostaglandins: Potential mediators of periodontal disease. J Dent Res 1972;51:375.
6. Goodson JM, Haffajee A, Socransky SS. Periodontal therapy by local delivery of tetracyclines. J Clin Periodontol 1979;6:83.
7. Hunter W. Oral sepsis as a cause of disease. Br Med J 1910;1:215.
8. Hunter W. The role of sepsis and antisepsis in medicine. Lancet 1910;1:79.
9. Kaigler D, Mooney D. Tissue engineering impact in dentistry. J Dent Educ 2001;65:456.
10. Lindhe J, Heijl L, Goodson M, Socransky SS. Local tetracycline delivery using hollow fiber devices in periodontal therapy. J Clin Periodontol 1979;6:141.
11. Matilla K, Niemeier M, Valtonen V, et al. Association between dental health and acute myocardial infarction. Br Med J 1989;298:770.
12. Miller WD. The human mouth as a focus of infection. Dent Cosmos 1891;33:689.
13. Miller WD. The Microorganisms of the Human Mouth. Philadelphia: S. S. White Dental, 1890. Reprinted, Basel: Karger, 1973.
14. Nyman S, Schroeder HE, Lindhe J. Suppression of inflammation and bone resorption by indomethacin during experimental periodontitis in dogs. J Periodontol 1979;50:450.
15. Paquette DW, Williams RC. Modulation of host inflammatory mediators as a treatment strategy for periodontal disease. Periodontol 2000 2000;24:239.
16. Schuessler CF, Fairchild JM, Stransky IM. Penicillin in the treatment of Vincent's infection. J Am Dent Assoc 1945;32:551.
17. Strock A. Penicillin in the treatment of Vincent's infection in naval recruits. Am J Surg 1944;50:23.
18. Vane JR. Inhibition of prostaglandin synthesis as a mechanism of action for aspirin-like drugs. Nature 1971; 231:232.
19. Williams RC. Periodontal disease. N Engl J Med 1990;332:373.

# *Illustration Credits*

Fig 1 Hoffmann-Axthelm W. History of Dentistry. Chicago: Quintessence, 1981.

Fig 2 Weinberger BW. An Introduction to the History of Dentistry. St Louis: Mosby, 1948. Reprinted with permission.

Fig 3 Hoffmann-Axthelm W. History of Dentistry. Chicago: Quintessence, 1981.

Fig 4 Ring ME. Dentistry: An Illustrated History. New York: Harry N. Abrams, 1985.

Fig 5 Ring ME. Dentistry: An Illustrated History. New York: Harry N. Abrams, 1985.

Fig 6 LeClerc L (trans). Albucasis. La Chirurgie. Paris: Balliere, 1861.

Fig 7 Hoffmann-Axthelm W. History of Dentistry. Chicago: Quintessence, 1981.

Fig 8 Lyons AS, Petrucelli RJ. Medicine: An Illustrated History. New York: Harry N. Abrams, 1978.

Fig 9 Hoffmann-Axthelm W. History of Dentistry. Chicago: Quintessence, 1981.

Fig 10 Ring ME. Dentistry: An Illustrated History. New York: Harry N. Abrams, 1985.

Fig 11 Dobell C. Antony van Leeuwenhoek and His "Little Animals." New York: Dover, 1960.

Fig 12 Collected Letters of Antoni van Leeuwenhoek, Amsterdam, 1938.

Fig 13 Fauchard P. Le Chirurgien Dentiste ou Traité des Dents (facsimile). Birmingham, AL: The Classics of Dentistry Library, 1980.

Fig 14 Fauchard P. Le Chirurgien Dentiste ou Traité des Dents, vol 2 (facsimile). Birmingham, AL: The Classics of Dentistry Library, 1980.

Fig 15 Collection of Gerald Shklar.

Fig 16 Hunter J. The Natural History of the Human Teeth, vol 1 (ed 2). London: Johnson, 1778.

Fig 17 Hoffmann-Axthelm W. History of Dentistry. Chicago: Quintessence, 1981.

Fig 18 Hoffmann-Axthelm W. History of Dentistry. Chicago: Quintessence, 1981.

Fig 19 Hoffmann-Axthelm W. History of Dentistry. Chicago: Quintessence, 1981.

Fig 20 Massachusetts General Hospital, Archives and Special Collections, Boston.

Fig 21 Latour B. Pasteur, une science, un style, un siécle. Paris: Librairie Academique Perrin, Institute Pasteur, 1994.

Fig 22 Courtesy of Institut für Mikrobiologie, Universitat Humboldt, Berlin.

Fig 23 Gay JL. A Time to Heal. Philadephia: American Philosophical Society, 1999.

Fig 24 Courtesy of Librairie Academique Perrin and Pasteur Institute, Paris.

Fig 25 Hoffmann-Axthelm W. History of Dentistry. Chicago: Quintessence, 1981.

Fig 26 Hoffmann-Axthelm W. History of Dentistry. Chicago: Quintessence, 1981.

Fig 27 Hoffmann-Axthelm W. History of Dentistry. Chicago: Quintessence, 1981.

Fig 28 Röntgen Rays Centennial, Exhibition on the Occasion of the Discovery of X Rays, November 8, 1995. Published by Würzburg University.

Fig 29 Röntgen Rays Centennial, Exhibition on the Occasion of the Discovery of X Rays, November 8, 1995. Published by Würzburg University.

Fig 30 Glenner RA. The Dental Office. Pictorial History. Missoula, MT: Pictorial Histories, 1984.

Fig 31 Glenner RA. The Dental Office. Pictorial History. Missoula, MT: Pictorial Histories, 1984.

Fig 32 Hoffmann-Axthelm W. History of Dentistry. Chicago: Quintessence, 1981.

Fig 33 Hoffmann-Axthelm W. History of Dentistry. Chicago: Quintessence, 1981.

Fig 34 Merritt AH. Biographical sketches. J Periodontol 1939;10:15.

Fig 35 Hoffmann-Axthelm W. History of Dentistry. Chicago: Quintessence, 1981.

Fig 36 Stern IB, Everett FG, Robicsek K. S. Robicsek—A pioneer in the surgical treatment of periodontal disease. J Periodontol 1965;36:264.

Fig 37 Courtesy of Berliner Medizinhistorische Museum an der Charité, Berlin.

Fig 38 Silverstein AM. A History of Immunology. San Diego: Academic Press, 1989.

Fig 39 Silverstein AM. A History of Immunology. San Diego: Academic Press, 1989.

Fig 40 Fox J. The History and Treatment of Diseases of the Teeth, the Gums and the Alveolar Processes (facsimile). Birmingham, AL: The Classics of Dentistry Library, 1981.

Fig 41 Hoffmann-Axthelm W. History of Dentistry. Chicago: Quintessence, 1981.

Fig 42 Hoffmann-Axthelm W. History of Dentistry. Chicago: Quintessence, 1981.

Fig 43 Orland FJ. William John Gies, his contributions to the advancement of dentistry. The William J. Gies Foundation for the Advancement of Dentistry, 1992.

Fig 44 Znamensky NN. Alveolar pyorrhea—Its pathological anatomy and its radical treatment. J Br Dent Assoc 1902;23:585.

Fig 45 Znamensky NN. Alveolar pyorrhea—Its pathological anatomy and its radical treatment. J Br Dent Assoc 1902;23:585.

Fig 46 Gold SI. Periodontics. The past. Part II. J Clin Periodontol 1985;12:171.

Fig 47 Gottlieb B. What is a normal pocket? J Am Dent Assoc 1926;13:1747.

Fig 48 J Periodontol 1960;31:266.

Fig 49 J Am Dent Assoc 1940;27:648.

Fig 50 J Periodontol 1960; 31:271.

Fig 51 Held A-J. Oskar Weski (1879–1952). Bull Hist Dent 1991;39:77.

Fig 52 J Am Dent Assoc 1961;62:460.

Fig 53 Simonton FV. Examination of the mouth–with special reference to pyorrhea. J Am Dent Assoc 1925; 12:287.

Fig 54 Glenner RA. The Dental Office. Pictorial History. Missoula, MT: Pictorial Histories, 1984. Reprinted with permission.

Fig 55 Ring ME. Dentistry: An Illustrated History. New York: Harry N. Abrams, 1985.

Fig 56 McCall JO. The evolution of the scaler and its influence on the development of Periodontia. J Periodontol 1939;10:69. Reprinted with permission.

Fig 57 McCall JO. The evolution of the scaler and its influence on the development of Periodontia. J Periodontol 1939;10:69. Reprinted with permission.

Fig 58 McCall JO. The evolution of the scaler and its influence on the development of Periodontia. J Periodontol 1939;10:69. Reprinted with permission.

Fig 59 J Periodontol 1965;36:94.

Fig 60 Ryan F. The Forgotten Plague. Boston: Little, Brown, and Co, 1992.

Fig 61 Christen AG. Charles C. Bass (1875–1975): That cantankerous genius of preventive dentistry. Bull Hist Dent 1990;38:8.

Fig 62 Gold SI. Robert Neumann: A pioneer in periodontal flap surgery. J Periodontol 1982;53:456.

Fig 63 Gold SI. Robert Neumann: A pioneer in periodontal flap surgery. J Periodontol 1982;53:456. Reprinted with permission.

Fig 64 Everett FG, Waerhaug J, Widman A. Leonard Widman: Surgical treatment of pyorrhea alveolaris. J Periodontol 1971;42:571.

Fig 65 J Periodontol 1974;45:273.

Fig 66 J Periodontol 1970;41:186.

Fig 67 Collection of Fermin Carranza, Jr.

Fig 68 Carranza F. Cuando y porque sacrificar hueso en el tratamiento de la paradentosis. Ateneo Inst Mun Odont Bs As 1941;1:311.

Fig 69 Collection of Fermin Carranza, Jr.

Fig 70 J Periodontol 1991;62:589.

Fig 71 Collection of Fermin Carranza, Jr.

Fig 72 J Periodontol 1992;63:236.

Fig 73 J Clin Periodontol 1980;7:534.

Fig 74 Collection of Fermin Carranza, Jr.

Fig 75 Pamphlet (1991), St. Mary's Hospital Medical School, London.

Fig 76 J Periodontol 1990;61:715.

Fig 77 J Periodontol 1990;61:661.

Fig 78 Ring ME. Dentistry: An Illustrated History. New York: Harry N. Abrams, 1985.

Fig 79 Hagy DM, Richards LW. Dental implants: Fact and fantasies. In: Steiner RB, Thompson RD (eds). Oral Surgery and Anesthesia. Philadelphia: Saunders, 1977.

Fig 80 Brånemark P-I. The Brånemark Novum Protocol for Same-Day Teeth: A Global Perspective. Berlin: Quintessence, 2001.

Fig 81 J Periodontol 1949;20:108.

Fig 82 Merritt AH. Biographical sketches. J Periodontol 1939;10:7.

Fig 83 Mustchelknauss RE. Lehrbuch der klinischen Paradontologie. Berlin: Quintessenz, 2000.

Fig 84 Mustchelknauss RE. Lehrbuch der klinischen Paradontologie. Berlin: Quintessenz, 2000.

Fig 85 Courtesy of Mrs. N. M. Keim.

Fig 86 Herschfeld JJ. Alfred C. Fones: Father of the dental hygiene movement. Bull Hist Dent 1989;37:129.

Fig 87 Herschfeld JJ. Alfred C. Fones: Father of the dental hygiene movement. Bull Hist Dent 1989;37:129.

# *Index to Persons*

# *Subject Index*

*Page numbers followed by "f" indicate figures*